John Brick, PhD
Editor

Handbook of the Medical Consequences of Alcohol and Drug Abuse

Pre-publication
REVIEWS,
COMMENTARIES,
EVALUATIONS . . .

"Whether they are used recreationally or addictively, alcohol and other drugs affect every organ system in the human body. Advances in medicine, toxicology, and epidemiology have been so rapid that periodic updates of the literature are an absolute necessity for the physician, the neuroscientist, the student, and the addiction treatment professional. That's what makes *Handbook of the Medical Consequences of Alcohol and Drug Abuse* a pleasure to read and a treasure on the bookshelf. John Brick has assembled a very readable guide to the most recent evidence on the medical consequences of substance abuse. Ranging from the practical to the theoretical, the chapters tell a compelling story about the burden of illness and disability that is caused by substance abuse."

Thomas F. Babor, PhD, MPH
Professor and Chair,
Department of Community Medicine,
University of Connecticut Health Center

"This book effectively incorporates the world literature and expert opinions on the medical outcomes of drug and alcohol abuse in our society, offering invaluable information for all health care providers as well as researchers and forensic investigators. The contributors have thoroughly covered a broad range of topics—from the common knowledge base of drug effects and drug-induced disease to the less well-known conditions such as holoprosencephaly in fetal alcohol syndrome and leukoencephalopathy associated with inhaled heroin. In a society that spends more on interdiction than treatment for drug abuse, this text will assist the development of the recently emerging disease model of substance abuse and pave the way for treatment as the medical norm."

Alan Clark, MD
Forensic Clinical Analyst and Educator,
InForum Reviews, LLC,
Carthage, Missouri

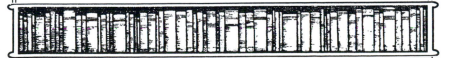

Handbook of the Medical Consequences of Alcohol and Drug Abuse

THE HAWORTH PRESS
Contemporary Issues in Neuropharmacology
John Brick, PhD, MA, FAPA
Senior Editor

Handbook of the Medical Consequences of Alcohol and Drug Abuse edited by John Brick

Other titles of related interest:

Drug Abuse and Social Policy in America: The War That Must Be Won by Barry Stimmel

Pain and Its Relief Without Addiction: Clinical Issues in the Use of Opioids and Other Analgesics by Barry Stimmel

Drugs, the Brain, and Behavior: The Pharmacology of Abuse and Dependence by John Brick and Carlton K. Erikson

The Love Drug: Marching to the Beat of Ecstasy by Richard S. Cohen

Alcoholism, Drug Addiction, and the Road to Recovery: Life on the Edge by Barry Stimmel

The Group Therapy of Substance Abuse edited by David W. Brook and Henry I. Spitz

Handbook of the Medical Consequences of Alcohol and Drug Abuse

John Brick, PhD
Editor

The Haworth Press®
New York • London • Oxford

The Haworth Press, Inc., 10 Alice Street, Binghamton, NY 13904-1580.

PUBLISHER'S NOTE:
This book has been published solely for educational purposes and is not intended to substitute for the medical advice of a treating physician. Medicine is an ever-changing science. As new research and clinical experience broaden our knowledge, changes in treatment may be required. While many potential treatment options are made herein, some or all of the options may not be applicable to a particular individual. Therefore, the author, editor, and publisher do not accept responsibility in the event of negative consequences incurred as a result of the information presented in this book. We do not claim that this information is necessarily accurate by the rigid scientific and regulatory standards applied for medical treatment. **No Warranty, Express or Implied, is furnished with respect to the material contained in this book. The reader is urged to consult with his/her personal physician with respect to the treatment of any medical condition.**

Cover design by Lora Wiggins.

Library of Congress Cataloging-in-Publication Data

Handbook of the medical consequences of alcohol and drug abuse / John Brick, editor.
    p. cm.
    Includes bibliographical references and index.
    ISBN 0-7890-1863-2 (hc : alk. paper)—ISBN 0-7890-1864-0 (sc : alk. paper)
    1. Substance abuse—Pathophysiology—Handbooks, manuals, etc. I. Brick, John, 1950-
RC564 .H3585 2003
616.86—dc21

                         2002015168

CONTENTS

ABOUT THE EDITOR

John Brick, PhD, MA, FAPA, a biological psychologist specializing in alcohol and drug studies for more than twenty-five years, is Executive Director of Intoxikon International, a company that provides multidisciplinary education, training, and consulting in alcohol and drug studies to governmental and other agencies. As a member of the research faculty of the Rutgers University Center of Alcohol Studies from 1980 to 1994, he held the positions of Laboratory Director of the Rutgers Alcohol Behavior Research Lab and Chief of Research at the Rutgers University Center of Alcohol Studies, Division of Education and Training. Dr. Brick was concurrently Associate Director of the Rutgers Summer School of Alcohol Studies and the Advanced School of Alcohol and Drug Studies where he has taught neuropharmacology and related subjects for more than fifteen years.

Dr. Brick is the author of nearly 100 scientific treatises, including the *President's Commission on Model State Drug Laws—Socioeconomic Evaluation of Addictions Treatment* (1993); *Drugs and the Brain*; and *Drugs, the Brain, and Behavior: The Pharmacology of Alcohol and Drug Abuse* (Haworth). He is a co-editor of *Stress and Alcohol Use* and has contributed to numerous other publications.

In 1990, Dr. Brick was one of only six Americans invited to address the Soviet National Academy of Medicine on their centenary anniversary. He is the only American scientist working in the field of alcohol studies to receive this distinct honor. In 1992, he co-organized and chaired the International Conference on Alcohol and Aggression and was made a Fellow of the American Psychological Association for his outstanding contributions to the science of psychology. In 2002, Dr. Brick became a visiting faculty member at the Peking University Institute of Mental Health International Center of Health Concerns in Beijing, China, where he taught a course titled Medical Consequences of Alcohol Abuse. Dr. Brick has been teaching at Rutgers–The State University of New Jersey for more than twenty years and has been in private practice in Yardley, Pennsylvania, since 1985.

CONTRIBUTORS

Alan J. Budney, PhD, Associate Professor, University of Vermont Treatment Research Center, South Burlington, Vermont.

Claire D. Coles, PhD, Emory University School of Medicine, Department of Psychiatry–Genetics, Georgia Mental Health Institute, Atlanta, Georgia.

Fulton T. Crews, PhD, Professor of Pharmacology and Psychiatry, Director, Center for Alcohol Studies, Bowles Center for Alcohol Studies, Pharmacology and Psychiatry School of Medicine, University of North Carolina at Chapel Hill, Chapel Hill, North Carolina.

Carlton K. Erickson, PhD, Director, Addiction Science Research and Education Center, and Pfizer Centennial Professor of Pharmacology, University of Texas at Austin College of Pharmacy, Austin, Texas.

Corinne E. Frantz, PhD, Clinical Neuropsychologist, Maplewood, New Jersey.

Karen K. Howell, PhD, Maternal Substance Abuse and Child Development Project, Emory University School of Medicine, Department of Psychiatry–Genetics, Georgia Mental Health Institute, Atlanta, Georgia.

Julie Kable, PhD, Emory University School of Medicine, Department of Psychiatry–Genetics, Georgia Mental Health Institute, Atlanta, Georgia.

Paul Kolecki, MD, Assistant Professor, Department of Surgery, Division of Emergency Medicine, Thomas Jefferson University, Philadelphia, Pennsylvania.

Mary Jeanne Kreek, MD, Professor and Head, Laboratory of the Biology of Addictive Diseases, The Rockefeller University, New York, New York.

Anthony S. Manoguerra, PharmD, DABAT, FAACT, Professor of Clinical Pharmacy, San Diego Program, School of Pharmacy, University of California at San Francisco, San Francisco, California, and Director, San Diego Division, California Poison Control System, San Diego, California.

Sarah N. Mattson, PhD, Associate Director, Center for Behavioral Teratology, San Diego, California.

Pauline F. McHugh, MD, Assistant Research Professor, Department of Psychiatry, New York University School of Medicine, Center for Brain Health, New York, New York.

Brent A. Moore, PhD, University of Vermont, Treatment Research Center, South Burlington, Vermont.

Rosemarie Scolaro Moser, PhD, ABPN, RSM Psychology Center LLC, Director, Lawrenceville, New Jersey.

Edward P. Riley, PhD, Director, Center for Behavioral Teratology, San Diego, California.

Aaron Schneir, MD, Medical Toxicology Fellow/Assistant Professor of Emergency Medicine, San Diego Division, California Poison Control System and Division of Medical Toxicology, Department of Emergency Medicine, University of California San Diego Medical Center, San Diego, California.

Richard Shih, MD, Emergency Medicine, Residency Director, Morristown Memorial Hospital, Morristown, New Jersey, and Medical Toxicologist, New Jersey Poison Information and Education Systems, Newark Beth Israel Medical Center, Newark, New Jersey.

Ryan Vandrey, BS, Treatment Research Center, University of Vermont, South Burlington, Vermont.

Tara S. Wass, PhD, Assistant Professor, University of Tennessee, Department of Child and Family Studies, Knoxville, Tennessee.

Foreword

Although the medical consequences of alcohol and drug abuse have been known for decades, new research is adding to the base of knowledge on this topic on a regular basis. Thus, recent and accurate information on such critical issues is always welcome. This peer-reviewed book is intended to provide the reader with such information.

The editor has gathered together an impressive mix of established scientists and young talent to write the ten chapters in this book. The scope of the topics is broad, ranging from effects of various drugs on peripheral organ systems from the fetus to the brain. Drugs discussed include alcohol (five chapters), and one chapter each on marijuana, opioids, cocaine, and inhalants. An additional chapter examines the medical consequences of prenatal exposure to many drugs.

The opening chapter provides basic information on alcohol, including definitions of alcohol (ethanol), use, abuse, and dependence. There is also a quick review of the measurement of alcohol concentrations in body products (along with an extremely helpful discussion of how to compare scientific notations of alcohol concentrations) and a brief discussion of what constitutes a drink. This chapter explains many of the terms used in the chapters that follow as well as the current literature.

Chapter 2 begins the scientific discussion of alcohol, with clear descriptions of the relationship between alcohol and accidental injuries (including driving, cycling, pedestrian, water sports, aircraft), and alcohol's effects on organ systems (skeletal, pancreas, liver, heart) and risk for certain cancers. This is an extremely detailed chapter, which is certain to answer many questions people have about the detrimental (and beneficial) effects of alcohol on the body.

Chapter 3 concerns the effects of alcohol and other drug use on neuropsychological function. This is the only chapter in the book to focus on brain-behavior relationships of abused drugs, and the authors indicate that, unlike the discrete effects on tissue and organs, drugs produce a more generalized, pervasive effect on the brain. These effects may be immediate and acute, or long-lasting and chronic. Most of the chapter deals with alcohol, and some overlap occurs with the following chapter with regard to discussions of alcohol's effects on brain pathways, brain damage, and neurotransmitter function. Brief but useful sections on polydrug abuse, cocaine, marijuana, LSD, phencyclidine, amphetamines, and ecstasy conclude the chapter.

Chapter 4 is an in-depth review of the involvement of alcohol on neuron signaling, neurotransmitter function (with a heavy emphasis on NMDA and GABA), and alcoholic brain damage and cognitive dysfunction. Information regarding recovery from long-term brain damage provides hope for suffering alcohol abusers and alcohol-dependent individuals. Also included is a brief discussion of treatment and recovery from alcohol dependence, not found in any other chapter. The basic neurobiological information in this chapter, written by a leading expert in alcohol research, is probably best suited to scientists or "budding scientists." Practitioners in the field will find it interesting in exposing the complexity of alcohol's actions in the brain.

Chapter 5 discusses the fetal effects of alcohol. "Everything you always wanted to know" about this topic is included. Topics include autopsy and brain-scan studies on affected children and neurobehavioral effects of heavy prenatal alcohol exposure. Readers will be especially interested in the descriptions of alcohol's prenatal effects on intelligence, language, learning and memory, attention and activity, executive function (decision making and judgment), and psychosocial functioning.

Marijuana is a difficult drug to review because of the relative paucity of solid scientific information on human psychological and physical health, particularly regarding marijuana's chronic effects. The authors of Chapter 6 have carefully studied the existing literature, however, and synthesized it into a clear review of available information. Particularly impressive are their comments on the strength and quality of data that support the effects of this drug on the respiratory system, immune system, cardiovascular system, hormones and fertility, and perinatal effects. There are also lucid discussions of the psychological and psychiatric effects of marijuana, effects on psychomotor performance, attention and memory, academic performance (not covered in many reviews of marijuana!), driving performance, motivation, and dependence ("addiction"). Finally, a fair and balanced discussion of the contemporary issue of medical marijuana helps make this chapter one of the highlights of the book.

Equally impressive is Chapter 7's examination of opioids (opium and its derivatives) and methadone pharmacotherapy. The issue of methadone and the need for broader use of this effective medication in the treatment of heroin-dependent individuals is of utmost importance. This is an interesting chapter because it begins with a discussion of the worst direct medical consequence of heroin (death) and ends with indirect causes of medical illness resulting from heroin use which many readers probably do not think about— such as infection and contamination with adulterants used to cut the drug. Methadone is compared with heroin throughout the chapter with respect to their effects on organ system function and dysfunction. This chapter is filled with interesting details. How many readers would know that opiates have negative pulmonary, renal, and skeletal effects when injected?

Chapter 8 focuses on the detrimental effects of cocaine, with a brief discussion of methamphetamine and phenylpropanolamine. A review is included of cocaine's history and the forms of cocaine, its physiologic effects, and finally the adverse effects of cocaine on the cardiovascular, neurologic, and pulmonary systems. Brief descriptions of cocaine's effects on other, usually neglected, systems (genitourinary, gastrointestinal, hepatic, pancreatic, ocular, for example) and on the fetus are highlights of this chapter.

Chapter 9 is an excellent review of the prenatal effects of nicotine, cocaine, marijuana, and opiate drugs. The chapter begins with an introduction to the principles of teratology and behavioral teratology, and then methodically covers the epidemiology and effects of each of the drugs on growth, cognition, language, auditory processing, attention and activity levels, motor and behavioral effects. As expected, these drugs produce temporary fetal changes and may have long-term effects that have not been completely researched.

One of the briefer chapters in the book, Chapter 10, involves the medical consequences of inhalants. There is a reason for this—not much is known about this broad class of chemicals. Inhalants constitute a category of abused substances that is very broad, ranging from nitrous oxide to gasoline. These compounds are extremely organotoxic, a fact nicely reviewed in this chapter. The authors cover the epidemiology of inhalant use and abuse (who uses them and why), a history of use of these substances, how they are administered, and how to treat their toxic effects. This is a wonderfully complete and up-to-date review of this class of abused substances.

The purpose of a foreword is to provide a critical review and summary of the contents of a book and to verify the importance of the book's contents. I also believe in trying to guide the reader toward specific chapters of interest. For this book, however, virtually every chapter is valuable for anyone interested in the medical consequences of drug use in adults and adolescents. Thus, this book is worth taking the time to read in its entirety. Furthermore, because the research on chemical abuse is relatively sparse, this information will remain "current" for many years to come.

Carlton K. Erickson, PhD
Pfizer Centennial Professor of Pharmacology
The University of Texas at Austin

Preface

The philosopher Thomas Hobbes (1588-1679) described the condition of humanity as "nasty, brutish and short." Interestingly, he was among the first proponents to write about the biological basis of behavior. In the ensuing 250 years or so, the great human condition and the quality of life have improved in most societies. Life is less nasty, less brutish, and far longer than it has ever been. With few exceptions, life as Hobbes knew it has changed dramatically, although then, as now, alcohol and other drugs were available and abused. Today, highly sophisticated neuroscientific research techniques enable scientists to study the neurophysiological and molecular changes that produce acute intoxication, and the increased longevity provided by advances in medical science allow the long-term consequences of alcohol and drug abuse to be more fully appreciated. Centuries ago, one was more likely to die from infectious diseases, other ailments, or occupational injuries before the pernicious medical consequences of alcohol or drug abuse presented themselves. That is no longer true.

Handbook of the Medical Consequences of Alcohol and Drug Abuse is part of a book series in neuropharmacology whose purpose is to bring the most recent findings to scientists, physicians, other clinicians, and advanced students of this fascinating and important topic. Alcohol scientists know more about the long-term consequences of alcohol and other drugs than at any other time in our history. Basic and clinical research in this area must continue, as must the efforts to educate physicians and other health care professionals, and increase public education and awareness of this problem. Included in this book are those drugs that generate the most interest and greatest consequences. Because of size constraints and deadlines, the exclusion of some drugs and the works of some outstanding researchers was unavoidable but will be addressed in future volumes in this series. No special significance should be given to the use of the phrase "alcohol and other drugs," which appears throughout this book. Alcohol is a drug and the use of the phrase is for heuristic convenience only.

The contributors have made this a pleasant and worthwhile endeavor and I thank them for taking time from their busy schedules to share their perspectives on this complicated problem. Several others whose names do not appear in the list of contributors have nonetheless been influential in this endeavor. Thanks to Dr. Mary E. Reuder, who has been a great teacher and a model mentor for many years, and to Jacquelyn Kaizar, my secretary, whose organization and hard work I greatly appreciate.

Finally, my deepest thanks to my wife, Laurie, and my daughters, Stephanie and Kyla, whose understanding, support, and inspiration are unending, and to my mother, Violet Holmes Treimanis, who always encouraged me to think with my head, not with my feet.

Chapter 1

Characteristics of Alcohol: Chemistry, Use, and Abuse

John Brick

Alcohol is one of the oldest and most widely used psychoactive drugs on earth. In an effort to provide a foundation for the interpretation of terms related to alcohol and its use throughout this text and elsewhere, this introductory chapter will define alcohol both as a chemical and as a drug, explain the scientific notation for reporting alcohol in blood or serum, and present an overview of the use of alcohol: how we currently define alcohol use, abuse, and dependence in American society.

WHAT IS ALCOHOL?

The term "alcohol" is used to define several types of alcohol, including the three most common: ethyl alcohol (ethanol), methyl alcohol (methanol), and isopropyl alcohol (isopropanol). All alcohols have a similar chemical structure and contain a hydroxyl group, OH, attached to a saturated carbon molecule. Methyl alcohol, also known as methanol or wood alcohol, is so highly toxic that even small amounts (less than an ounce) can cause retinal damage. Methanol's toxicity is the result of its metabolism to formaldehyde and then to formic acid, a cellular toxin that is about six times more poisonous than methanol. The accumulation of formic acid produces severe metabolic acidosis and six to seven ounces of methanol are lethal for most adults.

Isopropyl alcohol, also known as isopropanol or common rubbing alcohol, is also highly toxic. Small amounts, as little as several ounces, can also cause permanent damage to the visual system, and eight ounces is considered a lethal dose. Some alcoholics may consume methanol or isopropyl alcohol, intentionally or unknowingly, with potentially lethal consequences.

The alcohol that is the subject of this review, and the alcohol consumed as a beverage by most people is ethyl alcohol or ethanol, a clear, relatively odorless chemical. The lethal dose (LD:50) of acute ethanol is estimated to

1

be a blood alcohol concentration of about .40 percent, although death may occur at higher or lower concentrations depending upon factors such as tolerance. Given reasonable alcohol pharmacokinetics, a 150-pound male would reach LD:50 after consuming about four to five drinks per hour over a four-hour period. Sublethal doses are more insidious and are the primary focus of this review. Throughout this chapter and throughout this book, the term alcohol will be synonymous with ethanol.

Whether we are discussing alcohol as a chemical or psychoactive drug, alcohol is a relatively simple molecule, CH_3-CH_2-OH, formed during a process of fermentation that occurs when yeast combines with water and sugar. The yeast recombines carbon, hydrogen, oxygen, and water to form alcohol and carbon dioxide. The different types of alcoholic beverages are derived from the use of different fermenting ingredients. Wine manufacturing, for example, may utilize grapes, apricots, berries, and other fruits that are rich in sugars and provide the necessary oxygen for fermentation. Fermentation continues until a maximum alcohol concentration of about 15 percent is reached, at which point, the concentration of alcohol is so high the yeast dies. Beers are manufactured with a different source of sugar, namely, the starch found in cereal grains, which is enzymatically converted to sugar through a malting process. This process involves sprouting cereal, such as barley, in water. The dried sprouts are then mixed with water. The enzymes formed during sprouting convert starch to sugar, which allows fermentation to proceed. For beers, the process of fermentation is stopped when the alcohol concentration reaches about 3 to 6 percent. For wines, the process is stopped, or self-limiting, at higher concentrations (typically 11 to 13 percent). Distillation of fermented beverages allows exceptionally high alcohol concentrations (typically 50 to 60 percent in some beverages and up to nearly 100 percent in other products) to be obtained.

The range of alcohol concentration in alcoholic beverages is determined by biological processes, manufacturing design, or some combination of the two. Alcoholic beverage contents are usually expressed as a percentage of alcohol by volume, as in the case of beers and wines, or as "proof," an archaic term that is twice the alcohol concentration by volume. From a scientific perspective, the total amount of alcohol in a measured drink is for all practical purposes the same from drink to drink. However, the differences in alcohol concentrations among beverages may have medical consequences because of the direct action of alcohol on the tissues with which it comes in contact. Since peak alcohol absorption in blood takes from about 30 to 90 minutes in most social-drinking cases, and total absorption takes even longer, beverage type and beverage concentration may be a factor in determining some of the medical consequences of alcohol use. Therefore, studies regarding the acute effects of alcohol should be conducted, and the results interpreted with this fact in mind.

SCIENTIFIC NOTATION
FOR ALCOHOL CONCENTRATIONS

Throughout this book, alcohol concentrations are expressed using various scientific notations. When comparing the results within these chapters with other references, it may be necessary to convert from one scientific notation to another. The concentration of alcohol in blood, serum, water, or any other liquid is the quantity of absolute alcohol by weight in a fixed volume of fluid. When alcohol is measured in breath, most breath-testing instruments are calibrated to take a fixed breath sample size. Instruments are designed based upon certain physiological assumptions and calibrated so the results are reported as whole blood equivalents (e.g., .10 percent). In some literature, alcohol concentrations are reported as grams/2100 cc air, and in blood or other tissues or fluids, they are more commonly reported in milligrams per deciliter (mg/dl). In molecular biological studies of how alcohol affects tissues, alcohol is sometimes reported in millimolar concentrations (mM). In those studies, mg/dl alcohol = mM alcohol $\times$ 4.6 provides a good conversion to a more identifiable concentration. This will be helpful for interpreting some of the data presented in Chapter 4, for example.

When alcohol is measured in blood, the reported blood alcohol concentration (BAC) is the amount of alcohol by weight in a fixed volume of blood, which is usually 100 milliliters (ml) in the United States. BAC is usually expressed in grams per 100 ml or milligrams per 100 ml of whole blood or serum. The following BAC notations are identical with regard to the amount of alcohol expressed: .10 percent, .10 grams percent, .10 grams/100 ml, .10 grams/deciliter (g/dL), 100 mg/dl, 100 mg percent, 100 mg/100 cc or ml.

Clinical Measurement of Alcohol

Most hospital clinical laboratories measure alcohol in serum, rather than in whole blood. Since serum contains more alcohol than the whole blood from which it is derived, the concentration of alcohol in serum is proportionally higher than the equivalent whole blood concentration. In most cases, a serum alcohol value can be converted to its whole blood equivalent using a simple formula: Alcohol in Serum $\times$ .85 = BAC. The same result can be obtained by dividing the serum alcohol by the reciprocal of .85: Alcohol in Serum / 1.18 = BAC. For example, a serum alcohol concentration of .10 percent is equal, under normal physiological conditions, to a whole blood alcohol concentration of about 0.085 percent (Brick and Erickson, 1999). Variations between or within subjects due to hematocrit or other clinical chemical differences produce minor variations in the conversion of serum to whole blood alcohol.

DEFINING ALCOHOL USE

Alcohol has been used for thousands of years, but the medical consequences of alcohol abuse have only come to the attention of the medical/scientific community in the last 150 years or so. Alcohol consumption and related problems have been well documented (National Institute on Alcohol Abuse and Alcoholism, 2000). In the United States, for example, nearly half the adult population consumes alcohol, and alcohol-related medical problems account for a disproportionate number of hospital admissions. Data from the 1992 National Longitudinal Epidemiologic Survey indicate that nearly 9 percent of adults in the United States consume, on average, more than two drinks per day (Dawson et al., 1995), and the results of an ongoing national survey of high school students recently reported that 24 percent of eighth graders, 40 percent of tenth graders, and 51 percent of twelfth graders had used alcohol within the last month (Johnston et al., 1999). The use of alcohol and other drugs also has a profound economic impact. Estimates place the cost of addiction at more than $200 billion per year from direct effects on families and society through lost wages, absent or ineffectual parental models, and shared exposure to high risks and resulting injuries associated with intoxication.

Alcohol use is not always associated with deleterious medical consequences. In fact, some research suggests that alcohol use under some conditions has beneficial health effects. How alcohol exerts such biphasic effects has been the subject of considerable research and debate. However, we can define alcohol use in two ways: first, through current definitions of use, abuse, and dependence and, second, by defining what constitutes "a drink." The social use of alcohol is now generally described as a cold beer after a ball game, a glass of wine with meals, or a glass of champagne at festive occasions. Alcohol consumption is often defined as drug abuse (or misuse) whenever it places the drinker or others affected by the drinker's behavior at increased risk for injury. The term "moderate" drinking is sometimes used by clinicians, and often used by laypersons, to describe consumption that is neither abusive nor very infrequent, or that describes a constellation of behavioral or other factors that differentiate it from "light" or "heavy." However, these terms are relative. For example, a "moderate" drinker may drink heavily (e.g., more than six drinks a day on some days) but not be classified as a "heavy" drinker. On the other hand, the Department of Agriculture (USDA) and the U.S. Department of Health and Human Services in the *Dietary Guidelines for Americans* defines moderate drinking as one drink per day or less for women and two or fewer drinks per day for men (USDA, 1995). In addition, the NIAAA further recommends that people ages 65 and older limit their consumption of alcohol to one drink per day. The terms light, moderate, and heavy should be interpreted carefully based on the operational definition of the study since the definitions of these terms vary.

The *Diagnostic and Statistical Manual of Mental Disorders* (DSM-IV) (1996) defines two types of problem drinkers: (1) abusers, who intentionally drink too much, too often, and make wrong choices about their use of alcohol, and (2) dependent users (i.e., alcoholics), who lack control over their use of alcohol in lifestyle situations in which abusers would ordinarily stop drinking. Voluntary alcohol abuse is a significant problem that contributes to accidents, medical expenses, lost productivity, family problems, and, of course, a host of direct and indirect medical consequences. Drug dependence, whether the drug is alcohol or some other psychoactive substance, is a brain disease caused by a neurochemical imbalance. The addict has no control of his or her alcohol or other drug use (see Erickson and Wilcox, 2001 for a recent review). Both types of drinkers are overly represented as inpatients and as patients in hospital emergency rooms.

What Constitutes a Drink?

We can also define what is meant by a drink by standardizing this definition across beverage types so that the interpretation is meaningful and useful. Many epidemiological and empirical research studies define alcohol consumption in terms of the number of drinks consumed or the number of grams of absolute alcohol consumed. In many such studies, and certainly in terms of practical definitions, a drink can be defined as 1.5 ounces of 80-proof alcohol, 5 ounces of 12 percent wine or a 12-ounce standard beer (~4.8 percent v/v). Each of these contain approximately 14 grams of absolute alcohol and about 100 kilocalories. Outside of the laboratory, a mixed drink may contain more or less than 1.5 ounces of 80-proof alcohol (or the equivalent) and wine may be served in volumes larger or smaller than five ounces. Similarly, the concentration of alcohol in beers varies from an average of about 3.8 percent (v/v) for "lite" beers to about 4.75 to 4.9 percent (v/v) for most typical American beers. Imported or specialty beers may contain significantly more alcohol by volume.

Regardless of the type of alcoholic beverage consumed, it is the psychoactive drug ethanol that produces the effects on the brain, virtually all cells within the body, and behavior. The degree of those effects is determined by the concentration, amount and time of consumption, bioavailability due to factors such as absorption and the biotransformation of alcohol, and drinking experience. All of these factors ultimately result in the exposure and response of various cells to concentrations of alcohol.

REFERENCES

American Psychiatric Association (APA) (1996). *Diagnostic and Statistical Manual of Mental Disorders,* Fourth Edition. Washington, DC: APA, pp. 175-204.

Brick, J. and Erickson, C. (1999). *Drugs, the Brain, and Behavior: The Pharmacology of Abuse and Dependence.* Binghamton, NY: The Haworth Medical Press, p. 67.

Dawson, D.A., Grant, B.F., Chou, S.P., and Pickering, R.P. (1995). Subgroup variation in U.S. drinking patterns: Results of the 1992 national longitudinal alcohol epidemiologic study. *Journal of Substance Abuse 7*(3):331-344.

Erickson, C. and Wilcox, R. (2001). Neurobiological causes of addiction. *Journal of Social Work Practice in the Addictions 1*(3):7-22.

Johnston, L.D., O'Malley, P.M., and Bachman, J.G. (1999). Drug trends in 1999 are mixed. Retrieved from the University of Michigan Web site: <http://www.monitoringthefuture.org>.

National Institute on Alcohol Abuse and Alcoholism (2000). *Tenth Special Report to the U.S. Congress on Alcohol and Health.* Washington, DC: U.S. Department of Health and Human Services.

U.S. Department of Agriculture and U.S. Department of Health and Human Services (1995). *Home and Garden Bulletin* No. 232, Fourth Edition. Washington, DC: U.S. Department of Agriculture.

Chapter 2

Medical Consequences of Alcohol Abuse

John Brick

OVERVIEW

Alcohol is one of the oldest drugs known and it affects virtually every organ system in the body. The number of physiological systems affected by alcohol is staggering both in the scope of medical consequences and in terms of the economics of medical treatment of alcohol-related disorders. Alcohol damages the heart and can elevate blood pressure. It can increase the risk for heart failure and stroke. Excessive alcohol consumption can injure various tissues, produce diverse physiological changes, and impair and interfere with the hormonal and biochemical regulation of a variety of cellular and metabolic functions. Chronic alcohol exposure increases the risk for certain forms of cancer, and both acute and chronic alcohol use significantly increases the risk for accidental injuries and impairs the recovery from those injuries. However, not all of the medical consequences of alcohol use are deleterious. Substantial research indicates beneficial effects of this drug. Nonetheless, the economic and psychosocial costs of alcohol use in American society alone are estimated at more than $200 billion per year. This chapter will review the most significant and well-known medical consequences of alcohol use and abuse in four basic areas: accidental injuries, the skeletal system, the hepatic system, and the cardiovascular system.

ALCOHOL AND ACCIDENTAL INJURIES

Accidental injuries are a direct medical consequence of alcohol intoxication and it is well known that alcohol increases the risk for injuries through impairment of cognitive and psychomotor functioning while performing or engaging in a variety of behavioral activities. Among these, the effects of alcohol on automobile, bicycling, motorcycle, boating, aquatic and pedestrian injuries, as well as homicide, suicide, and death from fire have been examined.

7

Impaired Driving

Driving while intoxicated is probably the most well-studied injurious consequence of drinking. Whereas the older scientific literature on drinking and driving focused on the effects of high blood alcohol levels on simple reaction time, on the visual system, and on gross impairment, it is now known that the effects of alcohol are much broader and occur at relatively low blood alcohol levels. For example, alcohol use is coupled with increased risk taking and impulsivity, at least among young males (Cherpitel, 1993), and decreased seat belt use (CDC, 1991) which invariably places drinkers at increased risk for injury. Moreover, whereas high blood alcohol levels (>.15 percent) may produce obvious visible impairment in the absence of any testing (Brick and Carpenter, 2001), it is now known that very low levels of alcohol (.02 to .03 percent) impair the performance of complex divided attention tasks, at least in laboratory studies. Divided attention is believed to be a critical factor in a variety of tasks outside the laboratory, and divided attention failure is the most likely cause of motor vehicle collisions at blood alcohol levels above .05 percent, for it is at this level that impairment translates into actual highway statistics (in which the intoxicated driver is the cause of the accident). At higher blood alcohol levels (e.g., .15 percent or more), impairment in proprioception, visual perception, and lengthened simple reaction time are additional significant contributing factors to motor vehicle accidents.

Regardless of which functions are affected by alcohol, impaired drivers clearly present a public health risk because of the increased number of accidental injuries due to intoxication. About 16,000 people are killed each year as a result of drunk driving (NIAAA, 2000), and about 10 percent of all personal injury accidents and at least 180,000 to 200,000 property and personal injury crashes, respectively, are caused by alcohol intoxication per year (Wieczorek, 1995). The risk of injury as well as the responsibility for causing a collision when driving while intoxicated is proportional to the blood alcohol level. At the current legal definition of driving while intoxicated (.08 to .10 percent for most states), the relative risk for a crash is conservatively estimated to be five to six times greater than driving while sober (see Figure 2.1). More recent studies that examine the interaction between blood alcohol level, gender, and single versus multiple vehicle collision reveal the relative risk is many times greater than previously believed. For example, a recent study suggests the relative risk of a single car collision for a 16-to-20-year-old male with a blood alcohol level of .10 to .15 percent is about 49 to 1,187 times greater when compared to controls (Zador, Krawchuk, and Voas, 2000).

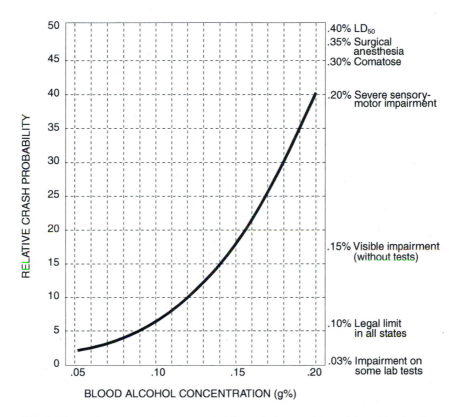

FIGURE 2.1. Relationship between BACs, relative accident risk, and behavior. Some effects may vary due to individual differences. Age and gender may also significantly alter (increase) risk at various BACs beyond what is indicated in figure. (*Source:* Brick and Erickson, 1999, p. 72.)

Pedestrian and Fall-Down Injuries

Although the relationship between alcohol intoxication and automobile accidents is by far the most well studied of alcohol-caused injuries, investigation of the role of alcohol intoxication in other types of injuries is growing. For example, pedestrian-like behaviors are also impaired by alcohol. Since driving and pedestrian activity rely on divided attention and visual-motor processes, it is reasonable to infer that they share similar alcohol-induced changes in relative risk.

Injuries related to falls are the second leading cause of accidents in the United States, and account for about 13,000 deaths per year. Most studies suggest that alcohol increases the risk for injuries due to falls, but one study in particular included a control group that allowed researchers to analyze increases in relative risk for a fall due to alcohol intoxication. Honkanen and colleagues evaluated 313 emergency room patients, more than half of whom had blood alcohol levels greater than .20 percent, and compared them with pedestrians who were at the same location of the accident one week later at the same time of day (Honkanen et al., 1983). The comparison revealed the relative risk for a fall was three times greater for patients with blood alcohol levels between .05 and .10 percent, ten times greater for patients with blood alcohol levels between .10 and .15 percent, and 60 times greater for patients with blood alcohol concentrations .16 percent or higher (Honkanen et al., 1983). More than two-thirds of drivers, pedestrians, and bicyclists who are killed each year are intoxicated (NHTSA, 1994).

Bicycling

Intoxication is believed to be a factor in other types of injuries as well. For example, Li and colleagues reported that fatally injured bicyclists were about twice as likely to be intoxicated as cyclists treated for nonfatal injuries (Li et al., 1996). Alcohol intoxication is a contributing factor in injuries from fires and burns, which account for an estimated 5,000 fatalities and about 1.4 million injuries a year, and is a leading cause of accidents and deaths in the United States (Baker et al., 1992). It is noteworthy that in a study of deaths due to fire, Hingson and Howland found that one-third to two-thirds of these victims had blood alcohol levels greater than .10 percent. At the time of the study, .10 percent represented the blood alcohol level that defined intoxicated driving in most states. The authors concluded from these data that alcohol intoxication is a risk factor for fire deaths (Hingson and Howland, 1993). More recent studies further revealed that alcohol was a factor in about 22 percent (Cherpitel, 1989) to 26 percent (Jones et al., 1991) of burn injuries. Moreover, intoxicated patients have a significantly higher fatality rate in severe burn cases. These data are more thoroughly reviewed in the *Ninth Special Report to the U.S. Congress on Alcohol and Health* (NIAAA, 1997).

Water Sports

The relationship between alcohol intoxication and leisure activities, such as swimming and boating, has been a subject of scientific interest for some time. For example, it can be reasonably predicted that since alcohol impairment causes errors in judgment, disorientation, hypothermia, impaired psychomotor skills, and a decrease in the ability to hold one's breath, it would increase drowning accidents. However, studies published prior to 1985 did not establish a causal relationship between these effects of alcohol intoxication and drowning. Hoxie and colleagues reported that 45 percent of drowning victims had some alcohol in their system and 22 percent were intoxicated with blood alcohol levels of .10 percent or more at the time of death (Hoxie et al., 1988). More recent studies suggest that alcohol consumption significantly increases risk for boating fatalities. In a review of the Boating Accident Report Files in Ohio from 1983-1986, Molberg and colleagues found that alcohol consumption was a factor in up to 21 percent of reported boating accidents (Molberg et al., 1993). Because alcohol deleteriously impairs balance, motor function, and judgment, intoxicated passengers, as well as vessel operators, are probably at risk for injury (Hingson and Howland, 1993).

In another water sport activity, diving, alcohol intoxication contributes to and aggravates spinal cord injuries that frequently follow diving accidents. In this context, Perrine and colleagues examined the effects of alcohol on the ability to perform shallow-water entry dives under experimental conditions (Perrine et al., 1994). The data revealed a progressive and significant impairment of specific aspects of diving performance at blood alcohol levels of .04 percent and higher. Interestingly, this study also correlated diving performance with psychomotor performance using the same standardized field sobriety tests used by many police to detect drunk drivers. Impaired diving correlated well with subjects who failed the validated scoring criteria for the detection of drivers with a blood alcohol level of more than .10 percent (Perrine et al., 1994).

Aircraft Operation

One of the more complex divided attention tasks to challenge persons outside of the laboratory is flying an aircraft. Pilots must attend to an array of instrumentation and make perceptual and cognitive decisions based on a large amount of information in an environment that changes in more than one plane. Although there have been few cases of fatal airline crashes due to pilot intoxication, sufficient data is available to raise concern about this issue of airline safety. For example, it is known from research in other fields that alcohol impairs skills such as divided attention that are believed necessary for safe motor vehicle operation. It is also known that alcohol deleteriously influences the ability of pilots to evaluate their performance (Morrow et al., 1991) and that low levels of alcohol (.025 to .04 percent) impair performance of trained pilots in flight simulators (Billings et al., 1991; Ross et al., 1992).

The effects of alcohol on piloting skills may exceed the direct pharmacological action of alcohol. It has also been suggested that alcohol can impair performance on flight simulators many hours after blood alcohol levels have returned to zero (Yesavage et al., 1994). Although these studies are based on known biobehavioral effects or on flight simulator results, rather than epidemiological data, it is clear more research is needed to understand this important relationship.

Miscellaneous Injuries

In a recent case-control study, Dawson examined the relationship between intoxication and the risk of death from external causes (e.g., suicide, homicide, and accidental injuries) and found that relative to lifetime abstainers and infrequent drinkers, the risk of death from external causes increased logarithmically among infrequent binge drinkers (Dawson, 2001). There was no evidence of reduced risk of death among light or moderate drinkers. The group at highest risk of death from external causes were drinkers who drank less than once a month, but when they did drink, consumed five or more drinks. Within this group, older subjects (defined as 65+ years) were at the highest risk, but younger drinkers (defined as 18 to 24 years of age) were also at high risk of death. Middle-aged drinkers (25 to 64 years of age) did not show the same increased mortality risk, which the author suggested was related to tolerance and experience. Although these data suggest that infrequent binge drinking, as defined, increases risk as a function of age, possible tolerance, and age-related experience, the blood alcohol level that would result from five drinks would be relatively low, allowing the other variables to have a measurable impact.

Intoxication and Injury Outcome

Not only does alcohol intoxication produce direct medical consequences as a result of injuries (e.g., fractures, traumatic amputations, etc.) sustained in a motor vehicle crash, for example, it may also affect injury outcome, particularly head injuries. This is highly significant since up to half of traumatic brain-injured patients have blood alcohol concentrations of .10 percent or more at the time of injury (Zink et al., 2001). For example, motorcycle riders with head injuries are about twice as likely to have fatal head injuries if they are intoxicated than similarly injured riders who are sober (Luna et al., 1984), and contrary to popular misconception, drunk drivers are more likely to be seriously or fatally injured than sober drivers (Waller et al., 1986). Alcohol-intoxicated accident victims with central nervous system injuries were more than twice as likely to die sooner than anatomically matched controls (Zink et al., 1996).

The mechanisms of the exacerbating effects of alcohol on central nervous system injuries are intriguing, but not well understood. Animal studies suggest that the mechanism may be due to the inhibition of free radical scavengers such as dimethyl sulfoxide (Albin and Bunegin, 1986), alcohol-induced cerebral edema as a result of lipid peroxidation (DeCrescito et al., 1974), or increases in plasma osmolality (Elmer et al., 1984; Steinbok and Thompson, 1978). However, Ward and colleagues found that hospitalized major trauma victims with average blood alcohol levels of about .15 percent were significantly less likely to die from injuries than victims in the sober control group (Ward et al., 1982). Similarly, Kraus and colleagues found that contrary to expectations, injury severity and mortality were inversely related to blood alcohol levels (Kraus et al., 1989). This may imply that the mechanisms through which alcohol exacerbates some injuries may be related to metabolic by-products as well as direct pharmacological actions of alcohol itself. In any case, these older study results support the commonly held belief that being intoxicated somehow protects against injuries. However, such a belief is not supported by the majority of more current research on this topic (e.g., Fell and Hertz, 1993). More recent studies suggest that the severity of hemorrhagic shock is greater when intoxicated and results in a higher mortality rate compared to sober controls (Molina et al., 2002). Hemorragic shock also induces acidosis with marked hypercarbia. In such cases, alcohol-induced acidosis would likely increase morbidity and mortality (Chen et al., 2000; Kinkaid et al., 1998; Molina et al., 2002) possibly because of the effects of acidosis on ventilatory responses. Although the literature is complex, some evidence suggests that the effects of alcohol on respiration are mediated through an opioid system. Zink and colleagues (and others) found that the opiate antagonist naloxone can improve hemodynamics and cerebral infusion following traumatic brain injury and hemorrhagic shock but not in alcohol-treated animals. However, alcohol-induced depression of hypercapic (carbon monoxide) ventilatory drive was reversed by naltrexone (Zink et al., 2001).

ALCOHOL AND THE SKELETAL SYSTEM

Although it is not difficult to appreciate the positive and causal relationship between alcohol intoxication and skeletal fractures—one need only look at the large number of motor vehicle and slip-and-fall injuries involving alcohol intoxication—this relationship is more complex and certainly did not start with current epidemiological studies. In fact, the relationship between alcohol abuse and increased risks for skeletal fractures was observed by the ancient Egyptians (Conn, 1985; Mathew, 1992; Seller, 1985). This relationship has since been confirmed by research that suggests alcoholics suffer from a generalized skeletal fragility and are prone to fracture.

Alcohol-Induced Fractures

Current scientific research on the prevalence of fractures in alcoholic subjects is based on epidemiological studies. Those results are generally inconsistent, but there is some evidence of a positive association between alcohol intake and fracture occurrence. For example, men hospitalized for alcohol-related problems are four times more likely to have rib fractures than nondrinking patients (Lindsell et al., 1982) and up to 14 times more likely to have spinal-crush fractures (Crilly et al., 1988; Israel et al., 1980).

In a prospective study, Tuppurainen et al. (1995) found alcohol intake higher among 3,140 perimenopausal women who experienced fractures than among those without fractures. Women who drank alcohol had a risk of a fracture that was about 50 percent higher than among women who did not drink. In another study, increased weekly alcohol intake was associated with greater risks for osteoporotic fractures in postmenopausal women (Paganini-Hill et al., 1981). In the Paganini-Hill study, osteoporotic fractures in women who consumed more than eight drinks per week were almost twice as likely as in nondrinkers. Similarly, a survey of 84,500 U.S. women (ages 34 to 59) who consumed 25 grams of alcohol per day was associated with a 133 percent increase in risk for hip fractures and a 38 percent increase in risk for wrist fractures (Hernandez-Avila et al., 1991). This effect is less common in other populations where the consumption of seven or more standard drinks per week was associated with a twofold increased risk of hip fractures in Japanese women (Fujiwara et al., 1997) and a 4.6-fold increased risk of fractures in a study of black women (Grisso et al., 1994).

Alcohol also increases the risk for fractures in men. In men under the age of 65, two to six drinks per week significantly increased the risk of fractures compared with the same injuries in subjects who consumed less than two drinks per week. For male heavy drinkers younger than age 65, there was almost ten times the risk of hip fractures as men in the same age group who drank lightly (Felson et al., 1988). As sobering as the results for men may be, other investigators have not identified any significant association between alcohol intake and risks for various fractures in women (Johnell et al., 1995; Cumming and Klineberg, 1994; Huang et al., 1996; Naves Diaz et al., 1997; O'Neill et al., 1996). Thus, evidence suggests that excessive alcohol intake increases the risk of fracture but the results are not unanimous. Further, the consequences of low levels of alcohol consumption on skeletal integrity are not well understood.

Studies involving older or intoxicated patients, two groups at high risk for fractures, have methodological limitations including but not limited to defining and quantifying alcohol use due to memory impairment. Despite these problems, including a host of confounding environmental factors such as diet, exercise, and general health, a thorough scientific investigation of the relationship between (moderate) alcohol intake and fracture risks would still have enormous public health implications.

Alcohol-Induced Osteoporosis

In addition to the risk of falls and related injuries previously reviewed, some evidence suggests that alcoholics may also suffer from a generalized skeletal fragility. Bone density is a predictor of fractures and the term osteoporosis is synonymous with low bone density or osteopenia (NIAAA, 2000). Saville was the first to demonstrate the association of osteopenia with alcohol abuse (Saville, 1965). Studying the bone mass of cadavers, Saville found marked reductions in the bone mass of persons with a history of alcoholism and further noted that the bone mass of young alcoholic males were comparable to elderly, postmenopausal females. Since those initial observations, numerous studies have confirmed this effect (Peris et al., 1995; Spencer et al., 1986). In a prospective case-control analysis of risk factors for the development of osteoporosis, Blaauw and colleagues found that average alcohol consumption was two to three times higher in both osteoporotic men and women than in age-matched controls (Blaauw et al., 1994). A similar finding was made in an earlier study in which premenopausal women who consumed more than two standard drinks per day exhibited 13 percent lower bone density of the hip, compared with women who consumed less than one standard drink per week (Gonzalez-Calvin et al., 1993).

Alcohol-reduced bone density is not universally reported within or between studies. Some studies have suggested that increasing alcohol consumption was positively, but anatomically and selectively correlated with bone density (Holbrook and Barrett-Connor, 1993; Lairinen et al., 1993; Lairinen et al., 1991). The Study of Osteoporotic Fractures (7,963 ambulatory, nonblack women ages 65 and older) revealed that modest alcohol intake, less than one drink per day in about 85 percent of the subjects, was associated with higher bone density (Orwoll et al., 1996).

Alcohol's contribution to osteopenia in the overall population is not known, although it is tempting to speculate that lower levels of consumption are less likely to be associated with low bone density and may even be associated with higher bone density. However, the evidence for a protective effect of moderate alcohol consumption is not entirely compelling and should be interpreted with caution as many confounding factors exist in and between many of these studies.

Microscopic Changes in Bone

Microscopic examination of bone (bone histomorphometry) from alcoholics has been helpful in understanding the etiology of skeletal disorders induced by alcohol. Bone mass is controlled by a remodeling cycle that begins with bone breakdown by cells called osteoclasts. This initial period of resorption is coupled with an equal amount of new bone formation by cells called osteoblasts. Bone mass remodeling is an ongoing process throughout most of the life cycle, but one that can be disrupted by alcohol. Alcoholics generally show a reduction in new bone formation with varying reports of increases (Schnitzler and Soloman, 1984) or no changes in bone resorption (Diamond et al., 1989). Overall, these studies suggest that alcoholic bone disease is characterized by considerable suppression of bone formation.

Although alcohol can disrupt the modeling cycle, these changes are reversible. Rapid recovery of osteoblast function occurs within two weeks of abstinence (Diamond et al., 1989; Feitelberg et al., 1987; Lairinen et al., 1992). Evidence also suggests that lost bone tissue is recovered following abstinence (Peris et al., 1994).

Potential Mechanisms of Alcohol-Induced Bone Disease

The normal growth of bone cells depends upon a variety of orchestrated factors, including adequate nutrition and the function and interaction of various hormones and intercellular regulating factors. Research in this area suggests that while the exact mechanism through which alcohol affects the integrity of the skeleton is not known, much has been learned. Even so, likely candidates have not been clearly identified.

Chronic consumption of relatively low amounts of alcohol (one to two drinks per day for women; three to four drinks per day for men) can interfere with the normal metabolism of nutrients. As a result of poor diets, impaired nutrient absorption, or increased renal excretion, alcoholics often have deficiencies in minerals such as calcium, phosphate, and magnesium (Bikle et al., 1985; Kalbfleisch et al., 1963; Lairinen et al., 1992; Tetrito and Tanaka, 1974), as well as low levels of vitamin D, which is necessary for the absorption of calcium from the intestinal system (Lalor et al., 1986; Morbarhan et al., 1984). However, there is little histomorphometric evidence that nutritional deficiencies related to alcohol use are a major cause of alcohol-induced bone disease.

Another candidate that may contribute to alcohol-induced bone disease is calcitonin, a peptide produced by the thyroid gland. Calcitonin inhibits bone resorption, in effect protecting bone. Some evidence suggests that the acute administration of alcohol (equal to about four drinks in a 150-pound male) increases calcitonin levels by about 38 percent three hours after consumption by nonalcoholic males (Williams et al., 1978). Such hypercalcitoninemia might explain why moderate intake of alcohol is associated with higher bone density. However, little is known about repeated alcohol use or how chronic alcohol affects calcitonin.

Blood calcium levels are regulated primarily through parathyroid hormone (PTH). When blood calcium levels drop, PTH induces the release of calcium from bone and reduces renal excretion of calcium. In nonalcoholic subjects, acute alcohol consumption decreased PTH levels three hours after drinking, but prolonged drinking for three weeks increased PTH levels as well as serum calcium (Lairinen et al., 1991). It is still unclear how alcohol might affect PTH and calcium in a clinical population where decreases in bone density are typically observed.

Gonadal hormones may also play a role in alcohol-induced bone disease since impaired gonadal function is a well-known risk factor for osteoporosis. Moreover, alcohol abuse has long been associated with impotence, sterility, testicular atrophy (Valimaki et al., 1982), and low testosterone (Van Thiel et al., 1974) in men, and menstrual disturbances, spontaneous abortions and miscarriages, impaired fertility, sexual function, and premature menopause in women (Gavaler, 1991; Hugues et al., 1980; Mello et al., 1993; Valimaki et al., 1984). Studies in women have yielded inconsistent results. Alcohol increases estradiol, a potent form of estrogen, but this effect has only been reported in postmenopausal women who are undergoing hormone replacement therapy. Nonetheless, if moderate alcohol consumption increases estrogen, it could explain the positive relationship between alcohol use and increased bone density in women (Orwoll et al., 1996; Holbrook and Barrett-Connor, 1993).

Chronic heavy drinking alters the growth and proliferation of many different cell types. In alcoholics, biochemical and histomorphometric studies reveal a significant impairment in osteoblastic, but not osteoclastic activity, suggesting that alcohol's primary adverse effects on bones is through osteoblasts. Since bone remodeling and mineralization both are dependent on osteoblasts, chronic heavy alcohol consumption will ultimately reduce bone mass and consequently lead to fractures.

Alcohol may decrease osteoblast proliferation through a direct toxic mechanism or by the inhibition of intracellular signaling processes that regulate cell replication. Preprogrammed cell death (apoptosis) of some cells is enhanced by alcohol (De et al., 1994; Ewald and Shao, 1993).

Alcohol reduces cell protein and deoxyribonucleic acid (DNA) synthesis in normal osteoblasts (Friday and Howard, 1991; Chavassieux et al., 1993) and impairs the induction of compounds called polyamines (Klein and Carlos, 1995) which regulate the synthesis of DNA. By disrupting the intracellular process that normally stimulates polyamine biosynthesis vital to osteoblast proliferation, alcohol even at low blood alcohol levels (.04 percent range) may inhibit cell division. Exogenous polyamines antagonize the inhibitory effect of alcohol on cell proliferation (NIAAA, 2000). Osteocalcin is a small peptide synthesized by osteoblasts. When released into the circulation, osteocalcin levels are positively correlated with histomorphometric parameters of bone formation in healthy individuals (Garcia-Carrasco et al., 1988) and patients with metabolic bone disease (Delmas et al., 1985). Alcohol produces a dose-dependent decrease in osteocalcin levels and chronic alcoholic patients have significantly lower osteocalcin levels than controls (Labib et al., 1989).

CANCERS

Gastrointestinal Diseases

Not all of the effects of alcohol occur rapidly, as in the cases of motor vehicle crashes, pedestrian falls, and subsequent skeletal injuries. Some medical consequences of alcohol are more insidious, taking years to unfold before any significant medical consequence is detected. Among these are cell damage caused by the direct or indirect toxic effects of alcohol. The first tissue that alcohol comes into contact with is, in most instances, the upper gastrointestinal system.* With the exception of minute quantities of alcohol that are directly absorbed through membranes in the buccal cavity and esophagus, when swallowed, alcohol goes directly to the stomach in high concentrations. Since the toxic effects of alcohol are directly related to dose and concentrations, one might reasonably predict that high concentrations of alcohol have potentially deleterious effects throughout the cells of the gastrointestinal system.

Alcohol inhibits smooth muscle contractions in the lower esophagus (Keshavarzian et al., 1994), which may cause chronic esophageal inflammation. Impaired contraction of the smooth muscles in the esophagus and in

---

*The author has received anecdotal reports from clinicians and recovering alcoholics about intravenous and rectal administration of alcohol, but it is believed that such experimental drug use is rare.

the stomach can also precipitate gastric acid reflux, resulting in a range of symptoms from the relatively benign but very uncomfortable heartburn, to severe esophagitis (inflammation of the esophagus). Prolonged gastric reflux may lead to a permanent tissue alteration, or metaplasia, of the esophageal lining that may progress to esophageal adenocarcinoma (Gray et al., 1993).

The relationship between alcohol consumption and various cancers of the gastrointestinal and other systems has been the subject of considerable research. Several studies have demonstrated a positive relationship between alcohol and esophageal cancer, for example. People who consume more than three drinks per day (21 drinks per week) have almost a tenfold higher risk of esophageal cancer than those who drink less than one drink per day (Vaughan et al., 1995). Esophageal cancers include adenocarcinomas as well as cancers that are derived from normal esophageal cells (i.e., squamous cell carcinomas). Both types of carcinomas are related by the local effects of alcohol metabolites or alcohol-metabolizing enzymes such as alcohol dehydrogenase (ADH) on esophageal cells (Yin et al., 1993). For example, acetaldehyde may alter normal DNA repair mechanisms in esophageal cells and lead to gene alterations and tumor formation (Wilson et al., 1994). Alcohol also increases levels of the CYP2E 1 isozyme in the esophageal mucosa, which can activate dietary carcinogens such as nitrosamines (Shimizu et al., 1990).

Despite the high concentrations of alcohol that reach the stomach from the esophagus, and the effects of alcohol consumption or alcohol metabolites on DNA, alcohol use is not clearly associated with a risk of stomach cancer (Franceschi and La Vecchia, 1994). Alcohol can cause gastritis, but other factors, such as bacterium, may be responsible for inflammation of the stomach. For example, gastritis and ulcer disease in nonalcoholics is often caused by *Helicobacter pylori*. Heavy drinkers have a higher incidence of *H. pylori* and gastritis, than do light drinkers (Paunio et al., 1994). Since alcoholic gastritis is not readily cured by abstinence but is improved by treatment with antibiotics, it has been quite reasonably suggested that gastritis is caused by bacterium (Uppal et al., 1991).

The nexus between gastritis and increased risk for stomach cancer is not well established, and the mechanism that leads the progression from chronic gastritis to neoplasia probably involves many factors besides alcohol. For example, nutritional factors, and in particular the deleterious effects of alcohol on the bioavailability of nutrients, probably play a role in alcohol-related colon cancer in humans. Alcohol in combination with diets low in essential nutrients such as methionine and folate, measurably increases the risk for colon cancer (Giovannucci and Willett, 1994; Giovannucci et al.,

1995). Alcohol also induces the formation of benign hyperplastic polyps in the colon and rectum in humans (Kearney et al., 1995).

The association between alcohol and cancers of the colon and rectum is positive, but weak (Doll et al., 1993; Longnecker, 1992; Longnecker et al., 1990; Seitz and Pöschl, 1997). Again, although alcohol probably plays some role, other mechanisms are probably involved. Recent studies indicate that smoking tobacco coupled with drinking alcohol may serve as a trigger-ing mechanism for colon cancer (Yamada et al., 1997). Acetaldehyde may also have a role as a cocarcinogen in cases of rectal cancer (Seitz and Pöschl, 1997). See NIAAA (2000) for further discussion of this topic.

Does Alcohol Increase the Risk for Breast Cancer?

Despite decades of research suggesting that alcohol increases the risk for breast cancer, reviews of this relationship suggest that the evidence for this relationship is not compelling (English et al., 1995; International Agency for Research on Cancer, 1988; McPherson et al., 1993; Longnecker, 1992, 1994; Longnecker, 1995; Smith-Warner et al., 1998). One factor may be that a complex alcohol-endocrine interaction exists that may be related to postmenopause hormone replacement therapy (Zumoff, 1997; Schatzkin and Longnecker, 1994; Colditz, 1990; Gapstur et al., 1992).

ALCOHOL-INDUCED PANCREATIC INJURY

It is well known that alcohol abuse can lead to chronic pancreatic inflam-mation, atrophy, and fibrosis, although only a small proportion of alcoholics develop pancreatic injury. Specific risk and mechanisms that lead to alco-holic pancreatitis have been difficult to identify (Haber et al., 1995; Doll et al., 1993), but research from animal models suggests that acetaldehyde may play some role in the development of alcoholic pancreatitis, as may di-ets high in polyunsaturated fat. Although alcohol is believed to be a cause of pancreatitis, a link between alcohol and pancreatic cancer has not been made (NIAAA, 2000).

ALCOHOL-INDUCED LIVER INJURY

As the majority of alcohol leaves the gastrointestinal tract, it travels via the hepatic portal vein from the small intestines to the liver, the largest organ in the body and the primary site of alcohol metabolism. Since some alcohol metabolites are toxic, and because the concentration of alcohol reaching the liver is so high and the liver is the primary site of alcohol metabolism, liver damage may be among the most likely and most serious physiological consequences of alcohol abuse. This is particularly significant because of the central role the liver plays in so many physiological activities. Epidemiological data clearly reveals that alcohol abuse is by far the leading cause of liver-related mortality in the United States. Excessive alcohol consumption leads to three serious types of liver injuries: fatty liver, hepatic inflammation (alcoholic hepatitis), and progressive liver scarring (fibrosis or cirrhosis). Chronic heavy drinking can alter normal metabolism and lead to an accumulation of fat in the liver. As a result, the liver cells become infiltrated and the liver itself becomes enlarged. The bad news is that extensive lipid infiltration may damage cells. The good news is that fatty liver is reversible with abstinence.

Hepatitis is a more serious medical condition, characterized by prolific inflammation and tissue damage. Hepatitis is life-threatening but there can be significant recovery following abstinence. The most serious form of liver damage is cirrhosis. This irreversible liver disease is characterized by scarring and cell death. Impaired liver functioning can cause primary hepatic encephalopathy, a brain disorder characterized by altered psychomotor, intellectual, and behavioral functioning.

Although chronic, heavy drinking may produce metabolic tolerance and unusually high rates of alcohol elimination, hepatitis and fibrosis ultimately will impair liver function and produce a reverse metabolic tolerance and impaired oxidation of alcohol. Underreporting of alcohol consumption makes the exact prevalence of alcoholic liver disease in the United States difficult to measure, but health statistics suggest that some form of alcoholic liver disease affects more than 2 million drinkers (Dufour et al., 1993). It is estimated that 900,000 Americans have cirrhosis, and of the 26,000 who die each year, 40 to 90 percent have a history of alcohol abuse (Dufour et al., 1993).

It is clear that the development of alcoholic liver disease is due to a combination of factors, most notably, prolonged alcohol consumption. One commonly asked question by both scientists and concerned drinkers is "How much alcohol does one need to drink before liver damage occurs?" Epidemiological studies suggest that reliable signs of injury begin after a "threshold" dose of alcohol is reached. Although there are always individual exceptions, the evidence suggests that the threshold is equal to a cumulative dose of about 600 kilograms for men, and between 150 and 300 kilograms for women. To place this in perspective, at the high end (for men), this is roughly equivalent to the average consumption of 10 to 12 drinks a day for ten years, and at the low end (for women), about three drinks per day (see Chapter 1). Below these doses, it is difficult (but certainly not impossible) to reliably detect liver injury (Lelbach, 1975; Marbet et al., 1987; Mezey et al., 1988; Tuyns and Pequignot, 1984), or the damage is not significant enough to warrant medical attention. The differences in threshold doses between men and women cannot be accounted for by anthropometrics or pharmacokinetics. In addition, many individuals who consume these amounts of alcohol never develop liver disease and less than one-half of heavy drinkers develop alcoholic hepatitis or liver fibrosis (Lelbach, 1975). This suggests that alcohol does not produce its effects independently and that hereditary and/or environmental factors interact with alcohol to affect the natural history of liver injury (Marbet et al., 1987). Marbet and colleagues suggested that other factors contribute to the pathogenesis of liver disease in alcoholics because even though a substantial amount of alcohol is required to induce liver injury, alcohol dose alone is not a good predictor of the severity of liver injury (Marbet et al., 1987).

Numerous possible mechanisms may affect the susceptibility of certain people to alcohol-induced liver damage, but the exact mechanisms by which chronic alcohol abuse leads to liver disease are not known. A number of mechanisms have been suggested which will be briefly reviewed below.

Mechanisms of Liver Injury

The metabolism of alcohol by hepatocytes requires oxygen, a process that produces free radicals, such as hydroxyl and 1-hydroxyethyl radicals and superoxide anions (Kukielka et al., 1994; Rashba-Step et al., 1993; Reinke et al., 1994). These highly reactive compounds can interact with proteins, lipids, and DNA to cause damage or death to liver cells (Fromenty et al., 1995; Nordmann et al., 1992). Chronic alcohol consumption also causes white blood cells (neutrophils) to migrate to the liver where they are activated by an inflammatory substance to release large amounts of superoxides which may contribute to liver pathology (Bautista et al., 1992).

Normal liver cells contain antioxidants that can neutralize free radicals. Chronic alcohol consumption decreases antioxidant levels in the liver resulting in a state of oxidative stress that makes liver cells more susceptible to free-radical-induced injury. One such antioxidant is glutathione, which is present at high concentrations in liver cytosol and mitochondria. Alcohol inhibits glutathione transport from the cytosol to the mitochondria of the cell, causing impaired mitochondrial functioning, which is believed to cause necrosis (Fernandez-Checa et al., 1991; Garcia-Ruiz et al., 1994).

Acetaldehyde is another highly reactive compound that may promote hepatic injury because high concentrations of this metabolite can become a substrate for aldehyde oxidase and other enzymes which produce free radicals as by-products of this reaction (Kato et al., 1990; Shaw and Jayatilleke, 1990, 1992; Tsukamoto et al., 1995). Since earlier studies have demonstrated that alcoholics accumulate high levels of acetaldehyde (Baraona et al., 1987), acetaldehyde may be part of the process by which the production of free radicals increase and injure liver cells. Acetaldehyde also can react with specific amino acid residues on cellular proteins to form acetaldehyde-protein adducts (Holstege et al., 1994; Niemela et al., 1991), which tend to be localized in sites of greatest liver injury. Acetaldehyde-protein adducts also may stimulate liver cells to produce collagen, which may result in fibrosis and, ultimately, cirrhosis (Bedossa et al., 1994; Casini et al., 1993). Eriksson (2001) recently pointed out that the most compelling evidence that acetaldehyde plays a role in alcoholic liver disease comes from a study of alcoholics who carry the ALDH2*2 and ADH2*2 alleles. In Asian, but not Caucasian alcoholics, there is an association between ADH2*2 alleles and cirrhosis. Interestingly, people with this allele drink less than those without it but are not protected from alcoholic liver disease. In fact, they may develop liver disease (i.e., cirrhosis) at lower levels of alcohol consumption (Eriksson, 2001).

Chronic alcohol use also depletes hepatic levels of vitamins A and E antioxidants (Hagen et al., 1989; Leo et al., 1993), which enhance alcohol-induced lipid peroxidation and exacerbates liver injury in animals (Kawase et al., 1989; Sadrzadeh and Nanji, 1994). However, health-supplement drinkers should note that neither vitamins A nor E have been shown to have any significant preventative effects against alcoholic liver injury (Sadrzadeh et al., 1995; Ahmed et al., 1994; Leo et al., 1992).

Cytokines are a diverse group of substances with inflammatory, fibrogenic, and growth-promoting properties. Many cytokines associated with alcohol-related liver disease are also believed to be mediators of liver injury because patients with alcohol-related hepatitis frequently have high circulating levels of cytokines such as interleukin-1 (IL-1), interleukin-6 (IL-6), interleukin-8 (IL-8), and tumor necrosis factor-alpha (TNF-alpha) (Bird et al., 1990; Hill et al., 1992, 1993; Khoruts et al., 1991; Ohlinger et al., 1993; Sheron et al., 1993; Tilg et al., 1992). Cytokines IL-8 and TNF-alpha, in particular, correlate negatively with prognosis of liver disease (Felver et al., 1990; Hill et al., 1992, 1993; Sheron et al., 1993). Another cytokine-transforming growth factor-beta (TGF-beta), which is found in the livers of alcoholics, is believed to be critical in the development of hepatic fibrosis.

Cirrhosis

Chronic alcohol consumption induces liver fibrosis (scarring) by stimulating the fat-storing cells of the liver to differentiate into collagen-producing stellate cells. It is believed this leads to irreversible cirrhosis. Alcoholic liver fibrosis may occur indirectly through acetaldehyde-protein adducts that can enhance collagen synthesis by stellate cells in vitro (Bedossa et al., 1994; Casini et al., 1993; Moshage et al., 1990). Products of lipid peroxidation also increase collagen synthesis which may lead to fibrosis (Maher et al., 1994; Parola et al., 1993; Tsukamoto, 1993).

Although there are a variety of biomechanical mechanisms through which alcohol or alcohol-metabolites may cause liver damage, the problem is more complex. Hereditary variations in enzymes may explain why only a small proportion of alcoholics develop serious liver disease. Although generic variants, polymorphisms in alcohol dehydrogenase (ADH), CYP2E1 isozyme, and aldehyde dehydrogenase (ALDH) result in various rates of alcohol metabolism among different ethnic groups, no single ADH allele has been causally linked to alcoholic liver injury (Chao et al., 1994; Day et al., 1991; Poupon et al., 1992).

ALDH polymorphisms may also play a role in the development of alcoholic liver injury. ALDHY, an allele which is present in about half of all Chinese and Japanese, encodes an enzyme that is completely nonreactive toward acetaldehyde. ALDHY homozygotic individuals (those who have two copies of this allele) generally have an aversion to alcohol because of the accumulation of acetaldehyde. However, chronic drinkers who are ALDHY heterozygotes (those who have one copy of the ALDHY allele) do not have an alcohol aversion and develop liver injury more frequently and at lower cumulative doses than people with normal ALDH (Enomoto et al., 1991; see Eriksson, 2001).

Finally, gender also may play a role in the development of alcohol-induced liver damage. Some evidence indicates that women are more susceptible than men to the cumulative effects of alcohol on the liver, even though women drink less than men (Becker et al., 1996; Gavaler and Arria, 1995; Hisatomi et al., 1997; Naveau et al., 1997; NIAAA, 1997). Compared with men, women who have alcoholic liver injuries remain at higher risk of disease progression even with abstinence (Galambos, 1972; Pares et al., 1986). This curious gender difference suggests that gastric ADH may be a causative factor. ADH is present at high levels in the liver in both men and women, but differences in gastrointestinal ADH between men and women may affect its bioavailability. Women have lower levels of gastric ADH activity than men (Frezia et al., 1990; Seitz et al., 1992) so their livers receive more concentrated levels of alcohol from the gut, thereby placing women at greater risk for liver damage. Although this is an interesting concept, other investigators have found no such gender differences in gastric ADH activity (Thuluvath et al., 1994), and some researchers question the significance of the stomach in the first-pass metabolism of alcohol (Levitt and Levitt, 1994).

Gender differences in alcohol-induced liver injury may be related to gender differences in the metabolism of fatty acids rather than alcohol itself. The accumulation of nonmetabolized fatty acids in the liver through alcohol inhibition of the oxidation of fatty acids by hepatic mitochondria has long been known to be part of the alcoholic disease process (Lieber et al., 1965; Lieber and DeCarli, 1970). It is believed the infiltration of fat impairs intracellular functioning and causes cell injury (NIAAA, 1997).

CARDIOVASCULAR DISEASES

Cardiovascular disease is the leading cause of death among Americans, followed by cancer and stroke (USDHHS, 1995). The role of alcohol as both a risk factor and a potential protective factor for cardiovascular disease has been the focus of intense investigation for many years (see NIAAA, 1997; Zakhari and Wassef, 1996). The results are clear: alcohol has both deleterious and beneficial effects, but the conditions under which alcohol exerts these unusual behavior effects and the mechanisms involved are complex at best.

Alcohol and Heart Disease

It has been known for nearly eighty years that heavy drinking decreases longevity. Pearl noted that moderate drinkers lived longer than either abstainers or heavy drinkers (Pearl, 1926). Over the life span, total alcohol consumption is inversely associated with heart damage. The deterioration of heart muscle, a condition known as alcoholic cardiomyopathy, is one of the most serious consequences of chronic heavy drinking. As cardiac cells deteriorate, the unique ability of these cells to contract is impaired. This is particularly significant in the heart's left ventricle which pumps freshly oxygenated blood throughout the body. Compensatory mechanisms result in an enlarged heart, but any benefit from such cardiac hypertrophy is temporary. Eventually the heart is unable to meet the body's demand for oxygen. Alcoholic cardiomyopathy is the most common cause of non-ischemic cardiomyopathy in Western societies and is a major source of heart failure and death (NIAAA, 1997, 2000).

As with other diseases, women may also be more sensitive to the toxic effects of alcohol on the heart, even though women drink less, or report drinking less, than men (Fernandez-Sola et al., 1997; Urbano-Marquez et al., 1995).

Possible Beneficial Effects of Alcohol on Coronary Heart Disease

Several prospective studies have reported a reduced risk of death from coronary heart disease across a wide range of alcohol consumption. These include studies among men in the United Kingdom (Doll et al., 1994), Germany (Keil et al., 1997), Japan (Kitamura et al., 1998), and the United States (Fuchs et al., 1995). The definitions of moderate drinking vary among studies; however, most, if not all, of the apparent protective effect against coronary heart disease (CHD) was realized at low to moderate levels of alcohol consumption. For example, in the Fuchs study of more than 85,000 U.S. women, "light to moderate" drinking ranging from one to three drinks *per week* to one to two drinks *per day* was associated with a reduced risk of death from cardiovascular diseases.

A meta-analysis of data from 19 cohort studies and six case-control studies found that the risk of death from CHD was reduced at all levels of alcohol consumption, but the maximum reduction in risk occurred when alcohol consumption was low (English et al., 1995). Other studies have suggested that the protective effects of alcohol are greatest in people already at risk for cardiovascular diseases. For example, an analysis of data from a nine-year follow-up of 490,000 Americans in the Cancer Prevention Study II (Thun et al., 1997) found that both men and women who consumed alcohol had a 30 to 40 percent lower risk of death from all cardiovascular diseases compared to those who abstained from drinking. This effect was greatest among people diagnosed as at risk and was not related to the amount of alcohol consumed.

Similarly, another large U.S. survey, the National Health and Nutrition Examination Survey I, found that the incidence of CHD in men who drank was lower across all levels of consumption than in nondrinkers (Rehm et al., 1997). CHD was also reduced among women, but only in those who consumed low to moderate levels of alcohol. In fact, an increased risk was observed in subjects who consumed more than 28 drinks per week, a finding that is not unique (see Hanna et al., 1997).

An association between moderate drinking and lower risk for CHD does not necessarily mean that alcohol itself is the protective agent. For example, a review of population studies indicates that the higher mortality risk among abstainers may be attributable to shared traits—socioeconomic and employment status, mental health, overall health, and health habits such as smoking—rather than participants' nonuse of alcohol (Fillmore et al., 1998).

It is also important to note that the apparent benefits of moderate drinking on CHD mortality are offset at higher drinking levels by increased risk of death from other types of heart disease, cancer, liver cirrhosis, and trauma (USDHHS, 1999). For these and other reasons, the U.S. Department of Agriculture (USDA) and the USDHHS have defined moderate drinking as one drink per day or less for women and two or fewer drinks per day for men (USDA, 1995). In addition, the NIAAA further recommends that people ages 65 and older limit their consumption of alcohol to one drink per day (NIAAA, 2000).

How Does Alcohol Protect Against Heart Disease?

The mechanisms through which alcohol may protect against CHD are diverse. Animal studies suggest that alcohol may impede uptake of fatty acids into the heart (Brick et al., 1987), the accumulation of fatty deposits, or atherosclerotic plaques in coronary arteries (Dai et al., 1997). Furthermore, the animals used in these studies showed increased levels of high-density lipoproteins (HDL), or "good cholesterol," that is clinically associated with lower risk of CHD.

Other studies have indicated that alcohol consumption increases HDL-cholesterol levels by decreasing the activity of cholesteryl ester transfer protein (CETP), which transfers cholesterol molecules from HDL particles to low (LDL) or very low (VLDL) density lipoprotein particles. High levels of LDL and VLDL are associated with increased risk of CHD (Fumeron et al., 1995). Drinking alcohol seems to alter the gene functioning to increase HDL-cholesterol. Researchers have confirmed the association between alcohol consumption and increased HDL-cholesterol in people through several large epidemiological studies (e.g., Sonnenberg et al., 1996; Marques-Vidal et al., 1995; Huijbregts et al., 1995). However, these changes in HDL-cholesterol and LDL-cholesterol levels contribute only about half of the observed protection against CHD with alcohol consumption. This suggests that other mechanisms may be contributory to the protective effects of alcohol. For example, alcohol may have antithrombotic effects, and may reduce platelet activation and clotting factor activity (Rubin and Rand, 1994). Indeed, evidence suggests that drinking 30 grams of alcohol (just over two drinks) per day for four weeks causes a reduction of platelet aggregation and a decrease in blood levels of fibrinogen, which stimulates clot formation (Pellegrini et al., 1996). Moderate alcohol consumption may

have other antithrombic effects by increasing blood levels of tissue plasminogen activator, an enzyme that breaks down blood clots (Ridker et al.,
1994), or it may suppress the production of substances that promote clotting
(Booyse, 1999).

Beverage Type and Pattern of Consumption

Wine may confer special protection against CHD (Goldberg et al., 1995)
or this protective effect may be due to the alcohol itself (Doll, 1997; Rimm
et al., 1996). Reviews of lipid-reducing effects of wines are available (see
Chadwick and Goode, 1998; Goldberg et al., 1995) and at least one recent
study of Chinese men revealed no additional reduction in overall mortality
associated with drinking rice-fermented wine (Yuan et al., 1997). However,
other factors besides wine may contribute to this effect. The pattern of
drinking, rather than the type of alcohol consumed, may help explain how
drinking wine might protect against CHD (Doll, 1997; Grønboek et al.,
1995; Klatsky and Armstrong, 1993). For example, wine drinkers tend to
consume small amounts of alcohol daily rather than consume larger amounts
of alcohol on weekends. It has been suggested that the pattern of frequent
drinking may confer some protection against CHD and that large amounts
are not needed to achieve a beneficial effect (Bondy, 1996). Similarly, alcohol consumed with meals was found to reduce the postprandial elevations of
blood lipids (Beenstra et al., 1990; Rubin and Rand, 1994). Other studies
have reported a reduced risk of coronary death or acute myocardial infarction with moderate, regular drinking and an increased risk associated with
binge drinking (McElduff and Dobson, 1997; Kauhanen et al., 1991, 1997).

Finally, because many of the epidemiological studies from which much
of the evidence is derived have involved middle-aged or older persons in stable social situations, the findings may not necessarily apply to younger
drinkers, whose risk of CHD is low to begin with, or to other social groups.

In summary, lowered CHD risk is most closely associated with a consistent pattern of drinking small amounts of alcohol. The apparent CHD benefit is largely, if not wholly, attributable to alcohol itself and not to specific
beverages or to other constituents of particular beverages such as red wine.
Future research should help bring clarity to this body of literature (Klatsky
et al., 1997; Rimm et al., 1996).

Alcohol and Blood Pressure

There is a well-documented association between heavy alcohol consumption and hypertension (Ascherio et al., 1996; Seppa et al., 1996; York

and Hirsch, 1997; Campbell et al., 1999). Heavy alcohol consumption elevates blood pressure and causes or exacerbates hypertension (Puddey et al., 1995; Ueshima et al., 1993). It is estimated that one drink per day can chronically increase blood pressure one millimeter of mercury in middle-aged individuals, and even more in the elderly and people with preexisting hypertension (Beilin et al., 1996). Controversy remains as to whether moderate alcohol consumption has any beneficial effects on blood pressure, but reducing alcohol intake may be one means of reducing blood pressure in people with hypertension (Lang et al., 1995; World Health Organization, 1996).

Despite the well-recognized association between alcohol and hypertension, the cellular mechanisms of alcohol's effect on blood pressure are not well understood and are made confusing by the fact that, initially, drinking alcohol dilates blood vessels, which lowers blood pressure. Studies looking to explain how long-term, heavy alcohol consumption reverses this effect and leads to elevated blood pressure have generally concluded that this effect is due to the actions of alcohol on the autonomic nervous system. For example, heavy alcohol consumption has been associated with increased release of the stress hormones adrenaline and norepinephrine, which constrict the blood vessels, increase blood pressure, and decrease sensitivity of baroreceptors. This may be one mechanism through which alcohol leads to hypertension.

Moderate alcohol consumption (about one to three drinks per day) is associated with a slight reduction in blood pressure and may protect against age-related development of hypertension (Gillman et al., 1995; Palmer et al., 1995). The significance of these findings may be offset by an increased risk of death from causes unrelated to cardiovascular disease (e.g., accidental injuries, liver disease, etc.). Heavy alcohol consumption also may alter peripheral regulation of blood pressure by affecting smooth muscle cells in the walls of blood vessels (see Altura and Altura, 1996).

Evidence indicates that the increased blood pressure associated with alcohol use is related to alcohol withdrawal rather than a direct effect of alcohol. Kawano and colleagues found that a single drink of alcohol depresses the blood pressure of patients with hypertension for several hours (Kawano et al., 1996). However, patients who consume one drink each evening for seven days have blood pressure that seesaws; it is low in the evening and increases in the morning, suggesting that regular consumption of alcohol can raise blood pressure during the hours that alcohol is not consumed (Abe et al., 1994). These findings are consistent with observations that sympathetic-nervous-system-induced increases in blood pressure occur during alcohol withdrawal (Denison et al., 1997).

Stroke Risk

There are two relevant forms of stroke: ischemic and hemorrhagic. Ischemic stroke occurs when a blood vessel in the brain is blocked. Hemorrhagic stroke occurs when a blood vessel in the brain ruptures. Alcohol-related hypertension, or high blood pressure, may increase the risk of both forms of stroke. Yet, in people with normal blood pressure, the risk of ischemic stroke may be decreased due to the apparent ability of alcohol to lessen damage to blood vessels due to lipid deposits and to reduce blood clotting. However, whereas alcohol's anticlotting effects may decrease the risk of ischemic stroke, alcohol-induced hypertension may increase the risk of hemorrhagic stroke (Hillbom and Juvela, 1996).

Two relatively recent reviews of the relationship between alcohol consumption and stroke risk revealed no differences in the risk patterns for ischemic or hemorrhagic stroke. One study found clear evidence that heavy drinking was associated with increased stroke risk, particularly in women. This evidence was inconsistent regarding a protective effect of low doses of alcohol against stroke (English et al., 1995). In the second review, the author concluded that although moderate drinking (defined in this review as usual consumption of fewer than two drinks daily for men and less than one drink daily for women) does not appear to increase the risk of ischemic stroke, it is not clear whether moderate drinking protects against this type of stroke (Camargo, 1996). Other studies also fail to offer clear evidence that moderate drinking protects against stroke (Knuiman and Vu, 1996; Yuan et al., 1997) and there is evidence, albeit inconsistent, that moderate drinking may actually increase the risk of hemorrhagic stroke (Camargo, 1996).

In contrast, the Cancer Prevention Study II found that all levels of drinking were associated with a significant decrease in the risk of stroke death in men, but in women, the decreased risk was significant only among those who consumed one drink or less per day (Thun et al., 1997). The Physicians' Health Study reported that male physicians who consumed more than one drink per week had a reduced overall risk of stroke compared with participants who had less than one drink per week (Berger et al., 1999). The authors concluded that the benefit was apparent with as little as one drink per week.

Among young people, long-term heavy alcohol consumption has been identified as an important risk factor for stroke (You et al., 1997). Very recent alcohol intoxication also has been found to be associated with a significant increase in the risk of ischemic stroke, especially in both men and women ages 16 through 40 (Hillbom et al., 1995). For example, researchers in another study reported that recent consumption of alcohol was associated with the onset of stroke in young people during weekends and holidays, possibly reflecting an association with heavy drinking (Haapaniemi et al., 1996).

In summary, heavy drinking appears to increase the risk of hypertension and, although the evidence is not entirely consistent, also may increase the risk of stroke. It remains uncertain whether lower levels of alcohol can help prevent ischemic stroke. In addition to examining how much alcohol is consumed, it may be important to consider drinking patterns in determining stroke risk.

Peripheral Vascular Disease

The possibility that alcohol may protect against CHD has led researchers to hypothesize that alcohol also may protect against peripheral vascular disease. In a 1985 analysis of data from the Framingham Heart Study, alcohol was not found to have a significant relationship, either harmful or protective, with regard to peripheral vascular disease (Kannel and McGee, 1985). Other studies have failed to find a significant relationship between alcohol consumption and the narrowing of blood vessels that define peripheral vascular disease as well. However, a recent study produced much more encouraging results. In an analysis of the 11-year follow-up data from more than 22,000 men enrolled in the Physicians' Health Study, researchers found that daily drinkers who consumed seven or more drinks per week had a 26 percent reduction in risk of peripheral vascular disease (Camargo et al., 1997). This study took into account the effects of smoking, exercise, diabetes, and parental history of myocardial infarction.

Two other studies found inconsistent results with regard to gender. One study of middle-aged and older men and women in Scotland showed that as alcohol consumption increased, the prevalence of peripheral vascular disease declined in men, but not in women (Jepson et al., 1995). In contrast, among people with non-insulin-dependent diabetes, alcohol was associated with a lower prevalence of peripheral vascular disease in women but not in men (Mingardi et al., 1997). Clearly, the relationship of alcohol consumption to peripheral vascular disease requires further study.

CONCLUSIONS

As a pharmacological agent, alcohol is a relatively simple compound. The ubiquitous nature of this drug on most, if not all major organ systems is consistent with its simple molecular structure and its widespread use. Alcohol affects the gastrointestinal, hepatic, cardiovascular, and skeletal systems included in this review, but these effects extend to the organism as a whole when accidental injuries due to intoxication are considered.

From the available alcohol research, several conclusions may be drawn regarding the medical consequences of alcohol use. Most notably and across physiological systems, alcohol's effects are multiphasic. Although the nature of the deleterious and possible protective effects of alcohol continues to emerge, the conditions under which these medical consequences present themselves is complex and will, in all probability, remain elusive for several years. Variables such as gender, diet, environment, lifestyle, genetics, dose and frequency of alcohol use, other drugs, and age interact in complex but sometimes visible ways. The majority of studies suggest that, overall, higher doses of alcohol are deleterious to many physiological systems and precipitate a range of psychosocial and biobehavioral problems. In some individuals and under some conditions, alcohol use seems to have a beneficial effect on health. Both experimental and clinical studies suggest that the protective effects of alcohol, when they do occur, are most often associated with low doses (the equivalent of about one to two drinks per day).

There are many other medical consequences beyond those selected for this review, some of which are presented elsewhere in this book. The exclusion of that body of literature was a function of the enormity of the topic and not the significance of that research. Also, whereas the research relied upon in this chapter focused on clinical studies, preclinical research has been helpful in testing and identifying many of the underlying mechanisms through which alcohol use and abuse causes pernicious as well as beneficial medical consequences. Finally, the importance of continued multidisciplinary research to identify the conditions under which, and the subjects in whom, alcohol produces medical consequences cannot be overstated.

REFERENCES

Abe, H.; Kawano, Y.; Kojima, S.; Ashida, T.; Kuramochi, M.; Matsuoka, H.; Omae, T. (1994). Biphasic effects of repeated alcohol intake on 24-hour blood pressure in hypertensive patients. *Circulation* 89(6):2626-2633.

Ahmed, S.; Leo, M.A.; Lieber, C.S. (1994). Interactions between alcohol and beta-carotene in patients with alcoholic liver disease. *Am Clin Nutr* 60(3):430-436.

Albin, M.; Bunegin, L. (1986). An experimental study of craniocerebral trauma during ethanol intoxication. *Crit Care Med* 14(10):841-846.

Altura, B.M.; Altura, B.T. (1996). Mechanisms of alcohol-induced hypertension: Importance of intracellular cations and magnesium. In Zakhari, S. and Wassef, J. (eds), *Alcohol and the Cardiovascular System*. National Institute on Alcohol Abuse and Alcoholism Research Monograph No. 31, Pub. No. 96-4133. Bethesda, MD: NIAAA, pp. 591-614.

Ascherio, A.; Hennekens, C.; Willett, W.C.; Sacks, F.; Rosner, B.; Manson, J.; Witteman, J.; Stampfer, M.J. (1996). Prospective study of nutritional factors, blood pressure, and hypertension among U.S. women. *Hypertension* 27(5):1065-1072.

Baker, S.P.; O'Neill, B.; Karpf, R. (1992). *The Injury Fact Book,* Second Edition. New York: Oxford University Press.

Baraona, E.; DiPadova, C.; Tabasco, I.; Lieber, C.S. (1987). Transport of acetaldehyde in red blood cells. *Alcohol Alcohol* (suppl):203-206.

Bautista, A.P.; D'Souza, N.B.; Lang, C.H.; Spitzer, I.I. (1992). Modulation of F-met-leu-phe induced chemotactic activity and superoxide production by neutrophils during chronic ethanol intoxication. *Alcohol Clin Exp Res* 16(4):788-794.

Becker, U.; Deis, A.; Sorensen, T.I.; Grønbaek, M.; Borch-Johnsen, K.; Muller, C.F.; Schnohr, P.; Jensen, G. (1996). Prediction of risk of liver disease by alcohol intake, sex, and age: A prospective population study. *Hepatology* 23(5):1025-1029.

Bedossa, P.; Houglum, K.; TrautWein, C.; Holstege, A.; Chojkier, M. (1994). Stimulation of collagen alpha 1 (I) gene expression is associated with lipid perioxidation in hepatocellular injury: A link to tissue fibrosis? *Hepatology* 19(5): 1262-1271.

Beenstra, J.; Ockhuizen, T.; Van de Pol, H.; Wedel, M.; Schaafsma, G. (1990). Effects of a moderate dose of alcohol on blood lipids and lipoproteins postprandially and in the fasting state. *Alcohol Alcohol* 25(4):371-377.

Beilin, L.J.; Puddey, I.B.; Burke, V. (1996). Alcohol and hypertension—Kill or cure? [Review]. *J Hum Hypertens* 10(suppl 2):S1-S5.

Berger, K.; Ajani, U.A.; Kase, C.S.; Gaziano, M.; Buring, J.E.; Glynn, R.J.; Hennekens, C.H. (1999). Light-to-moderate alcohol consumption and the risk of stroke among U.S. male physicians. *N Engl J Med* 341(21):1557-1564.

Bikle, D.D.; Genant, H.K.; Cann, C.E.; Recker, R.R.; Halloran, B.P.; Strewler, G.J. (1985). Bone disease in alcohol abuse. *Ann Intern Med* 103:42-48.

Billings, C.; Demosthesen, T.; White, T.; O'Hara, D. (1991). Effects of alcohol on pilot performance in simulated flight. *Aviat Space Environ Med* 62(3):2323-2335.

Bird, G.L.A.; Sheron, N.; Goka, A.K.; Alexander, G.J.; Williams, R.S. (1990). Increased plasma tumor necrosis factor in severe alcoholic hepatitis. *Ann Intern Med* 112(12):917-920.

Blaauw, R.; Albertse, E.C.; Beneke, T.; Lombard, C.J.; Laubscher, R.; Hough, F.S. (1994). Risk factors for the development of osteoporosis in a South African population: A prospective analysis. *S Afr Med J* 84:328-332.

Bondy, S. (1996). Overview of studies on drinking patterns and consequences. *Addiction* 91(11):1663-1674.

Booyse, F.M.; Aikens, M.L.; Grenett, H.E. (1999). Endothelial cell fibrinolysis: Transcriptional regulation of fibrinolytic protein gene expression (t-PA, u-PA, and PAI-1) by low alcohol. *Alcohol Clin Exp Res* 23(6):1119-1124.

Brick, J.; Carpenter, J.A. (2001). The identification of alcohol intoxication by police. *Alcohol Clin Exp Res* 25(6):850-855.

Brick, J.; Erickson, C. (1999). *Drugs, the Brain, and Behavior: The Pharmacology of Abuse and Dependence.* Binghamton, NY: The Haworth Medical Press, p. 72.

Brick, J.; Pohorecky, L.; DeTurck, K. (1987). Effect of ethanol and stress on cardiac lipase activity. *Life Sciences* 40:1897-1901.

Camargo, C.A. Jr. (1996). Case-control and cohort studies of moderate alcohol consumption and stroke. *Clin Chim Acta* 246(1-2):107-119.

Camargo, C.A. Jr.; Stampfer, M.J.; Glynn, R.J.; Gaziano, J.M.; Manson, J.E.; Goldhaber, S.Z.; Hennekens, C.H. (1997). Prospective study of moderate alcohol consumption and risk of peripheral arterial disease in U.S. male physicians. *Circulation* 95(3):577-580.

Campbell, N.R.; Ashley, M.J.; Carrurhers, S.G.; Lacourciere, Y.; McKay, D.W. (1999). Lifestyle modifications to prevent and control hypertension. 3. Recommendations on alcohol consumption. Canadian Hypertension Society, Canadian Coalition for High Blood Pressure Prevention and Control, Laboratory Centre for Disease Control at Health Canada, Heart and Stroke Foundation of Canada. *Can Med Assoc J* 160(suppl 9):513-520.

Casini, A.; Galli, G.; Salzano, R.; Rotella, C.M.; Surrenti, C. (1993). Acetaldehyde-protein adducts, but not lactate and pyruvate, stimulate gene transcription of collagen and fibronectin in hepatic fat-storing cells. *Hepatology* 19(3):385-392.

Center for Disease Control. (1991). *Morbidity and Mortality Weekly Report,* June 21.

Chadwick, D.J.; Goode, J.A. (eds.) (1998). *Alcohol and Cardiovascular Diseases. Novartis Foundation Symposium 216.* New York: John Wiley and Sons.

Chao, Y.C.; Liou, S.R.; Chung, Y.Y.; Tang, H.S.; Hsu, C.T.; Li, T.K.; Yin, S.J. (1994). Polymorphism of alcohol and aldehyde dehydrogenase genes and alcoholic cirrhosis in Chinese patients. *Hepatology* 19(2):360-366.

Chavassieux, P.; Serre, C.M.; Vernaud, P.; Delmas, P.D.; Meunier, P.J. (1993). In vitro evaluation of dose-effects of ethanol on human osteoblastic cells. *Bone Miner* 22:95-103.

Chen, R.J.; Fang, J.F.; Lin, B.C.; Hsu, Y.P.; Kao, J.L.; Chen, M.F. (2000). Factors determining operative mortality of grade V blunt hepatic trauma. *J Trauma* 49:886-891.

Cherpitel, C.J. (1989). Breath analysis and self reports as measures of alcohol-related emergency room admissions. *J Stud Alcohol* 50(2):155-161.

Cherpitel, C.J. (1993). Alcohol, injury, and risk-taking behavior: Data from a national sample. *Alcohol Clin Exp Res* 17(4):762-766.

Colditz, G.A. (1990). A prospective assessment of moderate alcohol intake and major chronic diseases. *Ann Epidemiol* 1(2):167-177.

Conn, H.O. (1985). Natural history of complications of alcoholic liver disease. *Acta Med Scand* 703(suppl):127-134.

Crilly, R.G.; Anderson, C.; Hogan, D.; Delaquerriére-Richardson, L. (1988). Bone histomorphometry, bone mass, and related parameters in alcoholic males. *Calcif Tissue Int* 43:269-276.

Criqui, M.H.; Ringel, B.L. (1994). Does diet or alcohol explain the French paradox? *Lancet* 344(8939-8940):1719-1723.

Cumming, R.G.; Klineberg, R.J. (1994). Case-control study of risk factors for hip fractures in the elderly. *Am J Epidemiol* 139:493-503.

Dai, J.; Miller, B.A.; Lin, R.C. (1997). Alcohol feeding impedes early atherosclerosis in low-density lipoprotein receptor knockout mice: Factors in addition to high-density lipoprotein-apolipoprotein A1 are involved. *Alcohol Clin Exp Res* 21(1):11-18.

Dawson, D. (2001). Alcohol and mortality from external cues. *J Stud Alcohol* 62: 790-797.

Day, C.P.; Bashir, R.; James, O.F.; Bassendine, M.F.; Crabb, D.W.; Thomasson, H.R.; Li, T.K.; Edenberg, H.J. (1991). Investigation of the role of polymorphisms at the alcohol and aldehyde dehydrogenase loci in genetic predisposition to alcohol-related end-organ damage. *Hepatology* 14(5):798-801.

De, A.; Boyadjieva, N.I.; Pastorcic, M.; Reddy, B.V.; Sarkar, D.K. (1994). Cyclic AMP and ethanol interact to control apoptosis and differentiation in hypothalamic-endorphin neurons. *J Biol Chem* 269:26697-26705.

DeCrescito, V.; Demopoulos, H.; Flamm, E.; Ransohoff, J. (1974). Ethanol potentiation of traumatic cerebral edema. *Surgical Forum* 25:438-440.

Delmas, P.D.; Malaval, L.; Arlot, M.E.; Meunier, P.J. (1985). Serum bone Gla-protein compared to bone histomorphometry in endocrine diseases. *Bone* 6:339-341.

Denison, J.; Jern, S.; Jagenburg, R.; Wandestam, C.; Wallerstedt, S. (1997). ST-segment changes and catecholamine-related myocardial enzyme release during alcohol withdrawal. *Alcohol Alcohol* 32(2):185-194.

Diamond, T.; Stiel, D.; Lunzer, M.; Wilkinson, M.; Posen, S. (1989). Ethanol reduces bone formation and may cause osteoporosis. *Am J Med* 86:282-288.

Doll, R. (1997). Cochrane and the benefits of wine. In Maynard, A.C. (ed.), *Non-random Reflections on Health Services Research on the 15th Anniversary of Archie Cochrane's Effectiveness and Efficiency.* London, UK: BMJ Publishing Group.

Doll, R.; Foreman, D.; La Vecchia, D.; Woutersen, R. (1993). Alcoholic beverages and cancers of the digestive tract and larynx. In Verschuren, P.M. (ed.), *Health Issues Related to Alcohol Consumption* (pp. 125-166). Washington, DC: International Life Sciences Institute Press.

Doll, R.; Peto, R.; Hall, E.; Wheatley, K.; Gray, R. (1994). Mortality in relation to consumption of alcohol: 13 years' observations on male British doctors. *BMJ* 309(6959):911-918.

Dufour, M.C.; Stinson, F.S.; Caces, M.F. (1993). Trends in cirrhosis morbidity and mortality: United States, 1979-1988. *Semin Liver Dis* 13(2):109-125.

Elmer, O.; Goransson, G.; Zoucas, E. (1984). Impairment of primary hemostasis and platelet function after alcohol ingestion in man. *Haemostasis* 14:223-228.

English, D.R.; Holman, C.D.J.; Milne, E.; Winter, M.J.; Hulse, G.K.; Codde, G.; Bower, C.I.; Cortu, B.; de Klerk, N.; Lewin, G.F.; et al. (1995). *The Quantification of Drug-Caused Morbidity and Mortality in Australia, 1992.* Canberra, Australia: Canberra Commonwealth Department of Human Services and Health.

Enomoto, N.; Takase, S.; Takada, N.; Takada, A. (1991). Alcoholic liver disease in heterozygotes of mutant and normal aldehyde dehydrogenase-2 genes. *Hepatology* 13(6):1071-1075.

Eriksson, C.J. (2001). The role of acetaldehyde in the actions of alcohol (update 2000). *Alcohol Clin Exp Res* 25(5):15S-33S.

Ewald, S.J.; Shao, H. (1993). Ethanol increases apoptotic cell death of thymocytes in vitro. *Alcohol Clin Exp Res* 17(2):359-365.

Feitelberg, S.; Epstein, S.; Ismail, F.; D'Amanda, C. (1987). Deranged bone mineral metabolism in chronic alcoholism. *Metabolism* 36:322-326.

Fell, J.; Hertz, E. (1993). The effects of blood alcohol concentration on time of death for fatal crash victims. *Alcohol Drugs and Driving* 9(2):97-106.

Felson, D.T.; Kiel, D.P.; Anderson, J.J.; Kannel, W.B. (1988). Alcohol consumption and hip fractures: The Framingham Study. *Am J Epidemiol* 128:1102-1110.

Felver, M.E.; Mezey, I.; McGuire, M.; Mitchell, M.C.; Herlong, H.F.; Veech, G.A.; Veech, R.L. (1990). Plasma tumor necrosis factor alpha predicts decreased long-term survival in severe alcoholic hepatitis. *Alcohol Clin Exp Res* 14(2):255-259.

Fernandez-Checa, I.C.; Garcia-Ruiz, C.; Ookhtens, M.; Kaplowitz, N. (1991). Impaired uptake of glutathione by hepatic mitochondria from chronic ethanol-fed rats: Tracer kinetic studies in vitro and in vivo and susceptibility to oxidant stress. *J Clin Invest* 87(2):397-405.

Fernandez-Sola, J.; Estruch, R.; Nicholas, J.M.; Pare, JC; Sacanella, E.; Antunex, E.; Urbano-Marquez, A. (1997). A comparison of alcohol cardiomyopathy in women versus men. *Am J Cardiol* 80(4):481-485.

Fillmore, K.M.; Golding, J.M.; Graves, K.L.; Kniep, S.; Leino, E.V.; Romelsjo, A.; Shoemaker, C.; Ager, C.R.; Allebeck, P.; Ferrer, H.P. (1998). Alcohol consumption and mortality. I. Characteristics of drinking groups. *Addiction* 93(2):183-203.

Franceschi, S.; La Vecchia, C. (1994). Alcohol and the risk of cancers of the stomach and colon-rectum. *Dig Dis* 12(5):276-289.

Frezia, M.; di Padova, C.; Pozzato, G.; Terpin, M.; Baraona, E.; Lieber, C.S. (1990). High blood alcohol levels in women: The role of decreased gastric alcohol dehydrogenase activity and first-pass metabolism. *N Engl J Med* 322(2):95-99.

Friday, K.; Howard, G.A. (1991). Ethanol inhibits human bone cell proliferation and function in vitro. *Metabolism* 40:562-565.

Fromenty, B.; Grimbert, S.; Mansouri, A.; Beaugrand, M.; Erlinger, S.; Rotig, A.; Pessayre, D. (1995). Hepatic mitochondrial DNA deletion in alcoholics: Association with microvesicular steatosis. *Gastroenterology* 108(1):193-200.

Fuchs, C.S.; Stampfer, M.J.; Colditz, G.A.; Giovannucci, E.L.; Manson, J.E.; Kawachi, I.; Hunter, D.J.; Hankinson, S.E.; Hennekens, C.H.; Rosner, B. (1995). Alcohol consumption and mortality among women. *N Engl J Med* 332(19): 1245-1250.

Fujiwara, S.; Kasagi, F.; Yamada, M.; Kodama, K. (1997). Risk factors for hip fracture in a Japanese cohort. *J Bone Miner Res* 12:998-1004.

Fumeron, F.; Betoulle, D.; Luc, G.; Behague, I.; Ricard, S.; Poirier, O.; Jemaa, R.; Evans, A.; Arveiler, D.; Marques-Vidal, P.; et al. (1995). Alcohol intake modulates the effect of a polymorphism of the cholesteryl ester transfer protein gene on plasma high density lipoprotein and the risk of myocardial infarction. *J Clin Invest* 96(3):1664-1671.

Galambos, I.T. (1972). Natural history of alcoholic hepatitis. 3: Histological changes. *Gastroenterology* 63(6):1026-1035.

Gapstur, S.M.; Potter, J.D.; Sellers, T.A.; Folsom, A.R. (1992). Increased risk of breast cancer with alcohol consumption in postmenopausal women. *Am J Epidemiol* 136(10):1221-1231.

Garcia-Carrasco, M.; Gruson, M.; De Vernejoul, C. (1988). Osteocalcin and bone histomorphometric parameters in adults without bone disease. *Calcif Tissue Int* 42:13-17.

Garcia-Ruiz, C.; Morales, A.; Ballesta, A.; Rodes, I.; Kaplowitz, N.; Fernandez-Checa, I.C. (1994). Effect of chronic ethanol feeding on glutathione and functional integrity of mitochondria in periportal and perivenous rat hepatocytes. *Clin Invest* 94(1):193-201.

Gavaler, J.S. (1991). Effects of alcohol on female endocrine function. *Alcohol Health Res World* 15:104-109.

Gavaler, J.S.; Arria, A.M. (1995). Increased susceptibility of women to alcoholic liver disease: Artifactual or real? In Hall, P.M. (ed.), *Alcoholic Liver Disease: Pathology and Pathogenesis,* Second Edition. London, UK: Edward Arnold, pp. 123-133.

Gillman, M.W.; Cook, N.R.; Evans, D.A.; Rosner, B.; Hennekens, C.H. (1995). Relationship of alcohol intake with blood pressure in young adults. *Hypertension* 25(5):1106-1110.

Giovannucci, E.; Rimm, E.B.; Ascherio, A.; Stampfer, M.J.; Colditz, G.A.; Willett, W.C. (1995). Alcohol, low-methionine, low-folate diets, and risk of colon cancer in men. *J Natl Cancer Inst* 87(4):265-273.

Giovannucci, E.; Willett, W.C. (1994). Dietary factors and risk of colon cancer. *Ann Med* 26(6):443-452.

Goldberg, D.M.; Hahn, S.E.; Parkes, J.G. (1995). Beyond alcohol beverage consumption and cardiovascular mortality. *Clin Chim Acta* 237(1-2):155-187.

Gonzalez-Calvin, J.L.; Garcia-Sanchez, A.; Bellot, V.; Munoz-Torres, M.; Raya-Alvarez, E.; Salvatierra-Rios, D. (1993). Mineral metabolism, osteoblastic function, and bone mass in chronic alcoholism. *Alcohol Alcohol* 28:571-579.

Gray, M.R.; Donnelly, R.I.; Kingsnorth, A.N. (1993). The role of smoking and alcohol in metaplasia and cancer risk in Barrett's columnar lined oesophagus. *Gut* 34(6):727-731.

Grisso, J.A.; Kelsey, J.L.; Strom, B.L.; O'Brien, L.A.; Maislin, G.; LaPann, K.; Samelson, L.; Hoffman, S. (1994). Risk factors for hip fracture in black women. The Northeast Hip Fracture Study Group. *N Engl J Med* 330:1555-1559.

Grønboek, D.A.; Deis, A.; Sørensen, T.I.; Becker, U.; Schnohr, P.; Jensen, G. (1995). Mortality associated with moderate intake of wine, beer, or spirits. *BMJ* 310(6988):1165-1169.

Haapaniemi, H.; Hillbom, M.; Juvela, S. (1996). Weekend and holiday increase in the onset of ischemic stroke in young women. *Stroke* 27(6):1023-1027.

Haber, P.; Wilson, I.; Apte, M.; Korsten, M.; Pirola, R. (1995). Individual susceptibility to alcoholic pancreatitis: Still an enigma. *J Lab Clin Med* 125(3):305-312.

Hagen, B.F.; Bjorneboe, A.; Bjorneboe, G.E.; Drevon, C.A. (1989). Effect of chronic ethanol consumption on the content of alpha-tocopherol in subcellular fractions of rat liver. *Alcohol Clin Exp Res* 13(2):246-251.

Hanna, F.Z.; Chou, S.P.; Grant, B.F. (1997). The relationship between drinking and heart disease morbidity in the United States: Results from the National Health Interview Survey. *Alcohol Clin Exp Res* 21(1):111-118.

Hernandez-Avila, M.; Colditz, G.A.; Stampfer, M.J.; Rosner, B.; Speizer, F.E.; Willett, W.C. (1991). Caffeine, moderate alcohol intake, and risk of fractures of the hip and forearm in middle-aged women. *Am J Clin Nutr* 54:157-163.

Hill, D.B.; Marsano, L.; Cohen, D.; Allen, I.; Shedlofsky, S.; McClain, C.I. (1992). Increased plasma interleukin-6 concentrations in alcoholic hepatitis. *J Lab Clin Med* 119(5):547-552.

Hill, D.B.; Marsano, L.S.; McClain, C.I. (1993). Increased plasma interleukin-8 concentrations in alcoholic hepatitis. *Hepatology* 18(3):576-580.

Hillbom, M.; Haapaniemi, H.; Juvela, S.; Palomaki, H.; Numminen, H.; Kaste, M. (1995). Recent alcohol consumption, cigarette smoking, and cerebral infarction in young adults. *Stroke* 26(1):40-45.

Hillbom, M.; Juvela, S. (1996). Alcohol and risk for stroke. In Zakhari, S. and Wassef, M. (eds.), *Alcohol and the Cardiovascular System.* NIAAA Research Monograph No. 31. Bethesda, MD: NIAAA, pp. 63-83.

Hingson, R.; Howland, J. (1993). Alcohol and non-traffic unintended injuries. *Addiction* 88(7):877-883.

Hisatomi, S.; Kumashiro, R.; Sata, M.; Ishii, K.; Tanikawa, K. (1997). Gender difference in alcoholic and liver disease in Japan: An analysis based on histological findings. *Hepatol Res* 8(2):113-120.

Holbrook, T.L.; Barrett-Connor, E. (1993). A prospective study of alcohol consumption and bone mineral density. *BMJ* 306:1506-1509.

Holstege, A.; Bedossa, P.; Poynard, T.; Kollinger, M.; Chaput, J.C.; Houglum, K.; Chojkier, M. (1994). Acetaldehyde-modified epitopes in liver biopsy specimens of alcoholic and nonalcoholic patients: Localization and association with progression of liver fibrosis. *Hepatology* 19(2):367-374.

Honkanen, R.; Ertoma, L.; Kuosmanen, P.; Linnoina, M.; Alah, A.; Visori, T. (1983). The role of alcohol in accident falls. *J Stud Alcohol* 44:231-245.

Hoxie, P.; Cardosi, K.; Stearns, M.; Mengert, P. (1988). *Alcohol in Fatal Recreational Boating Accidents.* Pub. No. DOT CGD 0488. Washington, DC: U.S. Department of Transportation, U.S. Coast Guard.

Huang, Y.S.; Chan, C.Y.; Wu, J.C.; Pai, C.H.; Chao, Y.; Lee, S.D. (1996). Serum levels of interleukin-8 in alcoholic liver disease: Relationship with disease stage, biochemical parameters, and survival. *J Hepatol* 24(4):377-384.

Hugues, J.N.; Coste, T.; Perret, G.; Jayle, M.F.; Sebaoun, J.; Modigliani, E. (1980). Hypothalamopituitary ovarian function in thirty-one women with chronic alcoholism. *Clin Endocrinol* 12:543-551.

Huijbregts, P.P.; Freskens, E.J.; Kromhout, D. (1995). Dietary patterns and cardiovascular risk factors in elderly men: The Zutphen Elderly Study. *Int J Epidemiol* 24(2):313-320.

International Agency for Research on Cancer (1988). *Alcohol Drinking.* Lyon, France: IARC.

Israel, Y.; Orrego, H.; Holt, S.; Macdonald, D.W.; Meema, H.E. (1980). Identification of alcohol abuse: Thoracic fractures on routine chest x-rays as indicators of alcoholism. *Alcoholism* 4:420-422.

Jepson, R.G.; Fowkes, F.G.; Donnan, P.T.; Housley, E. (1995). Alcohol intake as a risk factor for peripheral arterial disease in the general population in the Edinburgh Artery Study. *Eur J Epidemiol* 11(1):9-14.

Johnell, O.; Gullberg, B.; Kanis, J.A.; Allander, E.; Elffors, L.; Dequeker, J.; Dilsen, G.; Gennari, C.; Vaz, A.L.; Lyritis, G.; et al. (1995). Risk factors for hip fracture in European women: The MEDOS study. *J Bone Miner Res* 10:1802-1815.

Jones, J.D.; Barber, B.; Engrav, L.; Heimbach, D. (1991). Alcohol use and burn injury. *J Burn Care Rehabil* 12(2):148-152.

Kalbfleisch, J.M.; Lindeman, R.D.; Ginn, H.E.; Smith, W.O. (1963). Effects of ethanol administration on urinary excretion of magnesium and other electrolytes in alcoholic and normal subjects. *J Clin Invest* 42:1471-1475.

Kannel, W.B.; McGee, D.L. (1985). Update on some epidemiologic features of intermittent claudication: The Framingham study. *J Am Geriatr Soc* 33(1):13-18.

Kato, S.; Kawase, T.; Alderman, J.; Inatomi, N.; Lieber, C.S. (1990). Role of xanthine oxidase in ethanol-induced lipid peroxidation in rats. *Gastroenterology* 98(1):203-210.

Kauhanen, J.; Kaplan, G.A.; Goldberg, D.D.; Cohen, R.D.; Lakka, T.A.; Salonen, J.T. (1991). Frequent hangovers and cardiovascular mortality in middle-aged men. *Epidemiology* 8(3):310-314.

Kauhanen, J.; Kaplan, G.A.; Goldberg, D.E.; Salonen, J.T. (1997). Beer binging and mortality: Results from the Kuopio ischaemic heart disease risk factor study, a prospective population based study. *BMJ* 315(7112):846-851.

Kawano, Y.; Abe, H.; Imanishi, M.; Kojima, S.; Yoshimi, H.; Takishita, S.; Omae, T. (1996). Pressor and depressor hormones during alcohol-induced blood pressure reduction in hypertensive patients. *J Hum Hypertens* 10(9):595-599.

Kawase, T.; Kato, S.; Lieber, C.S. (1989). Lipid peroxidation and antioxidant defense systems in rat liver after chronic ethanol feeding. *Hepatology* 10(5):815-821.

Kearney, J.; Giovannucci, E.; Rimm, E.B.; Stampfer, M.J.; Colditz, G.A.; Ascherio, A.; Bleday, R.; Willett, W.C. (1995). Diet, alcohol, and smoking and the occurrence of hyperplastic polyps of the colon and rectum (United States). *Cancer Causes Control* 6(1):45-56.

Keil, U.; Chambless, L.E.; Doring, A.; Filipiak, B.; Stieber, J. (1997). The relation of alcohol intake to coronary heart disease and all-cause mortality in a beer-drinking population. *Epidemiology* 8(2):150-156.

Keshavarzian, A.; Zorub, O.; Sayeed, M.; Urban, G.; Sweeney, C.; Winship, D.; Fields, J. (1994). Acute ethanol inhibits calcium influxes into esophageal smooth but not striated muscle: A possible mechanism for ethanol-induced inhibition of esophageal contractility. *J Pharmacol Exp Ther* 270(3):1057-1062.

Khoruts, A.; Stahnke, L.; McClain, C.J.; Logan, G.; Allen, J.I. (1991). Circulating tumor necrosis factor, interleukin-1, and interleukin-6 concentrations in chronic alcoholic patients. *Hepatology* 13(2):267-276.

Kinkaid, E.H.; Miller, P.R.; Meredith, J.W.; Rahman, N.; Change, M.C. (1998). Elevated arterial base deficit in trauma patients: A marker of impaired oxygen utilization. *J Am Coll Surg* 187:384-392.

Kitamura, A.; Iso, H.; Sankai, T.; Naito, Y.; Sato, S.; Kiyama, M.; Okamura, T.; Nakagawa, Y.; Iida, M.; Shimamoro, T.; Komachi, Y. (1998). Alcohol intake and premature coronary heart disease in urban Japanese men. *Am J Epidemiol* 147(1):59-65.

Klatsky, A.L.; Armstrong, M.A. (1993). Alcoholic beverage choice and risk of coronary artery disease mortality: Do red wine drinkers fare best? *Am J Cardiol* 71(5):467-469.

Klatsky, A.L.; Armstrong, M.A.; Friedman, G.D. (1997). Red wine, white wine, liquor, beer, and risk for coronary artery disease hospitalization. *Am J Cardiol* 80(4):416-420.

Klein, R.F.; Carlos, A.S. (1995). Inhibition of osteoblastic cell proliferation and ornithine decarboxylase activity by ethanol. *Endocrinology* 136:3406-3411.

Knuiman, M.W.; Vu, H.T. (1996). Risk factors for stroke mortality in men and women: The Busselton Study. *J Cardiovasc Risk* 3(5):447-452.

Kraus, J.; Morgenstern, H.; Fife, D.; Conroy, C.; Nourjah, P. (1989). Blood alcohol tests, prevalence of involvement and outcomes following brain injury. *Am J Pub Health* 79(3):294-299.

Kukielka, E.; Dicker, E.; Cederbaum, A.I. (1994). Increased production of reactive oxygen species by rat liver mitochondria after chronic ethanol treatment. *Arch Biochem Biophys* 309(2):377-386.

Labib, M.; Abdel-Kader, M.; Ranganath, L.; Teale, D.; Marks, V. (1989). Bone disease in chronic alcoholism: The value of plasma osteocalcin measurement. *Alcohol Alcohol* 24:141-144.

Lairinen, K.; Karkkainen, M.; Lalla, M.; Lambergallardt, C.; Tunninen, R.; Tahtela, R.; Valimaki, M. (1993). Is alcohol an osteoporosis-inducing agent for young and middle-aged women? *Metabolism* 42(7):875-881.

Lairinen, K.; Lamberg-Allardt, C.; Tunninen, R.; Harkonen, M.; Valimaki, M. (1992). Bone mineral density and abstention-induced changes in bone and mineral metabolism in noncirrhotic male alcoholics. *Am J Med* 93:642-650.

Lairinen, K.; Valimaki, M.; Keto, P. (1991). Bone mineral density measured by dual-energy X-ray absorptiometry in healthy Finnish women. *Calcif Tissue Int* 48:224-231.

Lalor, B.C.; France, M.W.; Powell, D.; Adams, P.H.; Counihan, T.B. (1986). Bone and mineral metabolism and chronic alcohol abuse. *Q J Med* 59:497-511.

Lang, T.; Nicaud, V.; Darne, B.; Rueff, B. (1995). Improving hypertension control among excessive alcohol drinkers: A randomised controlled trial in France. The WALPA Group. *J Epidemiol Comm Health* 49(6):610-616.

Lelbach, W.K. (1975). Cirrhosis in the alcoholic and its relation to the volume of alcohol abuse. *Ann NY Acad Sci* 252:85-105.

Leo, M.A.; Kim, C.; Lowe, N.; Lieber, C.S. (1992). Interaction of ethanol with beta-carotene: Delayed blood clearance and enhanced hepatotoxicity. *Hepatology* 15(5):883-891.

Leo, M.A.; Rosman, A.S.; Lieber, C.S. (1993). Differential depletion of carotenoids and tocopherol in liver disease. *Hepatology* 17(6):977-986.

Levitt, M.D.; Levitt, D.G. (1994). The critical role of the rate of ethanol absorption in the interpretation of studies purporting to demonstrate gastric metabolism of ethanol. *Pharmacol Exp Ther* 269(1):297-304.

Li., G.; Baker, S.P.; Sterling, S.; Smialek, J.E.; Dischinger, P.C.; Soderstron, C. (1996). A comparative analysis of alcohol in fatal and non-fatal bicycling injuries. *Alcohol Clin Exp Res* 20:1553-1559.

Lieber, C.S.; DeCarli, L.M. (1970). Quantitative relationship between amount of dietary fat and severity of alcoholic fatty liver. *Am Clin Nutr* 23(4):474-478.

Lieber, C.S.; Jones, D.P.; DeCarli, L.M. (1965). Effects of prolonged ethanol intake: Production of fatty liver despite adequate diets. *Clin Invest* 44(6):1009-1021.

Lindsell, D.R.; Wilson, A.G.; Maxwell, J.D. (1982). Fractures on the chest radiograph in detection of alcoholic liver disease. *BMJ* 285:597-599.

Longnecker, M.P. (1992). Alcohol consumption in relation to risk of cancers of the breast and large bowel. *Alcohol Health Res World* 16:223-229.

Longnecker, M.P. (1994). Alcoholic beverage consumption in relation to risk of breast cancer: Meta-analysis and review. *Cancer Causes Control* 5(1):73-82.

Longnecker, M.P. (1995). Alcohol consumption and risk of cancer in humans: An overview. *Alcohol* 12(2):87-96.

Longnecker, M.P.; Orza, M.J.; Adams, M.E.; Vioque, J.; Chalmers, T.C. (1990). A meta-analysis of alcoholic beverage consumption in relation to risk of colorectal cancer. *Cancer Causes Control* 1(1):59-68.

Luna, G.K.; Maier, R.V.; Sowder, L.; Copass, M.K.; Oreskovich, M.R. (1984). The influence of ethanol intoxication on outcome of injured motorcyclists. *J Trauma* 24(8):695-700.

Maher, J.J.; Tzagarakis, C.; Gimenez, A. (1994). Malondialdehyde stimulates collagen production by hepatic lipocytes only upon activation in primary culture. *Alcohol* 29(5):605-610.

Marbet, U.A.; Bianchi, L.; Meury, U.; Stalder, G.A. (1987). Long-term histological evaluation of the natural history and prognostic factors of alcoholic liver disease. *J Hepatol* 4(3):364-372.

Marques-Vidal, P.; Cambou, J.P.; Nicaud, V.; Luc, G.; Evans, A.; Arveiler, D.; Bingham, A.; Cambien, F. (1995). Cardiovascular risk factors and alcohol consumption in France and Northern Ireland. *Atherosclerosis* 115(2):225-232.

Mathew, V.M. (1992). Alcoholism in biblical prophecy. *Alcohol* 27:89-90.

McElduff, P.; Dobson, A.J. (1997). How much alcohol and how often? Population based case-control study of alcohol consumption and risk of a major coronary event. *BMJ* 314(7088):1159-1164.

McPherson, K.; Engelsman, E.; Conning, D. (1993). Breast cancer. In Verschuren, P. (ed.), *Alcoholic Beverages and European Society: Annex 3. Health Issues Related to Alcohol Consumption* (pp. 221-244). Brussels, Belgium: International Life Sciences Institute.

Mello, N.K.; Mendelson, I.H.; Teoh, S.K. (1993). An overview of the effects of alcohol on neuroendocrine function in women. In Zakhari, S. (ed.), *Alcohol and the Endocrine System* (pp. 139-169). NIAAA Research Monograph No.23, National Institutes of Health Pub. No.93-3533. Bethesda, MD: NIH, NIAAA.

Mezey, E.; Kolman, C.I.; Diehl, A.M.; Mitchell, M.C.; Herlong, H.F. (1988). Alcohol and dietary intake in the development of chronic pancreatitis and liver disease in alcoholism. *Am Clin Nutr* 48(1):148-151.

Mingardi, R.; Avogaro, A.; Noventa, F.; Strazzabosco, M.; Stocchiero, C.; Tiengo, A.; Erie, G. (1997). Alcohol intake is associated with a lower prevalence of peripheral vascular disease in non-insulin-dependent diabetic women. *Nutr Metab Cardiovasc Dis* 7(4):301-308.

Mobarhan, S.A.; Russell, R.M.; Recker, R.R.; Posner, D.B.; Iber, F.L.; Miller, P. (1984). Metabolic bone disease in alcoholic cirrhosis: A comparison of the effect of Vitamin D, 25-hydroxyvitamin D, or supportive treatment. *Hepatology* 4:266-273.

Molberg, P.; Hopkins, R.; Paulson, J.; Gunn, R. (1993). Fatal incident risk factors in recreational boating in Ohio. *Pub Health Rep* 108(3):340-346.

Molina, P.E.; McClain, C.; Valla, D.; Guidot, D.; Diehl, A.M.; Lang, C.H.; Neuman, M. (2002). Molecular pathology and clinical aspects of alcohol-induced tissue injury. *Alcohol Clin Exp Res* 26(1):120-128.

Morrow, D.; Leirer, V.; Yesavage, J.; Tinklenberg, J. (1991). Alcohol, age, and piloting: Judgment, mood, and actual performance. *Int J Addict* 26(6):669-683.

Moshage, H.; Casini, A.; Lieber, C.S. (1990). Acetaldehyde selectively stimulates collagen production in cultured rat liver fat-storing cells but not in hepatocytes. *Hepatology* 12(3):511-518.

National Highway Traffic Safety Administration (1994). *Traffic Safety Facts 1993: Alcohol.* Washington, DC: U.S. Department of Transportation, National Center for Statistics and Analysis.

National Institute on Alcohol Abuse and Alcoholism (1997). *Ninth Special Report to the U.S. Congress on Alcohol and Health.* NIH Publication No. 97-4017. Bethesda, MD: NIAAA.

National Institute on Alcohol Abuse and Alcoholism (2000). *Tenth Special Report to the U.S. Congress on Alcohol and Health.* Washington, DC: U.S. Department of Health and Human Services.

Naveau, S.; Giraud, V.; Borocto, E.; Aubert, A.; Capron, F.; Chaput, J.C. (1997). Excess weight risk factor for alcoholic liver disease. *Hepatology* 25(1):108-111.

Naves Diaz, M.; O'Neill, T.W.; Silman, A.J. (1997). The influence of alcohol consumption on the risk of vertebral deformity. *Osteoporos Int* 7:65-71.

Niemela, O.; Juvonen, T.; Parkkila, S. (1991). Immunohistochemical demonstration of acetaldehyde-modified epitopes in human liver after alcohol consumption. *J Clin Invest* 87(4):1367-1374.

Nordmann, R.; Rjbiere, C.; Rouach, H. (1992). Implication of free radical mechanisms in ethanol-induced cellular injury. *Free Radical Biol Med* 12(3):219-240.

Ohlinger, W.; Dinges, H.P.; Zatloukal, K.; Mair, S.; Gollowitsch, F.; Denk, H. (1993). Immunohistochemical detection of tumor necrosis factor-alpha, other cytokines, and adhesion molecules in human livers with alcoholic hepatitis. *Virchows Arch A Pathol Anat Histopathol* 423(3):169-176.

O'Neill, T.W.; Marsden, D.; Adams, J.E.; Silman, A.J. (1996). Risk factors, falls, and fracture of the distal forearm in Manchester, UK. *J Epidemiol Comm Health* 50:288-292.

Orwoll, E.S.; Bauer, D.C.; Vogt, T.M.; Fox, K.M. (1996). Axial bone mass in older women: Study of osteoporotic fracture research group. *Ann Intern Med* 124:187-196.

Paganini-Hill, A.; Ross, R.K.; Gerkins, V.R. (1981). Menopausal estrogen therapy and hip fractures. *Ann Intern Med* 95:28-31.

Palmer, A.J.; Fletcher, A.E.; Bulpitt, C.J.; Beevers, D.G.; Coles, E.C.; Ledingham, J.G.; Petrie, J.C.; Webster, J.; Dollery, C.T. (1995). Alcohol intake and cardiovascular mortality in hypertensive patients: Report from the Department of Health Hypertension Care Computing Project. *J Hypertens* 13(9):957-964.

Pares, A.; Caballeria, J.; Bruguera, M.; Torres, M.; Rodes, J. (1986). Histological course of alcoholic hepatitis: Influence of abstinence, sex and extent of hepatic damage. *J Hepatol* 2(1):33-42.

Parola, M.; Pinzani, M.; Casini, A.; Albano, E.; Poli, G.; Gentilini, A.; Gentilini, P.; Dianzani, M.U. (1993). Stimulation of lipid peroxidation or 4-hydroxynonenal treatment increases procollagen alpha 1 (I) gene expression in human liver fat-storing cells. *Biochem Biophys Res Commun* 194(3):1044-1050.

Paunio, M.; Hook-Nikanne, J.; Kosunen, T.U.; Vainio, U.; Salaspuro, M.; Makinen, J.; Heinonen, O.P. (1994). Association of alcohol consumption and *Helicobacter pylori* infection in young adulthood and early middle age among patients with gastric complaints: A case-control study on Finnish conscripts officers and other military personnel. *Eur J Epidemiol* 10(2):205-209.

Pearl, R. (1926). *Alcohol and Longevity.* New York: Alfred Knopf.

Pellegrini, M.; Pareti, F.I.; Stabile, F.; Brusamolino, A.; Simonetti, P. (1996). Effects of moderate consumption of red wine on platelet aggregation and haemostatic variables in healthy volunteers. *Eur J Clin Nutr* 50(4):209-213.

Peris, P.; Guanabens, N.; Parés, A.; Pons, F.; Del Rio, L.; Monegal, A.; Suris, X.; Caballería, J.; Rodés, J.; Munoz-Gómez, J. (1995). Vertebral fractures and osteopenia in chronic alcoholic patients. *Calcif Tissue Int* 57:111-114.

Peris, P.; Pares, A.; Guanabens, N.; Del Rio, L.; Pons, F.; Deosaba, M.J.M.; Monegal, A.; Caballeria, J.; Rodes, J.; Munoz-Gómez, J. (1994). Bone mass improves in alcoholics after 2 years of abstinence. *J Bone Miner Res* 9(10):1607-1612.

Perrine, M.W.; Mundt, J.C.; Winer, R.I. (1994). When alcohol and water don't mix: Diving under the influence. *J Stud Alcohol* 55:517-524.

Poupon, R.E.; Nalpas, B.; Coutelle, C.; Fleury, B.; Couzigou, P.; Higueret, D. (1992). Polymorphism of alcohol dehydrogenase, alcohol and aldehyde dehydrogenase activities: Implication in alcoholic cirrhosis in white patients. The French Group for Research on Alcohol and Liver. *Hepatology* 15(6):1017-1022.

Puddey, I.B.; Beilin, L.J.; Vandongen, R.; Rouse, I.L.; Rogers, P. (1995). Evidence for a direct effect of alcohol consumption on blood pressure in normotensive men: A randomized controlled trial. *Hypertension* 7(5):707-713.

Rashba-Step, J.; Turro, N.J.; Cederbaum, A.I. (1993). Increased NADPH- and NADH-dependent production of superoxide and hydroxyl radical by microsomes after chronic ethanol treatment. *Arch Biochem Biophys* 300(1):401-408.

Rehm, J.T.; Bondy, S.J.; Sempos, C.T.; Vuong, C.V. (1997). Alcohol consumption and coronary heart disease morbidity and mortality. *Am J Epidemiol* 146(6): 495-501.

Reinke, L.A.; Moore, D.R.; Hague, C.M.; McCay, P.B. (1994). Metabolism of ethanol to *l-hydroxyethyl* radicals in rat liver microsomes: Comparative studies with three spin trapping agents. *Free Radic Res Commun* 21(4):213-222.

Ridker, P.M.; Vaughan, D.E.; Stampfer, M.J.; Glynn, R.J.; Hennekens, C.H. (1994). Association of moderate alcohol consumption and plasma concentration of endogenous tissue-type plasminogen activator. *JAMA* 272(12):929-933.

Rimm, E.B.; Klatsky, A.; Grobbee, D.; Stampfer, M.J. (1996). Review of moderate alcohol consumption and reduced risk of coronary heart disease: Is the effect due to beer, wine, or spirits? *BMJ* 312(7033):731-736.

Ross, L.; Yeazel, L.; Chau, A. (1992). Pilot performance with blood alcohol concentrations below 0.04 percent. *Aviat Space Environ Med* 63(11):951-956.

Rubin, R.; Rand, M.L. (1994). Alcohol and platelet function. *Alcohol Clin Exp Res* 18(1):105-110.

Sadrzadeh, S.M.; Meydani, M.; Khettry, U.; Nanji, A.A. (1995). High-dose vitamin E supplementation has no effect on ethanol-induced pathological liver injury. *J Pharmacol Exp Ther* 273(1):455-460.

Sadrzadeh, S.M.; Nanji, A.A. (1994). Detection of lipid peroxidation after acute alcohol administration is dependent on time of sampling. *Int J Vitam Nutr Res* 64(2):157-158.

Saville, P.D. (1965). Changes in bone mass with age and alcoholism. *J Bone Joint Surg* 47A:492-499.

Schatzkin, A.; Longnecker, M.P. (1994). Alcohol and breast cancer: Where are we now and where do we go from here? *Cancer* 74(suppl 3):1101-1110.

Schnitzler, C.M.; Solomon, L. (1984). Bone changes after alcohol abuse. *S Afr Med J* 66:730-734.

Seitz, H.; Pöschl, G. (1997). Alcohol and gastrointestinal cancer: Pathogenic mechanisms. *Addict Biol* 2(1):19-33.

Seitz, H.K.; Simanowski, U.A.; Egerer, G.; Waldherr, R.; Oertl, U. (1992). Human gastric alcohol dehydrogenase: In vitro characteristics and effect of cimetidine. *Digestion* 51(2):80-85.

Seller, S.C. (1985). Alcohol abuse in the Old Testament. *Alcohol* 20:69-76.

Seppa, K.; Laippala, P.; Sillanaukee, P. (1996). High diastolic blood pressure: Common among women who are heavy drinkers. *Alcohol Clin Exp Res* 20(1):47-51.

Shaw, S.; Jayatilleke, E. (1990). The role of aldehyde oxidase in ethanol-induced hepatic lipid peroxidation in the rat. *Biochem* 268(3):579-583.

Sheron, N.; Bird, G.; Koskinas, I.; Portmann, B.; Ceska, M.; Lindley, I.; Williams, R. (1993). Circulating and tissue levels of the neutrophil chemotaxin interleukin-8 are elevated in severe acute alcoholic hepatitis, and tissue levels correlate with neutrophil infiltration. *Hepatology* 18(1):41-46.

Shimizu, M.; Lasker, I.M.; Tsutsumi, M.; Lieber, C.S. (1990). Immunohisto-chemical localization of ethanol-inducible P450IIE1 in the rat alimentary tract. *Gastroenterology* 99(4):1044-1053.

Smith-Warner, S.A.; Spiegelman, D.; Yaun, S.-S.; van den Brandt, P.A.; Folsom, A.R.; Goldbohm, R.A.; Graham, S.; Holmberg, L.; Howe, G.R.; Marshall, J.R.; et al. (1998). Alcohol and breast cancer in women: A pooled analysis of cohort studies. *JAMA* 279(7):535-540.

Sonnenberg, L.M.; Quatromoni, P.A.; Gagnon, D.R.; Cupples, L.A.; Franz, M.M.; Ordovas, J.M.; Wilson, P.W.; Schaefer, E.J.; Millen, B.E. (1996). Diet and plasma lipids in women. II. Macronutrients and plasma triglycerides, high-density lipoprotein, and the ratio of total to high-density lipoprotein cholesterol in women: The Framingham Nutrition Studies. *J Clin Epidemiol* 49(6):665-672.

Spencer, H.; Rubio, N.; Rubio, E.; Indreika, M.; Seitam, A. (1986). Chronic alco-holism: Frequently overlooked cause of osteoporosis in men. *Am J Med* 80:393-397.

Steinbok, P.; Thompson, G.B. (1978). Metabolic disturbances after head injury: Abnormalities of sodium and water intoxication. *Neurosurgery* 3:9-15.

Tetrito, M.C.; Tanaka, K.R. (1974). Hypophosphatemia in chronic alcoholism. *Arch Intern Med* 134:445-447.

Thuluvath, P.; Wojno, K.; Yardley, J.H.; Mezey, E. (1994). Effects of *Helicobacter pylori* infection and gastritis on gastric alcohol dehydrogenase activity. *Alcohol Clin Exp Res* 18(4):795-798.

Thun, M.J.; Peto, R.; Lopez, A.D.; Monaco, J.H.; Henley, S.J.; Heath, C.W.; Doll, R. (1997). Alcohol consumption and mortality among middle-aged and elderly U.S. adults. *N Engl J Med* 337(24):1705-1714.

Tilg, H.; Wilmer, A.; Vogel, W.; Herold, M.; Nolchen, B.; Judmaier, G.; Huber, C. (1992). Serum levels of cytokines in chronic liver diseases. *Gastroenterology* 103(1):264-274.

Tsukamoto, H. (1993). Oxidative stress, antioxidants, and alcoholic liver fibro-genesis. *Alcohol* 10(6):465-467.

Tsukamoto, H.; Horne, W.; Kamimura, S.; Niemela, O.; Parkkila, S.; Yla-Herttuala, S.; Brittenham, G.M. (1995). Experimental liver cirrhosis induced by alcohol and iron. *J Clin Invest* 96(1):620-630.

Tuppurainen, M.; Kroger, H.; Honkanen, R.; Puntial, E.; Huopia, J.; Saarikoski, S.; Alhave, E. (1995). Risks of perimenopausal fractures: A prospective population-based study. *Acta Obstet Gynecol Scand* 74:624-628.

Tuyns, A.; Pequignot, G. (1984). Greater risk of ascitic cirrhosis in females in rela-tion to alcohol consumption. *Int J Epidemiol* 13(1):53-57.

Ueshima, H.; Mikawa, K.; Baba, S.; Sasaki, S.; Ozawa, H.; Tsushima, M.; Kawaguchi, A.; Omae, T.; Katayama, Y.; Kayemori, Y. (1993). Effect of re-duced alcohol consumption on blood pressure in untreated hypertensive men. *Hypertension* 21(2):248-252.

Uppal, R.; Lateef, S.K.; Korsten, M.A.; Paronetto, F.; Lieber, C.S. (1991). Chronic alcoholic gastritis: Roles of alcohol and *Helicobacter pylori*. *Arch Intern Med* 151(4):760-764.

Urbano-Marquez, A.; Estruck, R.; Ferandez-Sola, J.; Nicolas, J.M.; Pare, J.C.; Rubin, E. (1995). The greater risk of alcoholic cardiomyopathy and myopathy in women compared with men. *JAMA* 274(2):149-154.

U.S. Department of Agriculture; U.S. Department of Health and Human Services (1995). *Home and Garden Bulletin* No. 232, Fourth Edition. Washington, DC: U.S. Department of Agriculture.

U.S. Department of Health and Human Services (1995). *Healthy People 2000. Midcourse Review and 1995 Revisions.* Washington, DC: U.S. Department of Health and Human Services, U.S. Public Health Service.

U.S. Department of Health and Human Services (1999). *Alcohol and Coronary Heart Disease.* Alcohol Alert No. 45. Washington, DC: U.S. Department of Health and Human Services.

Valimaki, M.; Pelkonen, R.; Salaspuro, M.; Harkonen, J.; Hirvonen, E.; Ylikahri, R. (1984). Sex hormones in amenorrheic women with alcoholic liver disease. *J Clin Endocrinol Metab* 59:133-138.

Valimaki, M.; Salaspuro, M.; Ylikahri, R. (1982). Liver damage and sex hormones in chronic male alcoholics. *Clin Endocrinol* 17:469-477.

Van Thiel, D.H.; Lester, R.; Sherins, R.J. (1974). Hypogonadism in alcoholic liver disease: Evidence for a double defect. *Gastroenterology* 67:1188-1199.

Vaughan, T.I.; Davis, S.; Kristal, A.; Thomas, D.B. (1995). Obesity, alcohol, and tobacco as risk factors for cancers of the esophagus and gastric cardia: Adenocarcinoma versus squamous cell carcinoma. *Cancer Epidemiol Biomarkers Prev* 4(2):85-92.

Waller, P.; Steward, J.; Hansen, A.; Stutts, J.; Popkin, C.; Rodgman, E. (1986). The potentiating effects of alcohol on driver injury. *JAMA* 256(11):1461-1466.

Ward, R.; Flynn, T.; Miller, P. (1982). Effects of ethanol ingestion on the severity and outcome of trauma. *Am J Surg* 144:153-157.

Wieczorek, W.F. (1995). The role of treatment in reducing alcohol-related accidents involving DWI offenders. In Watson, R.R. (ed.), *Alcohol, Cocaine and Accidents. Drug Alcohol Abuse Rev* 7:105-129.

Williams, G.A.; Bowser, E.N.; Hargis, G.K.; Kukreja, S.C.; Shah, J.H.; Vora, N.M.; Henderson, W.J. (1978). Effect of ethanol on parathyroid hormone and calcitronin secretion in man. *Proc Soc Exp Biol Med* 159:187-191.

Wilson, D.M. III; Tenrler, J.J.; Carney, J.P.; Wilson, T.M.; Kelley, M.R. (1994). Acute ethanol exposure suppresses the repair of O^6-methylguanine DNA lesions in castrated adult male rats. *Alcohol Clin Exp Res* 18(5):1267-1271.

World Health Organization Ad Hoc Committee on Health Research Relating to Future Intervention Options (1996). *Investing in Health Research and Development.* Geneva, Switzerland: WHO, 1996.

Yamada, K.; Araki, S.: Tamura, M.; Sakai, I.; Takahashi, Y.; Kashihara, H.; Kono, S. (1997). Case-control study of colorectal carcinoma in situ and cancer in relation to cigarette smoking and alcohol use. *Cancer Causes Control* 8(5):780-785.

Yesavage, J.; Dolhert, N.; Taylor, J. (1994). Flight simulator performance of younger and older aircraft pilots. Effects of age and alcohol. *J Am Geriat Soc* 42(6):577-582.

Yin, S.J.; Chou, F.J.; Chao, S.F.; Tsai, S.F.; Liao, C.S.; Wang, S.L.; Wu, C.W.; Lee, S.C. (1993). Alcohol and aldehyde dehydrogenases in human esophagus: Comparison with the stomach enzyme activities. *Alcohol Clin Exp Res* 17(2):376-381.

York, J.L.; Hirsch, J.A. (1997). Association between blood pressure and lifetime drinking patterns in moderate drinkers. *J Stud Alcohol* 58(5):480-485.

You, R.X.; McNeil, J.J.; O'Malley, H.M.; Davis, S.M.; Thrift, A.G.; Donnan, G.A. (1997). Risk factors for stroke due to cerebral infarction in young adults. *Stroke* 28(10):1913-1918.

Yuan, J.-M.: Ross, R.K.; Gao, Y.-T.; Henderson, B.E.; Yu, M.C. (1997). Follow up study of moderate alcohol intake and mortality among middle-aged men in Shanghai, China. *BMJ* 314(7073):18-23.

Zador, P.L.; Krawchuk, S.A.; Voas, R.B. (2000). Alcohol-related risk of driver fatalities and driver involvement in fatal crashes in relation to driver age and gender: An update using 1996 data. *J Stud Alcohol* 61:387-395.

Zakhari, S.; Wassef, M. (eds.) (1996). *Alcohol and the Cardiovascular System.* NIAAA Research Monograph No. 31, Pub. No. 96-4133. Bethesda, MD: NIAAA.

Zink, B.; Maoi, R.; Chen, B. (1996). Alcohol, central nervous system injury, and time to death in fatal motor vehicle crashes. *Alcohol Clin Exp Res* 20(9):1518-1522.

Zink, B.J.; Schultz, C.H.; Stern, S.A.; Mertz, M.; Wang, X.; Johnston, P.; Keep, R.F. (2001). Effects of ethanol and naltrexone in a model of traumatic brain injury with hemorrhagic shock. *J Clin Exp Res* 25(6):916-923.

Zumoff, B. (1997). The critical role of alcohol consumption in determining the risk of breast cancer with postmenopausal estrogen administration. *J Clin Endocrinol Metab* 82(6):1656-1658.

Chapter 3

The Neuropsychological Consequences of Alcohol and Drug Abuse

Rosemarie Scolaro Moser
Corinne E. Frantz

OVERVIEW

The research and popular literature are replete with information discussing the physical mechanisms of addiction, theories of alcohol and drug action within the human body, and the psychosocial impact of substance abuse. We are gaining insight into the process of addiction and how the rewarding effects of certain substances are a result of dysregulation of the brain reward circuit (Leshner and Koob, 1999). However, the body of research linking the physical effects of substances of abuse to cognitive or neuropsychological functioning is less comprehensive. We are beginning to comprehend how physical changes in the brain due to substance abuse may lead to acute, transient, and permanent alterations in the way one thinks and processes information.

The purpose of this chapter is to provide the reader with a survey of research identifying the documented relationships between alcohol and drug abuse and neuropsychological functioning. Clearly, a significant portion of the research in this area has focused on alcohol abuse and this chapter will begin with an understanding of that body of research. Next will be a review of the research on polydrug abuse in which population samples are not distinguished by a particular drug, as is often the case. It is for this group of drug abusers that neurotoxicity has been most frequently observed (Hartman, 1995).

Few abusers commit to one substance alone, so it is difficult to find formidable research that represents each substance of abuse (Miller, 1985). Nonetheless, some specific research is available for a few drugs. The illegal drugs that have been more typically represented in neuropsychological research, including marijuana, cocaine, LSD, and PCP (phencyclidine), will be reviewed here. Opiates, solvents, and new designer drugs will also be mentioned despite the dearth of neuropsychological research pertaining to them.

Neuropsychology is the scientific study of brain-behavior relationships and how physiological brain function impacts neuropsychological processes such as "memory, language skills, sensory/perceptual/motor skills, visual/spatial skills, mental speed/efficiency/flexibility, physical and mental coordination, listening skills, attention and concentration, problem solving, and reasoning" (Moser, 1999, p. 2). Neuropsychologists, or cognitive scientists, utilize a variety of assessment tools to measure neuropsychological processes, a number of which will be referred to in this chapter.

When alcohol and other drugs have an effect on the brain, the effect tends not to be clear, lateralized, and focal in nature as seen in strokes, tumors, or other localized brain disorders. Rather, a more generalized, pervasive effect on the brain, with perhaps particular areas of concentration of dysfunction, may be observed. Thus, some drugs may specifically affect certain neuropsychological functions, although these functions may not be specific to a certain area of the brain. Effects may be immediate and acute, or long lasting and chronic.

Much controversy exists regarding the effects of repeated use of nonprescription drugs because of problems in the experimental design of the existing studies. With this in mind, the reader is cautioned to consider the limitations of current research in the area of the neuropsychology of alcohol and drug abuse. Nonetheless, the promise of future research may lie in the complementary use of neuroimaging and neuropsychological assessments that will offer greater insight into brain-behavior relationships.

BRAIN IMPAIRMENT AND ALCOHOL ABUSE

Alcohol ranks as one of the most serious substances of abuse due to the prevalence of abuse in the general population and the severity of its toxic effects. It has been estimated that between 5 and 12 million individuals abuse alcohol, with a significantly greater proportion being male (Hartman, 1995; Thompson, 2000). The acute effects of alcohol intoxication are well known. Some of the effects of chronic alcohol abuse are also well known and have been extensively reviewed, particularly the dramatic effect of alcohol on memory in the case of Korsakoff's syndrome (Butters, 1984; Butters and Miliotis, 1985). Less clear and still somewhat controversial are answers to the following questions:

1. What are the cognitive effects of chronic alcohol abuse in the absence of Korsakoff's syndrome?
2. What, if any, are the direct toxic effects of alcohol on brain tissue?
3. Are there cognitive predictive factors for individuals at high risk for alcohol abuse?
4. What is known about the recovery of cognitive functions after abstinence from chronic alcohol abuse?

As with all drugs of abuse, alcohol is initially sought out for its pleasurable effects which are mediated in the brain by its impact on the mesolimbic reward system (Leshner, 1997).

Recent evidence, however, points to alcohol's impact on the gamma-aminobutyric acid (GABA) receptor complex embedded in the membrane of neurons; in particular, the barbiturate site on the GABA (A) receptors (Thompson, 2000). Converging evidence from a variety of sources indicates that alcohol significantly alters GABA neurotransmission; may mediate many of the acute behavioral effects of alcohol, such as motor incoordination, anxiolysis, and sedation; and plays an important role in the development of alcohol tolerance and susceptibility to alcohol dependence (Mihic and Harris, 1997; Grobin et al., 1998). Thus, in addition to its common effects on the brain's reward system, which are shared by all substances of abuse, alcohol also affects those brain regions outside of the pleasure system that utilize GABA (Leshner, 1997; Thompson, 2000; see Chapter 4 for additional information).

Acute Effects of Alcohol Intoxication

Alcohol crosses the blood-brain barrier; therefore, the acute effects of alcohol intoxication are highly correlated with blood alcohol level (Hartman, 1995; Brick and Erickson, 1999). Studies of neuropsychological performance associated with acute alcohol intake have found impairments on a variety of cognitive tasks. Minocha and colleagues (1985), for example, found impairments in fine motor coordination, attention, concentration, auditory-verbal skills, and visuospatial skills. In a study comparing the acute effects of ethanol and temazepam ingestion on the formation of new semantic and episodic memories, Tiplady and colleagues (1999) found that the acquisition of new semantic and episodic memories, assessed with a test of learning-invented facts and by a measure of long-term learning of words on the Buschke test, were impaired by ingestion of both drugs. The effects of ethanol were more marked than the effects of temazapam on new learning. Psychomotor speed, assessed with the digit symbol subtest of the

Wechsler Adult Intelligence Scale, was equally impaired by both drugs. Semantic memory refers to recall of general knowledge that is not tagged to specific life experiences (e.g., knowledge of vocabulary and overlearned facts). Episodic memory, in contrast, refers to recall of events or facts that are related to an individual's specific life experiences. Both types of memory are considered to be declarative in nature, which will be defined later.

GABA exerts a prominent inhibitory effect on brain systems which it subserves. As already noted, this may account for the anxiolytic effect of alcohol intake. Similarly, the agitation and convulsions observed during alcohol withdrawal may be due to neuronal hypersensitivity. This is the hypersensitivity theory of withdrawal and addiction (Thompson, 2000).

Neuropsychological Findings in Chronic Alcoholism with Korsakoff's Amnesia

Considerable neuropsychological attention has been focused on the cognitive features of Korsakoff's syndrome. Afflicted individuals first undergo an acute encephalopathic crisis called Wernicke's encephalopathy which resolves into a persistent and severe amnesia referred to as Korsakoff's amnesia. The characteristics of this amnesia include a severe anterograde loss of memory during which the afflicted individual is unable to learn new verbal or nonverbal information that is declarative and episodic in nature. Declarative memory refers to knowledge of facts or events that can be consciously stated or declared by the individual. Episodic memory, as noted earlier, refers to recall of facts or events that occurred at a specific time in a person's life, such as recalling what one ate for breakfast in the morning. The anterograde amnesia in Korsakoff's syndrome is often accompanied by normal or near normal intellectual functions and a milder retrograde amnesia. Retrograde amnesia refers to difficulty retrieving facts or events from long-term memory that occurred before the onset of the illness. It is usually more pronounced for events that occurred just prior to the onset of the illness, while remote events, such as childhood memories, are relatively well preserved (Albert et al., 1981; Butters and Miliotis, 1985).

It has been known for some time that the damaging effects to the central nervous system, or brain, which give rise to Korsakoff's syndrome occur as an indirect effect of alcohol on the brain; namely, a severe nutritional deficiency that accompanies increasingly severe and protracted alcohol intake and results in a complete absence of thiamine in the diet. The immediate treatment for an individual suffering from Wernicke's encephalopathy is administration of large doses of thiamine. Although considered to be rare, there is evidence that Wernicke's encephalopathy is significantly underdiagnosed among chronic alcoholics (Hartman, 1995). Autopsy studies of individuals who have been afflicted with Wernicke-Korsakoff syndrome revealed pronounced damage to several limbic system structures, including the mammillary bodies of the hypothalamus and the medialis dorsalis nucleus of the thalamus. In addition, damage has been reported to the vermis of the cerebellum, the oculomotor nucleus which controls eye movements, and association areas in the cerebral cortex. Damage to the hippocampus has not been consistently reported (Butters, 1979; Butters and Miliotis, 1985). However, the mammillary bodies and the medialis dorsalis nucleus of the thalamus are known to have strong anatomical connections with the hippocampus, which is involved with memory functions.

Early investigations found that individuals with Korsakoff's syndrome were impaired in their retention of new information after delays of only a few seconds (Butters and Cermak, 1975; Kinsbourne and Wood, 1975; Piercy, 1978). Analysis of the nature of errors made in recall by Korsakoff patients revealed a high incidence of intrusions rather than errors of omission, suggesting that Korsakoff patients were highly vulnerable to distraction; in particular, they were vulnerable to the effects of proactive interference on recall (Butters, 1979; Butters and Miliotis, 1985). Proactive interference refers to the inability to acquire new information because of interference from previously learned material. Since distributed practice of new information has been known to be effective in reducing the effects of interference on recall, Butters and colleagues (1976) trained Korsakoff patients on new learning with distributed practice and found that patients' recall of new information was similar to that of control subjects who learned new information under conditions of mass practice.

Other studies have pointed to the possibility that the severe retention difficulties of Korsakoff patients reflect a failure to encode a sufficient number of attributes of the new information at the time of storage in order to facilitate adequate retrieval, thus making the new information more vulnerable to the effects of interference (Butters, 1979; Butters and Miliotis, 1985). In an early study, for example, Butters and Cermak (1974) found that semantic cues did not help Korsakoff patients retrieve new verbal information, even though phonemic cues did. They suggested that Korsakoff patients might be deficient in their ability to semantically analyze the material, which would limit the stored attributes of the material for later recall. This is consistent with studies in which patients were found to respond to irrelevant paraphenalia such as hats, etc., in attempting to recall faces in a facial matching task (Diamond and Carey, 1977; Dricker et al., 1978). These studies suggested that difficulty with retention and recall may be related to limited perceptual analysis. Additional work led to the formulation of the contextual encoding theory which posits that Korsakoff patients exhibit a specific failure to encode the contextual attributes of new information which gives rise to retrieval impairments (Butters, 1979; Butters and Miliotis, 1985).

Studies of the role of hippocampal neurons in memory and learning conducted with patients suffering from Korsakoff's amnesia and with animals have interesting points of convergence.

The mammillary bodies, an important site of damage in Korsakoff's syndrome, have strong anatomical connections to the hippocampus within the limbic system, a site known to be important in memory functions. For example, studies have found that rats with damaged hippocampi can learn which of two arms in a maze to run down for water in a conditioned brightness discrimination task, but have great difficulty unlearning it if the stimulus conditions change (Kimble, 1968). The animals appear to show behavioral perseveration which is similar to the phenomenon of proactive interference in the memory performance of Korsakoff patients. Other rat studies involving single cell recordings from the hippocampus have led to the discovery of "place cells" which appear to respond to particular locations in space (Thompson, 2000). This is consistent with decades of research indicating that the hippocampus plays a role in various learning paradigms (Graham, 1990). These findings suggest the hippocampus may play an important role in laying down contextual cues for the facilitation of recall of new information, and lend support to the clinical findings of vulnerability to distraction and interference due to a failure of contextual encoding of new information in Korsakoff patients.

It has been noted that Korsakoff patients demonstrate relative preservation of intellectual functions in the presence of their specific memory disturbance. Through extensive reviews of clinical research literature, Butters and colleagues (Butters, 1979; Butters and Miliotis, 1985) have noted that although overall IQ scores are indistinguishable from matched controls, Korsakoff patients manifest a number of specific cognitive deficits during formal neuropsychological testing. These deficits include: (1) a low symbol subtest score on the Wechsler Adult Intelligence Scale-Revised (WAIS-R); and (2) severely depressed Wechsler Memory Scale scores on logical memory (verbal passage recall), figural memory, and paired associate learning subtests. Hartman (1995) notes that Korsakoff patients also have difficulty on cognitive tasks such as the Halstead-Reitan Tactual Performance Test which involves the ability to create and utilize a visuospatial internal representation of the location of target stimuli through tactile-kinesthetic sensory input. Additional deficits are reported to be found in tests involving visuospatial and constructional abilities, and tests involving categorization, rule learning, and set shifting or mental flexibility (e.g., Wisconsin Card Sorting Test and Halstead-Reitan Category Test) (Hartman, 1995).

Despite the severity of impairment for new declarative memory in Korsakoff patients, these individuals are able to learn new motor tasks involving implicit, procedural memory (Butters and Miliotis, 1985). Support for this finding comes from a study by Beaunieux and colleagues (1998) who discovered a Korsakoff patient who was able to learn to solve the Tower of Hanoi puzzle, a test that involves cognitive procedural memory. Procedural memory is also known as nondeclarative or implicit memory and refers to memory of how a task is accomplished.

Neuropsychological Findings in Nonamnesic Chronic Alcoholism

More recently, neuropsychological interest has focused on documenting the chronic effects of alcoholism in the absence of Wernicke-Korsakoff syndrome. In 1971 Ryback proposed the continuity hypothesis, which posits that Korsakoff's syndrome is the end product of a gradual decline associated with chronic alcoholism (Hartman, 1995). In addition, chronic alcoholics without Korsakoff's syndrome have often been used as control subjects in studies on Korsakoff patients without a full understanding of the nature of their specific cognitive deficits.

Studies that have looked directly at the question of similarities or differences in cognitive functioning between Korsakoff amnesics and nonamnesic chronic alcoholics do not, in general, support the continuity hypothesis. In one study, Wilkinson and Carlen (1980) compared Korsakoff patients with non-Korsakoff alcoholics and found significant differences between the two groups on most subtests of the Wechsler Memory Scale, the digit symbol subtest of the Wechsler Adult Intelligence Scale (WAIS), and the memory score of the Halstead-Reitan Tactual Performance Test. Krabbendam and colleagues (2000) looked at neuropsychological data and magnetic resonance imaging (MRI) brain structure volumes in a group of Korsakoff patients and compared their findings with a group of chronic alcoholics and a normal control group. Significant differences in performance were found between the Korsakoff patients and the other two groups on tests of memory, visuoperceptual and executive functions, as well as in brain structure volumes, leading the investigators to conclude that the cognitive deficits seen in Korsakoff patients were unlikely to be accounted for by the mere chronic consumption of alcohol. In keeping with these findings, Hartman (1995) points out that current prevailing views regarding cognitive deficits in Korsakoff patients favor an additive model of acute traumatic effects arising out of avitaminosis superimposed on more chronic traumatic effects associated with long-term alcoholism.

In a recent review of studies that have found positive neuropsychological test results associated with chronic alcoholism, Hartman (1995) identified a number of important areas of demonstrable cognitive impairment. These areas include abstract thinking or flexible problem solving, visuospatial processing, and memory. A number of studies have found deficits on tests that assess conceptual problem solving and mental flexibility (e.g., Halstead-Reitan Category Test, Raven's Progressive Matrices Test, and Wisconsin Card Sorting Test) (Hartman, 1995). Impairments in visuospatial abilities have been repeatedly found throughout the literature. In addition, memory deficits in chronic alcoholics without Korsakoff's syndrome have been demonstrated through neuropsychological testing (Hartman, 1995).

Factors that appear to influence neuropsychological test performance include age at onset of drinking, pattern of drinking (i.e., frequency and amount consumed), handedness, predisposing risk factors such as family history, genetic vulnerability, and history of head injury (Hartman, 1995). In one study, DeBellis and colleagues (2000) used magnetic resonance imaging to ascertain hippocampal volume in a group of 12 adolescents with adolescent-onset alcohol abuse. A matched control group was also studied. DeBellis and colleagues found that both left-hemispheric and right-hemispheric hippocampal volumes were significantly smaller in adolescents who abused alcohol than in the control group. Other volume indices measured by MRI in this study, including intracranial, cerebral, cortical gray and white matter, as well as measures of the midsagittal area of the corpus callosum, were not significantly different between the two groups. Total hippocampal volume correlated positively with age at onset (i.e., younger age of onset of drinking was associated with smaller total hippocampal volumes), and correlated negatively with the duration of the alcohol-use disorder (i.e., shorter duration of alcohol-use disorder was associated with larger total hippocampal volumes). These results suggest that during adolescence, the hippocampus, an important site for memory functions, may be particularly vulnerable to the adverse effects of alcohol. Other studies suggest that older alcoholics may be more vulnerable to the negative impact of alcohol on brain-behavior functions than younger adult alcoholics. Pfefferbaum and colleagues (1997), for example, found that a younger group of alcoholic men (ages 26 to 44) had significant cortical gray matter volume deficits and sulcal and ventricular enlargement on magnetic resonance imaging when compared to a group of age-matched controls. However, a group of older alcoholic men (ages 45 to 63) showed volume deficits in both cortical gray and white matter in addition to sulcal and ventricular enlargement. When Pfefferbaum and colleagues looked closer at six cortical areas for MRI volume deficits, they found that the older alcoholic group had selectively more severe deficits in prefrontal gray matter compared to the younger alcoholic group. The two groups differed in age, but not in disease duration or estimated lifetime alcohol consumption.

Regarding pattern of drinking, at least one study found that a pattern of daily drinking, compared with "bout" drinking, was associated with lower scores on age-corrected Wechsler Adult Intelligence Scale Performance IQ measures, as well as on the Mental Control and Digit Span subtests of the Wechsler Memory Scale. "Bout" drinking refers to a pattern of periods of abstinence in between episodes of drinking for days, weeks, or months, compared with a pattern of drinking five or more days a week (Tarbox et al., 1986).

Some studies have suggested that left-handedness may be more highly represented among alcohol abusers than is seen in the general population. The exact significance of this finding, however, is uncertain in the absence of more carefully controlled, replicative studies (Hartman, 1995). Handedness has important implications for the interpretation of certain neuropsychological test findings and may represent a sign, in some cases, of co-existing vulnerability to other disorders that may contribute to or may be part of a predisposing risk factor.

Given the high correlation between alcohol abuse and a family history of alcoholism, a number of studies have looked at children in an effort to identify possible patterns of preexisting neuropsychological vulnerabilities in family members of alcoholics (Hartman, 1995). These studies have been able to differentiate the sons of alcoholics from control subjects on the basis of poorer performance on selected neuropsychological tests such as the Rey-Osterreith Complex Figure Test, the hard (unfamiliar) paired associates from the Wechsler Memory Scale, and the information subtest of the WAIS-R (Peterson et al., 1992), as well as on tasks of verbal and nonverbal abstraction and perceptual-motor skill (Schaeffer et al., 1984). Insufficient research exists to form a clear consensus about the interpretation or significance of these findings; however, the strong possibility of preexisting cognitive vulnerabilities in certain individuals who may be at risk for developing an alcohol-use disorder represents an important direction for future research.

Demographic data point to a high association between alcohol abuse and head injury (see Chapter 2 for a review). Dikmen and colleagues (1993) note:

> Alcohol use shortly before injury is the most commonly cited and best established predisposing factor in head trauma, having a high level of direct and indirect involvement in motor vehicle accidents, falls, and assaults, which represent the most common causes of such injuries. (p. 296)

According to a variety of sources cited by Dikmen and colleagues (1993), "Up to two thirds of head trauma victims have a detectable alcohol level . . . and from a third to a half are intoxicated when they arrive at the emergency room; . . . a third of head trauma victims [are] diagnosed as alcohol dependent" (p. 296). (For more information on alcohol-related injuries, see Chapter 2.) The latter data indicate a much higher percentage of chronic alcohol abuse in the premorbid history of head trauma victims than in the general population. Thus, chronic alcohol abuse represents a serious complicating factor in the neuropsychological profile of head trauma patients, and vice versa. Dikmen and colleagues (1993) studied the question of whether a premorbid history of alcohol abuse leads to an increase in neuropsychological deficits associated with head injuries in a group of diverse head-injured patients compared with a group of demographically matched and preexisting-condition-matched body trauma controls. They found that severity of head injury and degree of alcohol problems were both related to neuropsychological test performance; however, an interaction between head injury and alcohol problems was not able to be demonstrated. In other words, a head injury sustained by an individual who had a history of heavy drinking was not more detrimental on neuropsychological test performance than a head injury sustained in the absence of a history of heavy drinking (Dikmen et al., 1993). A subgroup of head-injured patients seen in this study was characterized by lower levels of education, poor neuropsychological test performance (including lower verbal/intellectual skills), and a lifestyle pattern of heavy drinking. Dikmen and colleagues raised the possibility that this subgroup may be similar to another subgroup that has been identified in the literature as meeting diagnostic criteria for antisocial personality disorder with a high incidence of alcohol abuse, a history of poorer verbal cognitive abilities possibly associated with premorbid attention deficit disorder or minimal brain dysfunction, and an increased risk for head injuries (Malloy et al., 1990; Tarter, 1988; Tarter and Edwards, 1988).

According to Hartman (1995), three neuropathological possibilities have been proposed in the literature to account for neurological and cognitive findings associated with nonamnesic chronic alcoholism. The first neuropathological explanation is that chronic alcoholism gives rise to diffuse brain injury. Neuroradiological studies, for example, have found bilateral enlargement of the lateral ventricles, the third ventricle, and cerebral sulci (Hartman, 1995), suggesting the presence of widespread cerebral atrophy. The second neuropathological explanation is that chronic alcoholism gives rise to lateralized damage involving the right hemisphere. This is based on observations of visuospatial and constructional deficits in the test performances of chronic alcoholics. However, the localizing value of these findings and the lack of consistent clinical research support for this neuropathological conclusion have called this explanation into question (Hartman, 1995). The third neuropathological explanation is that chronic alcoholism gives rise to brain damage or neural compromise in frontal-limbic-diencephalic brain regions. In a recent study, Dao-Castellana and colleagues (1998) used MRI and positron emission tomography (PET) scans to examine a group of chronic alcoholics with no known neurological or psychiatric complications. They found metabolic abnormalities in the mediofrontal and left dorsolateral prefrontal cortex, which correlated with impairment on neuropsychological tests assessing verbal fluency and mental flexibility (Stroop test: Interference condition). In another study, Ratti et al. (1999) looked at standard computerized axial tomography (CAT) scan data in a group of male alcoholic inpatients and a matched control group. Atrophy of the frontal region was found significantly more frequently among the alcoholic inpatient group than among the controls. Davila et al. (1994) looked at MRI images of the mammillary bodies, cerebellar hemispheres, and cerebellar vermis in a group of middle-aged and older chronic alcoholics (ages 40 to 65 years), who had no history of Korsakoff's amnesia, alcoholic dementia, or diagnosed cerebellar degeneration. Tissue volume ratings were evaluated along with performance on neuropsychological tests of long-term declarative memory and measures of balance. They found that the alcoholics were more impaired on measures of balance than they were on measures of declarative memory, and that the difficulty with balance (in particular, ataxia while eyes are closed) showed a modest relationship with volume reduction in cerebellar vermis tissue. A high percentage of the alcoholic group also showed clinically abnormal mammillary body tissue ratings despite a relative absence of significant deficits on measures of declarative memory, consistent with expectations for nonamnesic chronic alcoholics. Evidence of compromise to the mammillary bodies is in keeping with the hypothesis of frontal-limbic-diencephalic brain involvement in chronic alcohol abuse. Davila and colleagues noted that brain tissue volume reductions might not represent atrophy (i.e., cell loss), but rather tissue shrinkage due to possible intracellular fluid shifts or other factors that may be partly or totally reversible (Davila et al., 1994).

In summary, individuals who present with nonamnesic chronic alcohol abuse have been found to exhibit a significant picture of neuropsychological deficit affecting abstract thinking, perceptual processing, memory and learning, attention and concentration, and psychomotor skills, even though the continuity hypothesis that neuropsychological deficits are in a simple relationship with the amount of alcohol consumed over time has not been supported by clinical research.

Mechanisms of Indirect and Direct Toxic Effects from Alcohol Abuse

Several studies have noted the indirect toxic effects of alcohol on brain memory systems due to severe nutritional depletion. Marchiafava-Bignami syndrome, a rare condition associated with severe malnourishment in chronic alcoholism involves demyelination or necrosis of the corpus callosum with accompanying damage to pericallosal white matter. Symptoms include dementia, dysarthria, spasticity, and inability to ambulate (Hartman, 1995). Liver disease represents an additional indirect toxic effect of alcohol that can give rise to hepatic encephalopathy (Hartman, 1995). Hepatic encephalopathy is associated with brain damage in widespread areas including the basal ganglia, thalamus, red nucleus, pons, and cerebellum (Charness, 1994; cited in Hartman, 1995, p. 235; also see Chapter 4 for additional review). Studies by Tarter and colleagues (1990) have found that alcoholics who also suffer liver damage are more compromised than alcoholics without demonstrated liver damage on tasks involving short-term memory, visual tracking, and eye-finger coordination (cited in Hartman, 1995, p. 236).

In addition to indirect toxic effects, growing evidence suggests that alcohol is also a direct neurotoxin in the central nervous system. Various studies have documented important neurochemical changes affecting the functioning of cell membranes, neurotransmission, and the availability of certain neurotransmitter substances necessary for the integrity of important brain circuits (Hartman, 1995). Numerous studies have documented cerebral atrophy, including loss of both cortical gray matter and subcortical white matter (Jernigan et al., 1991; Pfefferbaum et al., 1992). Korbo (1999) studied the total number of neuron and glial cells in the hippocampus in a small group of severely affected alcoholics and a group of controls. A statistically significant loss of glial cells, but not neurons, differentiated the severe alcoholics from the controls. Glial cells provide important support functions to help maintain the health of neurons. These functions include taking up excess chemical transmitters, cleaning away cellular debris after neuronal damage or death, myelinating axons for effective neurotransmission along the axon, and establishing the blood-brain barrier. In addition, recent discoveries indicate that some glial cells can transmit information between themselves within the immediate environment and may play a role in certain memory processes (Thompson, 2000). Thus, the finding that hippocampal glial cell loss is associated with severe alcoholism may have important implications for the cognitive finding of memory loss in afflicted individuals.

Risk Factors for Alcohol Abuse
and Neuropsychological Dysfunction

The issue of predicting risk among adolescent boys for future drug involvement was raised by Aytaclar et al. (1999), who looked at the predictive value of executive cognitive functioning deficiency, measured by neuropsychological tests, and high levels of behavioral activity in a group of high-risk preadolescent boys whose fathers had a history of lifetime psychoactive substance-abuse disorder. The boys were compared with a low-to-average-risk control group of boys whose fathers had neither psychoactive substance-use disorder nor a history of any other psychiatric diagnosis. Total number of drugs ever tried, severity of drug involvement, and presence of tobacco and cannabis use two years later were predicted by the presence of measurable executive cognitive dysfunction but not by behavioral activity levels. Another recent study, conducted by Hammoumi et al. (1999), looked at the relationship of alcohol dependence and dysfunction of the serotonin 5-hydroxytryptamine (5-HT) system based on recent research that suggests that the serotonin system's transporter chemical and receptor may be important in the etiology of alcohol dependence (Lovinger, 1997). Hammoumi et al. (1999) found a significant difference between alcohol-dependent patients and control subjects in the frequency of a genetic variant of serotonin transmission that might be predictive of a genetic vulnerability for alcohol dependence.

Recovery of Function after Chronic Alcohol Abuse

The importance of abstinence for the recovery of functions in chronic alcohol abusers cannot be more strongly emphasized, given the severity of the risk for permanent brain damage associated with long-term, protracted abuse and given recent studies that show some recovery of neuropsychological functioning is possible in abstinent chronic alcohol abusers who have not suffered Korsakoff's syndrome, cerebellar degeneration, or irreversibly damaging encephalopathic conditions. Rourke and Grant (1999) found that chronic male alcoholics who maintained interim abstinence for a period of two years following initial detoxification showed improvement on neuropsychological tests of abstracting ability compared with a group of chronic male alcoholics who resumed drinking during the two-year post-detoxification period, and compared with a control group of long-term abstinent alcoholics and a control group of nonalcoholics. The latter two groups were comparable in their neuropsychological performances on measures of abstracting ability, complex perceptual-motor integration, and simple motor skills. The group of relapsed chronic male alcoholics showed deterioration in their performance on the motor tests.

In another study that looked at perfusion images in frontal brain systems of abstinent long-term alcoholics using single photon emission computerized tomography (SPECT), Gansler et al. (2000) found an increased level of perfusion in the left inferior frontal brain region associated with greater years of sobriety in recovering alcoholics. Alcoholics with less than four years of sobriety showed a significantly reduced left inferior-frontal perfusion when compared with a group of nonalcoholic controls and a group of recovering alcoholics who had been abstinent for a longer period of time. These findings not only support the hypothesis of the negative impact of chronic alcohol intake on frontal-limbic-diencephalic brain systems, but also the possibility for some recovery of function in these brain systems with prolonged abstinence.

Studies which have looked at the recovery of cognitive functions have found that maintaining prolonged abstinence is a crucial requirement for any recovery of cognitive functions. Even with abstinence, however, not all cognitive functions show recovery or recover to levels equal to the control subjects. Age at onset of drinking, premorbid intellectual status, history of head injury, and age at which abstinence begins appear to be important modifying factors in determining cognitive function recovery (Hartman, 1995).

Despite evidence that chronic alcohol abuse, even in the absence of an amnesic syndrome, is associated with neuropsychological deficits that are indicative of moderate to severe cerebral dysfunction (Morris and Lawson, 1998), few treatment programs for recovering alcoholics routinely include neuropsychological evaluation and consultation as a standard treatment modality or offer rehabilitation for cognitive deficits as an integral part of their treatment program. Such deficits can present a significant obstacle to an individual's ability to fully participate and benefit from various aspects of the prescribed treatment program. The need for further research into the efficacy of such an integrated treatment program for recovering alcoholics has been recently called for (Allen et al., 1997).

BRAIN IMPAIRMENT AND ILLICIT DRUG ABUSE

Studies of General and Polydrug Abuse

Our more recent understanding of how drug addiction occurs involves the interference of brain reward circuits, resulting in an increase in the desire to use. In particular, it is posited that the amygdala and subregions of the basal forebrain are involved in a mesolimbic dopamine system that activate mesolimbic dopamine function. Repeated use alters dopamine production, resulting in a dysregulation of the brain reward circuitry. The result is a biological addiction to the drug (Leshner and Koob, 1999).

With such brain involvement and alteration of the brain circuitry, alterations in neuropsychological functioning is likely. A preliminary report of neuropsychological functioning in polydrug abusers by Grant and colleagues (1977) noted a study in which 15 polydrug users were administered a comprehensive neuropsychological battery including neuropsychological tests from the Halstead-Reitan Neuropsychological Test Battery, as well as the Wechsler Adult Intelligence Scale and the Minnesota Multiphasic Personality Inventory (MMPI). The 15 polydrug users were compared to a group of 66 psychiatric inpatients. Although both groups demonstrated severe psychopathology, as measured by the MMPI, the patterns of neuropsychological impairment that were observed in both groups were diverse. The pattern of impairment suggested differences between the two groups in terms of sensory, motor, perceptual, and verbal abilities. Although no significant difference occurred between the *level* of neuropsychological functioning, there were significant differences in the *pattern* of functioning in those ability areas. The polydrug group appeared to rely upon spatial/perceptual/motor abilities in problem solving and exhibited weakness in verbal abilities. The converse was true for the psychiatric patients whose *pattern* of neuropsychological functioning, although impaired, resembled that of normal adults. Further results from this research suggested that greater neuropsychological impairment was related to the use of opiates and depressants rather than to alcohol, stimulants, or marijuana.

In a later study of polydrug users, Carlin and colleagues (1980) sought to discern whether any differences occurred in neuropsychological functioning between two groups of polydrug users: "streetwise" users "whose lifestyle and value orientation reflect the drug culture underworld" (p. 229) and "straight" users whose lifestyle was more associated with traditional values. Seventy-nine polydrug users were studied and grouped into one of the two categories. The Halstead-Reitan Neuropsychological Test Battery was administered and neuropsychological impairment was statistically related to heavy alcohol and opiate abuse in the streetwise abusers. In contrast, straight abusers who were identified with neuropsychological dysfunction tended to use fewer drugs in general with the exception of depressants. These straight abusers were also found to have more medical problems that were associated with greater events of drug toxicity. It was suggested that neuropsychological impairment in the straight abusers could be associated with medical risk that is secondary to developmental history or greater vulnerability to drug toxicity, and that for the streetwise users, impairment could be associated with heavy drug intake resulting in toxicity. The meaning of these results is not very clear although the authors also posited that alcohol, opiates, and "perhaps the depressants" were most related to brain impairment.

Cognitive or neuropsychological impairment clearly affects behavioral functioning in polysubstance abusers. Schafer et al. (1994) observed that the emotional and marital functioning of male polysubstance abusers was directly related to their level of neuropsychological impairment. In a study of 31 married couples, the cognitive functioning of the husband was related to a pattern of negative communication behaviors, fewer positive behaviors, and increased events of violence.

Traditional testing of neuropsychological or cognitive performance has been called into question in a recent study by Beatty and Borrell (2000). It was suggested that some of the deficits identified by testing drug abusers could be accounted for by the knowledge these abusers acquire due to their lifestyle, and that this knowledge may be different than the knowledge acquired by nondrug abusers. Beatty and Borrell compared the test results of 63 methadone clinic clients with 24 nonabusing participants. They devised a task that included identifying the title, artist, year, and meaning of a song. There were no significant differences in task performance between the abusers and nonabusers except that the abusers tended to relate the song to drug addiction. Beatty and Borrell offered an interesting hypothesis, although the extent of cognitive assessment in their study was both narrow and limited.

Not surprisingly, drug abusers have been shown to demonstrate impaired decision-making skills. An interesting study employed a gambling task to assess decision-making skills, choice, and planning (Grant et al., 2000). Thirty polysubstance abusers and 24 nonabusers were compared using the Wisconsin Card Sorting Task, a measure of executive functioning and planning, as well as on the Gambling Task, which assessed judgment regarding short-term and long-term losses. There was no significant difference between the two groups on the Wisconsin Card Sorting Task. However, the groups demonstrated differences on the Gambling Task, suggesting that the drug abusers were more likely to use poor decision-making skills.

The questions of whether drug abuse results in deficits in executive functioning and whether individuals with such deficits are predisposed to substance abuse was investigated by Giancola and Tarter (1999). Giancola and Tarter identified children who were at high risk for drug abuse by selecting those children whose parents exhibited a substance-use disorder. High-risk children tended to exhibit greater dysfunction of the prefrontal cortex as identified through electrophysiological studies that documented attenuated amplitudes of the P300 event-related potential. Since the attenuated amplitude measure has been associated with the prefontal cortex, which is believed to be involved in executive cognitive functioning, the authors hypothesized that individuals with dysfunction in the prefrontal cortex tend to experience deficits in executive cognitive functioning that would then leave them more vulnerable to substance-use disorders. This finding is important to consider when attempting to infer causality from correlational data regarding drug abusers' cognitive functioning.

The comorbidity of substance abuse, neuropsychological dysfunction, and violent behavior have been identified as mediated by executive functioning and the prefrontal cortex (Fishbein, 2000). Bauer and Hesselbrock (1999) related the decrease in P300 amplitude in teenagers to a coincidence of family alcohol/drug dependence and the prevalence of conduct disorder problems. In this study, 57 participants (15 to 20 years old) were evaluated. Smaller P300 amplitudes in the posterior region were associated with increased conduct problems in the teenagers who were younger than 16.5 years. For older teenagers, the effect was seen in the frontal region.

The more recent use of imaging of the brain has been helpful in relating neuropsychological findings to structural and anatomic functioning in the substance-abuse population. Gatley and Volkow (1998) noted the value of PET and SPECT in research designs that employ neuropsychological measures. Indeed, functional-imaging and brain-imaging studies have contributed to the understanding of maladaptive behavior as it is associated with orbitofrontal cortex connections (London et al., 2000). Studies such as Liu and colleagues' (1998) have documented the reduced volume of prefrontal lobe area in polysubstance abusers through the use of magnetic resonance imaging.

Cognitive functioning is especially important in the patient's ability to benefit from rehabilitation. In a study by Blume et al. (1999), 22 dually diagnosed inpatients were administered intellectual-executive, and memory-functioning tests, as well as an assessment of their readiness to change. The authors reported that, especially for those who are dually diagnosed with both a substance-abuse and psychiatric disorder, cognitive impairment was related to a lowered likelihood of motivation to change their substance-abuse behaviors.

Drug abuse may leave its mark on brain functioning. However, the synergistic effect of drug abuse on an individual who already suffers from a history of traumatic brain injury can be devastating. The interaction of traumatic brain injury and substance abuse has been documented. In a study of 119 participants with severe closed-head traumatic brain injuries, those who tested positively for drug use at the time of head injury performed significantly lower on testing than those patients with a normal drug screening at the time of trauma. It is suggested that there is an additive effect of substance abuse on the neuropsychological outcome of those with traumatic brain injuries (Kelly et al., 1997).

Cocaine

Cocaine, a derivative of the coca plant, was first noted for its use among South American Indians sometime between 3000 and 1500 B.C. (Bolla, Cadet, et al., 1998; Hartman, 1995). Cocaine became popular for pharmacological use in medicine in the late 1800s since it offered both anesthetic and mood-altering properties. In the 1980s, estimated use of cocaine on at least one occasion affected more than 22 million Americans (Washton and Gold, 1984). With the introduction of "crack" in 1985, a resurgence of cocaine use was observed. By the mid-1990s, it was estimated that 1.5 million Americans used cocaine (Bolla, Cadet, et al., 1998).

The effects of chronic cocaine use include irritability, fatigue, depression, impotence, and loss of libido. Neurotoxic reactions resulting in cardiac arrhythmia, convulsions, and respiratory failure have also been noted. Cocaine has been documented for its powerful psychologically addictive qualities with a question as to the extent to which there is an actual physical addiction or associated withdrawal syndrome (Washton and Gold, 1984; Brick and Erickson, 1999). The neuropsychological studies that have focused on cocaine use have not been as forthcoming as the studies that have focused on neuroimaging (Hartman, 1995). Although neuropsychological impairment has been documented in cocaine abusers, studies have not been able to support differential diagnoses of specific structural abnormalities (Hartman, 1995). Thus, the mechanism for the impairment, whether vascular, metabolic, etc., is not clear. In adults under the age of 45, cocaine abuse has been reported as a significant risk factor for stroke (Lacayo, 1995). Particular subgroups of cocaine abusers may reveal abnormalities in brain perfusion that are related to cognitive deficits (Strickland and Stein, 1995).

In a review by Strickland and colleagues (1998), the authors noted how cerebral metabolic and hypoperfusion irregularities are seen in the neuroimaging of the cocaine abuser. In particular, techniques such as computerized axial tomography (CAT) and MRI may show significant cerebral events, although newer techniques such as PET, SPECT, and quantitative electroencephalography (QEEG) are revealing a greater frequency of changes in brain functioning that may have initially gone unnoticed.

Findings of these neuroimaging studies have been validated by neuropsychological evaluations. For example, in a study of eight long-term cocaine abusers who were abstinent for six months, the use of SPECT revealed significant differences between abusers and normal subjects. Neuropsychological impairment was documented in users, particularly in the areas of learning, memory, and executive functioning. Interestingly, the use of MRI was unremarkable for seven out of the eight patients. The pattern of multifocal hypoperfusion seen on SPECT exam was associated with deficits in neuropsychological test performance (Strickland et al., 1993).

In another study pairing diagnostic imaging with neuropsychological testing, Bolla, Cadet, et al. (1998) revealed that use of PET and MRI with neuropsychological evaluation revealed that those who abuse cocaine experience specific difficulties in executive functioning, judgment, and decision making. It is suggested that structures of the prefrontal, orbitofrontal, and anterior cingulate gyrus are affected in cocaine abusers (Bolla, Cadet, et al., 1998).

The use of MRI to determine premorbid brain size or intracranial volume in abstinent crack/cocaine- and crack/cocaine and alcohol-dependent individuals has been studied (Di Sclafani et al., 1998). Findings concluded that crack- and crack-and-alcohol-dependent individuals appeared similar both in neuropsychological performance and in brain size. However, intracranial volume appeared to account for the variability in neuropsychological test performance. It was suggested that individuals with larger brains are better able to maintain cognitive functioning in spite of substance abuse or other cerebral insult. Thus, it appears that the more brain reserves one has, the more one can afford to lose.

Although cocaine use has been related to numerous structural brain complications including seizure, stroke, hemorrhage, transient ischemic attacks, and cerebral vasculitis/spasms, as well as changes in cerebral blood flow and metabolism, we are still beginning to explore the specific ways in which cocaine abuse affects neuropsychological or cognitive functioning (Horner, 1999). In a study of 37 crack abusers, Ardila et al. (1991) observed overall lower neuropsychological test performance in abusers with regard to short-term verbal memory and attention abilities. In particular, the "lifetime amount" of cocaine use was related to neuropsychological test performance, implicating a direct relationship between cognitive impairment and long-term use of cocaine.

A subsequent study by Mittenberg and Motta (1993) also examined attention and learning. Sixteen chronic abstinent cocaine abusers were tested on tasks of verbal learning, word knowledge, and nonverbal visual-motor perceptual reasoning. When compared to controls, the cocaine abusers demonstrated significantly greater problems with learning and recall of words. However, there was no significant difference regarding intellectual ability. The authors concluded from their findings that cognitive impairment related to chronic cocaine use may be associated more with memory storage difficulties than with problems of attention or general intellectual functioning.

A study by Horner (1997) further explored memory abilities. An examination of the neuropsychological functioning of 32 cocaine-dependent alcoholic patients versus 52 alcoholic patients who did not engage in cocaine abuse supported poor performance on tests of immediate and delayed verbal memory for the cocaine-dependent individuals. Although all of the patients in the study abused alcohol, those who also abused cocaine demonstrated specific deficits in the area of verbal memory. An assessment of attention, visual-spatial abilities, and reasoning and judgment skills revealed no significant differences between the groups. This study supports the review by Horner (1999) in which he reported that in seventeen research studies examining attention skills in cocaine abusers, he observed inconsistent findings and insufficient evidence regarding the implication of impaired attention in cocaine abusers. This study also appears to support the previously discussed findings of Mittenberg and Motta (1993) with regard to inconsiderable impairment of attention.

Instead of examining alcohol abusers with and without cocaine abuse, Robinson et al. (1999) studied cocaine abusers with and without alcohol dependence. Overall, subjects who abused both cocaine and alcohol demonstrated few differences on neuropsychological testing measures when compared to nonabusers. However, mild cognitive dysfunction was noted in those individuals who abused cocaine. Importantly, those young abusers of both alcohol and cocaine appeared to be less neuropsychologically impaired than those who abused cocaine only. These findings may well be a function of the mediating factor of age.

Few studies have been able to follow substance abusers on a long-term basis. However, the chronicity of abnormal QEEG profiles in crack cocaine users has been noted even after six months of abstinence (Alper et al., 1998). Five to ten days, one month, and six months after last cocaine use, QEEG measures of seventeen subjects revealed no significant changes over time. The implications of these findings are not clear. Relating such electrophysiological studies to neuropsychological test data may provide greater insight into the functional long-term effects of cocaine abuse.

Marijuana

Although the use of marijuana became especially popular during the 1960s, its use since then has appeared to decline significantly (Hartman, 1995). THC, or tetrahydrocannabinol, is the psychoactive ingredient in marijuana that is now used for experimental medical use and for its anti-emetic and appetite-enhancing effects in cancer patients. As with cocaine, the neuropsychological research has been mixed regarding the effects of marijuana use on long-term cognitive functioning. An early study of long-term effects (Carlin and Tupin, 1977) examined a group of ten individuals who smoked marijuana daily for an average of five years. The authors concluded that when compared to nonusers, minimal differences in cognitive functioning were observed with no support for any differences between groups on complex cognitive tasks.

As with most substance-abuse research, the short-term effects of marijuana have received greater attention in the research literature. The allegation that marijuana in some way enhances creative or associational thinking was tested by Tinklenberg and colleagues (1978). In this study, 16 male subjects were tested while under the influence of marijuana. Contrary to myth and popular belief, the authors concluded that marijuana did not increase fluency, flexibility, elaboration, or uniqueness in responses to a creative-thinking task.

Other popular beliefs of enhanced attention and greater access to long-term memory have also been explored and challenged. Some studies support that speed in visual scanning is negatively affected in those who begin use of cannabis at an early age (Ehrenreich et al., 1999). Casswell and Marks (1973) documented problems with attention on a visual task testing both experienced and nonexperienced users who were under the influence of cannabis. The authors reported that the results of this study were similar to those that would be found in one of alcohol intoxication and that there was no evidence to support the idea that experienced cannabis users are better able to negotiate visual stimuli (such as during driving) than nonusers.

Similarly, the idea that marijuana may enhance access to information in long-term memory has not received much scientific support. To the contrary, impairment of memory has been noted as the "single most consistently reported psychological deficit produced by cannabinoids" (Miller and Branconnier, 1983, p. 453).

The phenomenon of thought disorder and memory intrusions during marijuana intoxication was tested during a word list learning task (Pfefferbaum et al., 1997). Sixteen males were each evaluated under intoxicated and nonintoxicated conditions. Results suggested that while under the influence of marijuana, one may be subjected to memory intrusions. Marijuana use was associated with poor correctly-called list items and increased intrusions, or incorrect word recall. These findings suggested the possibility that marijuana results in disinhibition or intrusive thoughts.

Melges and colleagues (1970) discussed a similar phenomenon called "temporal incoordination," suggesting that marijuana use disorganizes sequential thought and cognitive processes. Eight male graduate students were tested on four different days while under the influence of marijuana extract or a placebo. Performance on serial subtraction of sevens did not appear to be impaired by THC consumption. However, performance on forward and backward digit span revealed differences in short-term memory related to THC. A more complicated goal-directed serial alternation task, which required more complex serial addition and subtraction, was administered to assess for temporal disintegration. Significant differences in performance, with greater disorganization and disintegration while under the influence of THC, were observed. This increased disorganization is reminiscent of the problems with complex attention and concentration described earlier.

Indeed, discontinuity of thought and disorganization were related to marijuana in a study where the thought processes of 72 male volunteers were analyzed based on their responses to the Thematic Apperception Test (TAT) (Roth et al., 1975). The TAT is a projective test in which pictures of scenes are presented to the subject and the subject provides a response in the form of a story. Subjects' written stories were evaluated with regard to three components: (1) events preceding the scene in the picture, (2) a description of what was happening in the picture, and what each of the characters were thinking and feeling, and (3) the resolution or outcome of the story. The researchers concluded that while subjects were under the influence of marijuana, greater discontinuity of thought and contradictory ideas were observed, as well as a tendency toward unusual ideas.

Neuroimaging has also begun to help researchers understand the effects of marijuana use. In a recent study, 18 young adult (mean age of 22 years) frequent marijuana users were compared to nonusers with regard to evidence of tissue volume on MRI (Block et al., 2000). No significant differences or abnormalities in MRIs were noted between the two groups. Interestingly, ventricular cerebrospinal fluid volumes were lower in marijuana users despite no differences in tissue volume and composition.

Another neuroimaging procedure, SPECT, has been used to study marijuana users with attention deficit hyperactivity disorder (ADHD) (Amen and Waugh, 1998). Thirty heavy marijuana users with ADHD were compared to ten nonusers with ADHD who served as the control group. The authors concluded that chronic marijuana use results in decreased cerebral perfusion particularly in the temporal lobe areas of the brain. The temporal lobe has been commonly associated with memory abilities.

LSD

Lysergic acid diethylamide (LSD-25) is a natural substance and hallucinogen that made its appearance in modern times during the mid-1900s. Its use peaked in the American culture in the 1950s and 1960s. LSD became most popular for its mind altering effects, which include visual distortion and hallucinations, a distorted sense of time, feelings of detachment, alterations in sensory perception, emotional lability, and mystical experiences (Strassman, 1984). There has been a question as to whether LSD use results in organic brain damage. An early study by McGlothlin et al. (1969) examined sixteen subjects who had received LSD in either an experimental or psychotherapeutic setting. These subjects and controls, who were matched for sex, age, and education, were administered a number of spatial and visual tests including the Trail Making Test, which assesses the speed and accuracy of visual scanning and cognitive flexibility. Also, a measure of general intelligence, a verbal fluency test, and tests from the Halstead-Reitan Neuropsychological Test Battery were administered. Results revealed that only the category test, which assesses nonverbal reasoning and abstract problem solving, demonstrated a significant difference in performance between the two groups. Otherwise, there was no support for generalized brain damage related to the amount of LSD ingestion. Although mean performances for the LSD group on a number of visual perception tests was lower, none of the differences reached statistical significance. The authors noted limitations to their research with concern that premorbid factors might have accounted for the difference in category test scores between the two groups.

A later study by Wright and Hogan (1972) concluded that there was no significant difference between a group of 20 LSD users and a control group matched for age, sex, education, and intelligence when compared on the Halstead-Reitan Neuropsychological Test Battery. A more comprehensive evaluation of LSD users was conducted by Culver and King (1974) who studied undergraduate seniors over a period of two years, comparing a control group with a marijuana-using group and an LSD-using group. Subjects were matched on intellectual and personality dimensions, as well as comparative drug use. Although LSD users performed within normal limits on the Trail Making Test, their performances were statistically significantly lower than either the marijuana users or normal controls. The authors concluded that although such differences were observed, a clear argument for organic dysfunction could not be made.

Phencyclidine

Phencyclidine was originally synthesized for use as an anesthetic agent in the late 1950s (Burns et al., 1975). However, it was taken off the market due to its side effects that include disorientation, hallucinations, and excitatory activity. Insufflation or "snorting" low doses of phencyclidine (PCP, also called angel dust or crystal) can produce mild agitation, catatonic rigidity, and possible lack of verbal communication. Higher doses can result in coma, apnea, hypertension, and fatality.

The possibility that PCP produces organic mental impairment was studied by Carlin and colleagues (1979). PCP abusers who had been abstinent for an average length of 27 months were compared on a number of neuropsychological measures to polydrug users who had never used PCP and to controls who were neither alcohol nor substance abusers. Neuropsychological impairment was demonstrated for six of the 12 PCP users, five of the 12 polydrug users, and none of the controls. Neuropsychological test protocols of the Halstead-Reitan Neuropsychological Test Battery and MMPI were rated on overall level of performance on a scale of 1 to 6. Subjects were matched for age, education, sex, and ethnicity. The authors found that 50 percent of the PCP users demonstrated neuropsychological deficits in the range of mild organic mental impairment.

A comprehensive review by Ellison (1995) documented animal studies that revealed the neurotoxic effects in, and neuronal degeneration of, limbic structures. Increased glucose metabolism in the areas of degeneration was noted. These changes in the limbic circuit with degeneration and alteration in glucose metabolism appeared to be similar to that seen in "some schizophrenics and most Alzheimers patients" (Ellison, 1995, p. 250). Thus, increased glucose utilization and neuronal degeneration from neurotoxicity in the limbic structures is seen as the reason for memory disturbances in schizophrenics, Alzheimers patients, and chronic PCP users. Animal studies have also suggested that PCP is involved in a number of different brain neurotransmitter systems (Sircar and Li, 1994). Compared to the illegal drug studies already discussed, the PCP research seems to most clearly demonstrate its deleterious effects.

Amphetamines and MDMA (Ecstasy)

Although amphetamine use can result in neurological findings such as hypertension, stroke, brain hemorrhage, or other neuropathy, neuropsychological findings in human subjects have not been well documented, except in the cases of infant and developmental exposure (Hartman, 1995). With the increase of methamphetamine use in the United States, patients are presenting with chronic psychotic illnesses likely to be related to vasoconstriction and neurotoxicity resulting in brain damage (Buffenstein et al., 1999).

The decision-making abilities of chronic amphetamine abusers were studied by Rogers and others (1999). In a computerized decision-making task, chronic amphetamine abusers tended to exhibit longer response times before making their decisions when compared to opiate abusers. In general, the research data suggested that decision-making performances of chronic amphetamine abusers was similar to the performances of patients with focal damage of the prefrontal cortex. In addition, it was found that the chronic amphetamine abusers' performances were also similar to that of the performances of normal volunteers with induced decreases in plasma tryptophan. This finding helped support the notion that amphetamine abusers may experience reduced levels of serotonin (5-hydroxytryptamine, 5-HT) in the orbital regions of the brain. The authors suggested that the results supported the likelihood that amphetamines affect the orbitofrontal/prefrontal cortex.

With the introduction of "designer drugs," there seems to have been a shift in the research focus with fewer investigations into the effects of classic amphetamines per se. One of these new designer drugs is Ecstasy (3,4-methylenedioxymethamphetamine or MDMA). MDMA is considered a psychedelic compound that is chemically related to methamphetamine and results in problems similar to those found in amphetamine and cocaine usage (Campagna, 1986). This synthetic amphetamine derivative has been shown to produce effects such as cerebral venous sinus thrombosis (Rothwell and Grant, 1993) and Parkinsonism (Mintzer et al., 1999). The neurotoxicity of MDMA has been well documented (McCann and Ricuarte, 1995). Despite the frightening popularity of MDMA in the U.S. college student population, insidious effects of serotonin toxicity may go unnoticed until significant brain damage has occurred.

With the benefit of neuroimaging, the effects of MDMA can be more critically documented. In a study of 21 abstinent MDMA users and 21 age-and-gender-matched nonusers, both SPECT and MRI studies were reviewed to detect any changes in cerebral blood flow (Chang et al., 2000). Abstinent MDMA users initially demonstrated no significant differences in cerebral blood flow when compared to nonusers. Overall results indicated that persistent changes in cerebral blood flow were not observed in low-dose users. However, higher dosages of MDMA resulted in decreased regional cerebral blood flow within three weeks post-MDMA administration, in the visual cortex, the caudate, and the superior parietal and dorsolateral frontal regions of the brain. In a study of long-term effects on the brain, PET was employed for seven Ecstasy users and seven controls (Obrocki et al., 1999). The authors concluded that users' glucose metabolic uptake was altered within the areas of the amygdala, hippocampus, and Brodmann's area II (part of the primary somatosensory cortex on the postcentral gyrus) when compared with control subjects. Thus, it is possible that cerebral glucose metabolic rate is altered by MDMA.

A computerized cognitive performance test battery was administered to 22 MDMA users and 23 control subjects to assess differences in cognitive performance (McCann et al., 1999). Although controls and MDMA users performed similarly on some neuropsychological tasks, MDMA users demonstrated weaker sustained attention, short-term memory, and verbal reasoning. Results were thought to support "subtle but significant" neuropsychological deficits.

Memory disturbances are also noted in a study by Reneman and colleagues (2000). To assess for memory disturbance in five abstinent MDMA users versus nine nonusers, the Rey Auditory Verbal Learning Test was administered. SPECT studies of the subjects were compared revealing preliminary results that suggested altered functioning of the occipital cortex associated with memory impairment. A previous study conducted by Bolla, McCann, et al. (1998) documented memory impairment associated with greater MDMA use. In particular, immediate verbal memory and delayed visual memory were most affected. The authors concluded that even abstinent users could show these pervasive cognitive effects and that impairment was correlated with serotonin neurotoxicity and degree of exposure to MDMA. Thus, the research confirms the clear toxicity and deleterious effects of MDMA, especially in the area of memory.

Other Illegal Drug Use

Although the research on neuropsychological (neurophysiological) consequences of polysubstance abuse, cocaine, marijuana, LSD, phencyclidine, and amphetamines is, overall, quite limited, research on the remaining illicit drugs is even more sparse. Use of solvent inhalants, such as toluene, has been demonstrated to result in dementia and cerebral white-matter deterioration (Filley et al., 1990). Idiopathic Parkinsonism in a case of solvent abuse has also been documented (Uitti et al., 1994).

Amyl nitrite may have an extensive body of literature associated with documentation of physiological changes, however, neuropsychological investigation has not been very forthcoming. Amyl nitrite inhalation has been found to be related to increases in cerebral blood flood (Mathew et al., 1989). It also has been employed in medical applications as a coronary vasodilator (Hartman, 1995). Its recreational use has been documented in male homosexuals to facilitate intercourse and heighten sexual experience.

Neuropsychological deficits from chronic use of heroin and other opiates have not been consistently demonstrated (Hartman, 1995). Furthermore, it is not clear whether these substances result in any medical neurotoxicity.

SUMMARY

With regard to the neuropsychological consequences of alcohol abuse, the research indicates that chronic alcohol abuse gives rise to not only severe indirect toxic effects on brain and behavior functioning, but it also is a source of direct toxic effects on brain functions. In addition to the well-known and extensively studied syndrome of Korsakoff amnesia arising from severe nutritional depletion associated with chronic alcoholism, a history of nonamnesic chronic alcohol abuse is also associated with well-documented evidence of neuropsychological deficits which include impairments in abstraction and mental flexibility, perceptual skills, memory and learning functions, attention and concentration, and fine motor skills. Evidence appears to favor the hypothesis of dysfunction in the frontal-limbic-diencephalon brain regions in addition to involvement of the cerebellum, even in the absence of evidence of cerebellar degeneration. With prolonged abstinence, some recovery of cognitive functioning can occur for some individuals. Because of the high prevalence of neuropsychological deficits indicative of moderate to severe cerebral dysfunction in individuals who chronically abuse alcohol and because of the impediment that such cognitive deficits can present in an individual's ability to benefit from certain aspects of an alcohol treatment or rehabilitation program, neuropsychological evaluation and consultation and rehabilitation of cognitive deficits is strongly recommended to form an integral part of such intervention programs.

Research regarding the neuropsychological consequences of illegal drug use is especially sparse, limited, or in some cases, nonexistent. A review of the literature indicates some type of neuropsychological impairment in polydrug abusers, memory difficulties in cocaine abusers, attention and disorganizational problems in users of marijuana, and more serious brain consequences in those who abuse amphetamines and newer, synthetic drugs. However, available studies tend to be inconclusive, small in size, unable to control for, or take into account, premorbid functioning or other factors, or tend to be focused on immediate rather than long-term effects. It is well known that some neuropsychological effects may be possible with abuse of any type of drug, especially depending on the dosage administration. However, the identification of enduring, long-term effects is complicated by the lack of well-controlled research as well as a myriad of subject and research factors. Much of the research is correlational, and therefore, it is difficult to determine causality and the role of premorbid predisposition to substance abuse.

In the assessment of neuropsychological/cognitive functioning of any individual, it is important to identify and recognize preexisting or constitutional factors that may account, in part or in whole, for the individual's symptoms and test performance. The value of a thorough developmental, intellectual, academic, medical, vocational, social, and psychiatric history cannot be underestimated in the interpretation of current cognitive impairment.

REFERENCES

Albert, M. S., Butters, N., and Brandt, J. (1981). Patterns of remote memory in amnesic and demented patients. *Archives of Neurology, 38,* 495-500.

Allen, D. N., Goldstein, G., and Seaton, B. E. (1997). Cognitive rehabilitation of chronic alcohol abusers. *Neuropsychology Review, 7*(1), 21-39.

Alper, K. R., Prichep, L. S., Kowalik, S., Rosenthal, M. S., and John, E. R. (1998). Persistent QEEG abnormality in crack cocaine users at 6 months of drug abstinence. *Neuropsychopharmacology, 19*(1), 1-9.

Amen, D. G. and Waugh, M. (1998). High resolution brain SPECT imaging of marijuana smokers with AD/HD. *Journal of Psychoactive Drugs, 30*(2), 209-214.

Ardila, A., Rosselli, M., and Strumwasser, S. (1991). Neuropsychological deficits in chronic cocaine abusers. *International Journal of Neuroscience, 57,* 73-79.

Aytaclar, S., Tarter, R. E., Kirisci, L., and Lu, S. (1999). Association between hyperactivity and executive cognitive functioning in childhood and substance use in early adolescence. *Journal of the American Academy of Child and Adolescent Psychiatry, 38*(2), 172-178.

Bauer, L. O. and Hesselbrock, V. M. (1999). P300 decrements in teenagers with conduct problems: Implications for substance abuse risk and brain development. *Biological Psychiatry, 46*(2), 263-272.

Beatty, W. W. and Borrell, G. K. (2000). Forms of knowledge, cognitive impairment, and drug abuse: A demonstration. *Progress in Neuropsychopharmacology and Biological Psychiatry, 24*(1), 17-22.

Beaunieux, H., Desgranges, B., LaLevee, C., de la Sayette, V., Lechevalier, B., Eustache, F. (1998). Preservation of cognitive procedural memory in a case of Korsakoff's syndrome: Methodological and theoretical insights. *Perceptual and Motor Skills, 86*(3), 1267-1287.

Block, R. I., O'Leary, D. S., Ehrhardt, J. C., Augustinack, J. C., Ghoneim, M. M., Arndt, S., and Hall, J. A. (2000). Effects of frequent marijuana use on brain tissue volume and composition. *Neuroreport: For Rapid Communication of Neuroscience Research, 11*(3), 491-496.

Blume, A. W., Davis, J. M., and Schmaling, K. B. (1999). Neurocognitive dysfunction in dually-diagnosed patients: A potential roadblock to motivating behavior change. *Journal of Psychoactive Drugs, 31*(2), 111-115.

Bolla, K. I., Cadet, J., and London, E. D. (1998). The neuropsychiatry of chronic cocaine abuse. *Journal of Neuropsychiatry and Clinical Neurosciences, 10*(3), 280-289.

Bolla, K. I., McCann, U. D., and Ricuarte, G. A. (1998). Memory impairment in abstinent MDMA (Ecstasy) users. *Neurology, 51*(6), 1532-1537.

Brick, J. and Erickson, C. (1999). *Drugs, the Brain, and Behavior: The Pharmacology of Abuse and Dependence.* Binghamton, NY: The Haworth Medical Press.

Buffenstein, A., Heaster, J., and Ko, P. (1999). Chronic psychotic illness methamphetamine. *American Journal of Psychiatry, 156*(4), 662.

Burns, R. S., Lerner, S. E., Corrado, R., James, S., and Schnoll, S. (1975). Phencyclidine: States of acute intoxications and fatalities. *The Western Journal of Medicine, 123,* 345-349.

Butters, N. (1984). Alcoholic Korsakoff's syndrome: An update. *Seminars in Neurology 4*(2), 229-247.

Butters, N. and Cermak, L. S. (1974). The role of cognitive factors in the memory disorder of alcoholic patients with the Korsakoff syndrome. *Annals of the New York Academy of Science, 233,* 61-75.

Butters, N. and Cermak, L. S. (1975). Some analyses of amnesic syndromes in brain-damaged patients. In Pribram, K. and Isaacson, R. (Eds.), *The Hippocampus* (pp. 377-410). New York: Plenum Press.

Butters, N. and Miliotis, P. (1985). Amnestic Disorders. In Heilman, K. and Valenstein, E. (Eds.), *Clinical Neuropsychology,* Second Edition (pp. 403-451). New York: Oxford University Press.

Butters, N., Tarlow, S., Cermak, L. S., and Sax, D. (1976). A comparison of the information processing deficits of patients with Huntington's chorea and Korsakoff's syndrome. *Cortex, 12,* 134-144.

Campagna, K. D. (1986). Drug information forum: What are designer drugs? *U.S. Pharmacist, 11*(5), 16-17.

Carlin, A. S., Grant, I., Reed, R., and Adams, K. (1979). Is phencyclidine (PCP) abuse associated with organic mental impairment? *American Journal of Drug and Alcohol Abuse, 6,* 273-281.

Carlin, A. S., Stauss, F. F., Grant, I., and Adams, K.M. (1980). Drug abuse style, drug use type, and neuropsychological deficit in polydrug users. *Addictive Behaviors, 5*(3), 229-234.

Carlin, A. S. and Tupin, E. W. (1977). The effect of long-term chronic marijuana use on neuropsychological functioning. *International Journal of the Addictions, 12*(5), 617-624.

Casswell, S. and Marks, D. (1973). Cannabis induced impairment of performance of a divided attention task. *Nature, 241,* 60-61.

Chang, L., Grob, C. S., Ernst, T., Itti, L., Mishkin, F. S., Jose-Melchor, R., and Poland, R. (2000). Effect of ecstasy3,4-methylenedioxymethamphetamin (MDMA) on cerebral blood flow: A co-registered SPECT and MRI study. *Psychiatry Research: Neuroimaging, 98*(1), 15-28.

Charness, M. E. (1994). Brain lesions in alcoholics. *Alcoholism: Clinical and Experimental Research, 17,* 2-11.

Culver, C. M. and King, F. W. (1974). Neuropsychological assessment of under-graduate marihuana and LSD Users. *Archives of General Psychiatry, 31,* 707-711.

Dao-Castellana, M. H., Samson, Y., Legault, F., Martinot, J. L., Aubin, H.J., Crouzel, C., Feldman, L., Barrucand, D., Rancurel, G., Feline, A., et al. (1998). Frontal dysfunction in neurologically normal chronic alcoholic subjects: Metabolic and neuropsychological findings. *Psychological Medicine, 28*(5), 1039-1048.

Davila, M. D., Shear, P. K., Lane, B., Sullivan, E. V., and Pfefferbaum, A. (1994). Mamillary body and cerebellar shrinkage in chronic alcoholics: An MRI and neuropsychological study. *Neuropsychology, 8*(3), 433-444.

DeBellis, M. D., Clark, D. B., Beers, S. R., Soloff, P. H., Boring, A. M., Hall, J., Kersh, A., and Keshavan, M. S. (2000). Hippocampal volume in adolescent-onset alcohol use disorders. *American Journal of Psychiatry, 157*(5),737-744.

Di Sclafani, V., Clark, J. W., Tolou-Shams, M., Bloomer, C., Salas, G. A., Norman, D., and Fein, G. (1998). Premorbid brain size is a determinant of functional reserve in abstinent crack-cocaine and crack-cocaine-alcohol dependent adults. *Journal of the International Neuropsychological Society, 4*(6), 559-565.

Diamond, R., and Carey, S. (1977). Developmental changes in the representation of faces. *Journal of Experimental Child Psychology, 23,* 1-22.

Dikmen, S. S., Donovan, D. M., Loberg, T., Machamer, J. E., and Temkin, N. R. (1993). Alcohol use and its effects on neuropsychological outcome in head injury. *Neuropsychology, 7*(3), 296-305.

Dricker, J., Butters, N., Berman, G., Samuels, I., and Carey, S. (1978). Recognition and encoding of faces by alcoholic Korsakoff and right hemisphere patients. *Neuropsychologia, 16,* 683-695.

Ehrenreich, H., Rinn, T., Kunert, H. J., Moeller, M. R., Poser, W., Schilling, L., Gigerenzer, G., and Hoehe, M. R. (1999). Specific attentional dysfunction in adults following early start of cannabis use. *Psychopharmacology, 142*(3), 295-301.

Ellison, G. (1995). The *N*-methyl-D-aspartate antagonists phencyclidine, ketamine, and dizocilpine as both behavioral and anatomical models of the dementias. *Brain Research Reviews, 20*(2), 250-267.

Filley, C. M., Heaton, R. K., and Rosenberg, N. L. (1990). White matter dementia in chronic toluene abuse. *Neurology, 40*(3), 532-534.

Fishbein, D. (2000). Neuropsychological function, drug abuse, and violence: A conceptual framework. *Criminal Justice and Behavior, 27*(2), 139-159.

Gansler, D. A., Harris, G. J., Oscar-Berman, M., Streeter, C., Lewis, R. F., Ahmed, I., and Achong, D. (2000). Hypoperfusion of the inferior frontal brain regions in abstinent alcoholics: A pilot SPECT study. *Journal of Studies on Alcohol, 61*(1), 32-37.

Gatley, S. J. and Volkow, N. D. (1998). Addiction and imaging of the living human brain. *Drug and Alcohol Dependence, 51*(1-2), 97-108.

Giancola, P. R. and Tarter, R. E. (1999). Executive cognitive functioning and risk for substance abuse. *Psychological Science, 10*(3), 203-205.

Graham, R. B. (1990). *Physiological Psychology.* California: Wadsworth Publishing Company.

Grant, I., Adams, K. M., Carlin, A. S., and Rennick, P. M. (1977). Neuropsychological deficit in polydrug users. A preliminary report of the findings of the collaborative neuropsychological study of polydrug users. *Drug and Alcohol Dependence, 2*(2), 91-108.

Grant, S., Contoreggi, C., and London, E. D. (2000). Drug abusers show impaired performance in a laboratory test of decision making. *Neuropsychologia, 38*(8), 1180-1187.

Grobin, A. C., Matthews, D. B., Devaud, L. L., and Morrow, A. L. (1998). The role of GABA(A) receptors in the acute and chronic effects of ethanol. *Psychopharmacology, 139*(1-2), 2-19.

Hammoumi, S., Pyen, A., Favre, J.-D., Balmes, J.-L., Bernard, J.-Y., Husson, M., Ferrand, J.-P., Martin, J.-P., and Daoust, M. (1999). Does the short variant of the serotonin transporter linked polymorphic region constitute a marker of alcohol dependence? *Alcohol, 17*(2), 107-112.

Hartman, D. E. (1995). *Neuropsychological Toxicology.* New York: Plenum Press.

Horner, M. D. (1997). Cognitive functioning in alcoholic patients with and without cocaine dependence. *Archives of Clinical Neuropsychology, 12*(7), 667-676.

Horner, M. D. (1999). Attentional functioning in abstinent cocaine abusers. *Drug and Alcohol Dependence, 54*(1), 19-33.

Jernigan, T. L., Butters, N., DiTraglia, G., Schafer, K., Smith, T., Irwin, M., Grant, I., Schuckit, K., and Cermak, L. (1991). Reduced cerebral gray matter observed in alcoholics using magnetic resonance imaging. *Alcoholism: Clinical and Experimental Research, 15*(3), 418-427.

Kelly, M. P., Johnson, C. T., Knoller, N., and Drubach, D. A. (1997). Substance abuse, traumatic brain injury, and neuropsychological outcome. *Brain Injury, 11*(6):391-402.

Kimble, D. P. (1968). Hippocampus and internal inhibition. *Psychological Bulletin, 70,* 285-295.

Kinsbourne, M. and Wood, F. (1975). Short-term memory processes and the amnesic syndrome. In Deutsch, D. and Deutsch, J.A. (Eds.), *Short-Term Memory* (pp. 288-291). New York: Academic Press.

Korbo, L. (1999). Glial cell loss in the hippocampus of alcoholics. *Alcoholism: Clinical and Experimental Research, 23*(1), 164-168.

Krabbendam, L., Visser, P. J., Derix, M. M. A., Verhey, F., Hofman, P., Verhoeven, W., Tuinier, S., and Jolles, J. (2000). Normal cognitive performance in patients with chronic alcoholism in contrast to patients with Korsakoff's syndrome. *Journal of Neuropsychiatry and Clinical Neurosciences, 12*(1), 44-50.

Lacayo, A. (1995). Neurologic and psychiatric complications of cocaine abuse. *Neuropsychiatry, Neuropsychology, and Behavioral Neurology, 8*(1), 53-60.

Leshner, A. I. (1997). Addiction is a brain disease, and it matters. *Science, 278*(5335), 45-47.

Leshner, A. I. and Koob, G. F. (1999). Drugs of abuse and the brain. *Proceedings of the Association of American Physicians, 111*(2), 99-108.

Liu, X., Matochik, J. A., Cadet, J., and London, E. D. (1998). Smaller volume of prefrontal lobe in polysubstance abuser: A magnetic resonance imaging study. *Neuropsychopharmacology, 18*(4), 243-252.

London, E. D., Ernst, M., Grant, S., Bonson, K., and Weinstein, A. (2000). Orbitofrontal cortex and human drug abuse: Functional imaging. *Cerebral Cortex, 10*(3), 334-342.

Lovinger, D. M. (1997). Serotonin's role in alcohol's effects on the brain. *Alcohol Health and Research World, 21*(2), 114-120.

Malloy, P., Noel, N., Longabaugh, R., and Beattie, M. (1990). Determinants of neuro-psychological impairment in anti-social substance abusers. *Addictive Behaviors, 15,* 431-438.

Mathew, R. J., Wilson, W. H., and Tant, S. R. (1989). Regional cerebral blood flow changes associated with amyl nitrite inhalation. *British Journal of Addiction, 84*(3), 293-299.

McCann, U. D., Mertl, M., Eligulashvili, V., and Ricuarte, G. A. (1999). Cognitive performance in 3,4-methylenedioxymenthamphetamine (MDMA, ecstasy) users: A controlled study. *Psychopharmacology, 143*(4), 417-425.

McCann, U. D. and Ricuarte, G. A. (1995). On the neurotoxicity of MDMA and related amphetamine derivatives. *Journal of Clinical Psychopharmacology, 15*(4), 295-296.

McGlothin, W., Arnold, D. O., and Freedman, D. X. (1969). Organicity measures following repeated LSD ingestion. *Archives of General Psychiatry, 21*(6), 704-709.

Melges, F. T., Tinklenberg, J. R., Hollister, L. E., and Gillespie, H. K. (1970). Marihuana and temporal disintegration. *Science, 168,* 1118-1120.

Mihic, S. J. and Harris, R. A. (1997). GABA and the GABA (A) receptor. *Alcohol Health and Research World, 21*(2), 127-131.

Miller, L. (1985). Neuropsychological assessment of substance abusers: Review and recommendations. *Journal of Substance Abuse Treatment, 2,* 5-17.

Miller, L. L. and Branconnier, R. J. (1983). Cannabis: Effects on memory and the cholinergic limbic system. *Psychological Bulletin, 93,* 441-456.

Minocha, A., Barth, J. T., Roberson, D. G., Herold, D. A., and Spyker, D. A. (1985). Impairment of cognitive and psychomotor function by ethanol in social drinkers. *Veterinary and Human Toxicology, 27,* 533-536.

Mintzer, S., Hickenbottom, S., and Gilman, S. (1999). Parkinsonism after taking ecstasy. *New England Journal of Medicine, 340*(18), 1443.

Mittenberg, W. and Motta, S. (1993). Effects of chronic cocaine abuse on memory and learning. *Archives of Clinical Neuropsychology, 8,* 477-483.

Morris, J. A., and Lawson, W. M. (1998). Neuropsychological deficits in patients with alcohol and other psychoactive substance abuse and dependency: A pilot study. *Alcoholism Treatment Quarterly, 16*(4), 101-111.

Moser, R. S. (1999). *Practice Information Clearinghouse of Knowledge (PICK 42): Clinical Neuropsychology.* Washington, DC: American Psychological Association.

Obrocki, J., Buchert, R., Vaeterlein, O., Thomasius, R., Beyer, W., and Shiermann, T. (1999). Ecstasy—long-term effects on the human central nervous system revealed by positron emission tomography. *British Journal of Psychiatry, 175,* 186-188.

Petersen, J. B., Finn, P. R., and Pihl, R. O. (1992). Cognitive dysfunction and inherited predisposition to alcoholism. *Journal of Studies on Alcohol, 53,* 154-160.

Pfefferbaum, A., Darley, C. F., Tinklenberg, J. R., Roth, W. T., and Kopell, B. S. (1977). Marijuana and memory intrusions. *Journal of Nervous and Mental Disease, 165*(6), 381-386.

Pfefferbaum, A., Lim, K. O., Zipursky, R. B., Mathalon, D. H., Lane, B., Ha, C. N., Rosenbloom, M. J., and Sullivan, E. V. (1992). Brain gray and white matter volume loss accelerates with aging in chronic alcoholics: A quantitative MRI study. *Alcoholism: Clinical and Experimental Research, 16,* 1078-1089.

Pfefferbaum, A., Sullivan, E. V., Mathalon, D. H., and Lim, K. O. (1997). Frontal lobe volume loss observed with magnetic resonance imaging in older chronic alcoholics. *Alcoholism: Clinical and Experimental Research, 21*(3), 521-529.

Piercy, M. F. (1978). Experimental studies of the organic amnesic syndrome. In Whitty, C. W. M. and Zangwill, O. L. (Eds.), *Amnesia,* Second Edition (pp. 1-51). London: Butterworths.

Ratti, M. T., Soragna, D., Sibilla, L., Giardini, A., Albergati, A., Savoldi, F., and Bo, P. (1999). Cognitive impairment and cerebral atrophy in "heavy drinkers." *Progress in Neuro-Psychopharmacology and Biological Psychiatry, 23*(2), 243-258.

Reneman, L., Booij, J., Schmand, B., van der Brink, W., and Gunning, B. (2000). Memory disturbances in Ecstasy users are correlated with an altered brain serotonin neurotransmission. *Psychopharmacology, 148*(3), 322-324.

Robinson, J. E., Heaton, R. K., and O'Malley, S. S. (1999). Neuropsychological functioning in cocaine abusers with and without alcohol dependence. *Journal of International Neuropsychological Society, 5*(1), 10-19.

Rogers, R. D., Everitt, B. J., Baldacchino, A., Blackshaw, A. J., Swainson, R., Wynne, K., Baker, N. B., Hunter, J., Carthy, T., Booker, E., et al. (1999). Dissociable deficits in the decision-making cognition of chronic amphetamine abuser, opiate abusers, patients with focal damage to prefrontal cortex, and tryptophan-depleted normal volunteers: Evidence for monoaminergic mechanisms. *Neuropsychopharmacology, 20*(4), 322-339.

Roth, W. T., Rosenbloom, M. J., Darley, C. F., Tinklenberg, J. R., and Kopell, B. S. (1975). Marihuana effects on TAT form and content. *Psychopharmacologia, 43*(3), 261-266.

Rothwell, P. M. and Grant, R. (1993). Cerebral venus sinus thrombosis induced by "ecstasy." *Journal of Neurology, Neurosurgery, and Psychiatry, 56*(9), 1035.

Rourke, S. B. and Grant, I. (1999). The interactive effects of age and length of abstinence on the recovery of neuropsychological functioning in chronic male alcoholics: A 2-year follow-up study. *Journal of the International Neuropsychological Society, 5*(3), 234-246.

Ryback, R. (1971). The continuum and specificity of the effects of alcohol on memory: A review. *Quarterly Journal of Studies on Alcohol, 32,* 995-1016.

Schaeffer, K. W., Parsons, O. A., and Yohman, J. R. (1984). Neuropsychological differences between male familial and nonfamilial alcoholics and nonalcoholics. *Alcoholism: Clinical and Experimental Research, 8,* 347-351.

Schafer, J., Birchler, G. R., and Fals-Stewart, W. (1994). Cognitive affective, and marital functioning of recovering male polysubstance abusers. *Neuropsychology, 8*(1), 100-109.

Sircar, R. and Li, C. (1994). PCP/NMDA receptor-channel complex and brain development. *Neurotoxicology and Teratology, 16*(4), 369-375.

Strassman, R. J. (1984). Adverse reactions to psychedelic drugs. *Journal of Nervous and Mental Disease, 172,* 577-595.

Strickland, T. L., Mena, I., Villanueva-Meyer, J., Miller, B., Cummings, J., Mehringer, C. M., Satz, P., and Myers, H. (1993). Cerebral perfusion and neuropsychological consequences of chronic cocaine use. *Journal of Neuropsychiatry and Clinical Neurosciences, 5,* 419-427.

Strickland, T. L., Miller, B. L., Kowell, A., and Stein, R. (1998). Neurobiology of cocaine-induced organic brain impairment: Contributions from functional neuroimaging. *Neuropsychology Review, 8*(1), 1-9.

Strickland, T. L. and Stein, R. (1995). Cocaine-induced cerebrovascular impairment: Challenges to neuropsychological assessment. *Neuropsychology Review, 5*(1), 69-79.

Tarbox, A. R., Connors, G. J., and McLauglin, E. J. (1986). Effects of drinking pattern on neuropsychological performance among alcohol misusers. *Journal of Studies on Alcohol, 47,* 176-179.

Tarter, R. E. (1988). Are there inherited behavioral traits that predispose to substance abuse? *Journal of Consulting and Clinical Psychology, 56,* 189-196.

Tarter, R. E. and Edwards, K. (1988). Psychological factors associated with the risk for alcoholism. *Alcoholism, Clinical and Experimental Research, 12,* 471-480.

Tarter, R. E., Moss, H., Arria, A., and Van Thiel, D. (1990). Hepatic, nutritional, and genetic influences on cognitive processes in alcoholics. *National Institute on Drug Abuse Research Monograph Series: 1990 Research Monograph, 101,* 124-135.

Thompson, R. F. (2000). *The Brain: A Neuroscience Primer,* Third Edition. New York: Worth Publishers.

Tinklenberg, J. R., Darley, C. F., Roth, W. T., Pfefferbaum, A., and Kopell, B.S. (1978). Marijuana effects on associations to novel stimuli. *Journal of Nervous and Mental Disease, 166*(5), 362-364.

Tiplady, B., Harding, C., McLean, D., Ortner, C., Porter, K., and Wright, P. (1999). Effects of ethanol and temazepan on episodic and semantic memory: A dose-response comparison. *Human Psychopharmacology Clinical and Experimental, 14*(4), 263-269.

Uitti, R. J., Snow, B. J., Shinotoh, H., Vingerhoets, F.J., Hayward, M., Hashimoto, S., Richmond, J., Markey, S., Markey, C., and Calne, D. (1994). Parkinsonism induced by solvent abuse. *Annals of Neurology, 35,* 616-619.

Washton, A. and Gold, M. (1984). Chronic cocaine abuse. *Psychiatric Annals, 14,* 733-743.

Wilkinson, D. A. and Carlen, P. L. (1980). Relationship of neuropsychological test performance to brain morphology in amnesic and non-amnesic chronic alcoholics. *Acta Psychiatrica Scandinavica, 62*(Suppl. 286), 89-101.

Wright, M. and Hogan, T. (1972). Repeated LSD ingestion and performance on neuropsychological tests. *Journal of Nervous and Mental Disease, 154*(6), 432-438.

Chapter 4

Effects of Alcohol Abuse on the Brain

Fulton T. Crews

OVERVIEW

Alcohol is a major drug of use and abuse by Americans. An estimated 15 million Americans are alcohol abusers or are alcohol dependent (Massey et al., 1989). Lifetime prevalence of alcohol dependence is estimated at 13 percent and 4 percent for American men and women over 18 years of age respectively (Grant and Dawson, 1997). According to the National Drug and Alcoholism Treatment Unit Survey (Massey et al., 1989), 1.8 million individuals were treated for alcoholism in the United States in 1989. It is well established that chronic excessive ethanol consumption produces deficits in cognitive and motor abilities (Crews, 1999; Sullivan, Rosenbloom, and Pfefferbaum, 2000; also see Chapters 2 and 3 of this book). Alcoholic dementia is a leading cause of adult dementia in the United States, accounting for approximately 10 percent of cases (Alzheimer's disease is the leading cause, accounting for 40 to 60 percent of cases) (Martin et al., 1986). Although evidence suggests reversibility of deficits with sobriety (Sullivan, Rosenbloom, Lim, et al., 2000), studies report that 50 to 75 percent of sober, detoxified, long-term alcohol-dependent individuals suffer from some degree of detectable cognitive impairment, with approximately 10 percent being seriously demented (Martin et al., 1986). The effects of alcohol appear as a continuum, with moderate deficits in the majority of long-term alcoholics, progressing to the more severe deficits of Wernicke's disease and Wernicke's encephalopathy with Korsakoff's amnestic syndrome (Butterworth, 1995; Pfefferbaum et al., 1996). A variety of lifestyle factors, including nutrition, are implicated in the more severe cases. However, all alcohol-induced deficits appear to be related to alcohol consumption and to the amount of alcohol consumed, i.e., the more severe cases of brain damage are associated with more severe and long-term alcoholism (Butterworth,

The author thanks Jen Obernier for her editorial and research contributions to this chapter.

1995; Pfefferbaum et al., 1996). Thus, alcohol can be neurotoxic when abused. The acute and chronic effects as well as the neurotoxic actions of alcohol appear to be due to changes in neuronal signaling. Our understanding of the effects of ethanol on the brain has increased tremendously in the past decade and will likely continue to increase as researchers investigate the specific sites of action of ethanol on the brain.

Ethanol Effects on Neuronal Signaling

A review of all of the actions of ethanol on neuronal signaling is not addressed in this chapter due to the extensive number of studies and a poor understanding of how changes in neuronal signaling relate to the effects of ethanol. This chapter will focus on the glutamate and GABA (γ-aminobutyric acid) neurotransmitter systems because they are the major excitatory and inhibitory neurotransmitters in the brain, respectively, and appear to be the predominant neurotransmitters involved in the actions of ethanol on the brain.

ETHANOL EFFECTS ON GLUTAMATE RECEPTOR ION CHANNELS

Glutamate receptors are altered by ethanol and represent major excitatory receptors in the brain. The three classes of ionotropic glutamate receptors include the NMDA (*N*-methyl-D-aspartic acid), kainate, and AMPA (L-α-amino-3-hydroxy-5-methyl-4-isoxazole proportionate) receptor subtypes (Bettler and Mulle, 1995; Hollmann and Heineman, 1994; Sommer and Seeburg, 1992; Sprengel and Seeburg, 1993). There is also a group of metabotropic receptors that couple to secondary messengers, e.g., G-protein-coupled receptors. While there is some evidence that ethanol directly or indirectly affects all types of glutamate receptors, overwhelming evidence and a vast literature document ethanol's direct effects on NMDA receptors and the radical changes in neuronal signaling and cognitive function that result. As such, the focus of this section will be on NMDA receptors with a brief discussion of other glutamate receptors.

NMDA Receptors

Late in 1991, a report appeared in *Nature* that an NMDA-receptor complementary DNA (cDNA) had been cloned from a rat brain (Moriyoshi et al., 1991). The protein described by Moriyoshi and colleagues was designated as NMDAR-1 and had significant sequence homology with previously identified AMPA/kainate receptors (Hollmann et al., 1989). It is now clear that this cDNA was associated with the classic NMDA receptor previously identified pharmacologically (Davies et al., 1981; Watkins, 1962). NMDAR-1 was immediately recognized to have a ubiquitous distribution in the brain (Monyer et al., 1994; Moriyoshi et al., 1991) and later to have eight splice variants generated from the presence of three cassettes—two on the C terminal and one on the N terminal (Durand et al., 1992; Nakanishi et al., 1992; Sugihara et al., 1992). The discovery of the splice variants for the NMDAR-1 subunit provided the potential for heterogeneity among NMDA receptors. Partial probes of these NMDAR-1 variants showed by in situ hybridization that these variants were differentially distributed in the brain (Laurie and Seeburg, 1994; Monyer et al., 1994; Standaert et al., 1993). Pharmacologically, the type "A" splice variants (lacking the N-terminal cassette) possess greater agonist potencies, lower antagonist associations and are potentiated by Zn^{2+} (Hollmann et al., 1993). The converse is true for type "B" variants (with the N-terminal insert).

Other NMDA subunits homologous to the NMDAR-1 subunit were subsequently cloned and are referred to as NMDAR-2A, -2B, -2C, and -2D (Meguro et al., 1992; Monyer et al., 1992; Nakanishi et al., 1992; Yamazaki et al., 1992), although another classification system based upon cloning from mouse brains refers to these same subunits as ξ1-4 (Kutsuwada et al., 1992; Meguro et al., 1992; Yamazaki et al., 1992). All NMDAR-2 subunits must be expressed with an NMDAR-1 subunit for maximal sensitivity to NMDA (Monyer et al., 1992; Nakanishi et al., 1992). As was found for the variants of the NMDAR-1 subunit, the NMDAR-2 subunits have a discrete neuroanatomical localization in the brain (Ishii et al., 1993; Monyer et al., 1992). Comparisons with other ion channel receptors and a variety of other direct NMDA receptor studies have led to the conclusion that endogenous NMDA receptors are heteromeric multisubunit complexes of NMDAR-1 and NMDAR-2 subunits with a wide variety of combinations in different brain regions.

NMDA receptor heterogeneity has also been demonstrated with Mg^{2+} (Mayer et al., 1984; Nowak et al., 1984), redox manipulations (Sullivan et al., 1994), polyamines (Bowe and Nadler, 1995; Ransom and Stec, 1988; Reynolds, 1990; Reynolds and Miller, 1989; Rock and Macdonald, 1995), glycine (Igarashi and Williams, 1995; Johnson and Ascher, 1987; Kleckner and Dingledine, 1988; Reynolds et al., 1987), Zn^{2+} (Peters et al., 1987; Westbrook and Mayer, 1987), and noncompetitive NMDA antagonists (Reynolds and Miller, 1989; Williams et al., 1993; Williams et al., 1994). The variants of the NMDAR-1 subunit and the four NMDAR-2 subunits provide the potential for considerable heterogeneity among NMDA receptor isoforms (Buller et al., 1994; Durand et al., 1992; Ishii et al., 1993;

Kumar et al., 1991; Meguro et al., 1992; Monaghan, 1991; Monyer et al., 1994; Monyer et al., 1992; Moriyoshi et al., 1991; Nakanishi et al., 1992; Sugihara et al., 1992). Pharmacological studies of the noncompetitive NMDA antagonist, ifenprodil, provide evidence that multiple NMDA receptor isoforms exist in the brain (Williams et al., 1993). The action and binding of ifenprodil appear to be selective for the NMDAR-2B subunit (Lovinger, 1995; Nicolas and Carter, 1994; Williams et al., 1993; Williams et al., 1994). Ifenprodil inhibition of NMDA receptors through the NMDAR-2B subunit was hypothesized from research that ifenprodil inhibited NMDA responses from a recombinant receptor formed by the NMDAR-1A and NMDAR-2B subunits, but was found to be relatively inactive against the combination of NMDAR-1A and NMDAR-2A subunits (Lynch et al., 1995; Williams et al., 1993; Williams et al., 1994). When developmental expression of NMDA subunits was evaluated, an association was also found between ifenprodil binding and the presence of the NMDAR-1A and NMDAR-2B subunits, but not the NMDAR-2A subunits (Molinoff et al., 1994; Zhong et al., 1994). Since the NMDAR-2B subunit has a variable distribution in the brain (Monyer et al., 1994; Monyer et al., 1992), it was presumed that ifenprodil would affect responses to NMDA in vivo in a subset of neurons which expressed the NMDAR-2B subunit, and this was indeed found to be the case (Yang et al., 1996). Although the basic molecular mechanism of ifenprodil antagonism has yet to be determined, evidence is convincing that the NMDAR-2B receptor subunit is important to the action of this drug. The particular importance of ifenprodil to the pharmacological action of ethanol on NMDA responses will become clear later in this discussion.

Ethanol's Physiological Actions Mediated Through Changes in NMDA Receptor Function

Initial evidence that ethanol antagonizes NMDA-induced responses came from electrophysiological studies (Lima-Landman and Albuquerque, 1989; Lovinger et al., 1989, 1990; Weight, 1992), as well as in vitro experiments which show that ethanol inhibits NMDA activation of calcium flux and cGMP formation (Dildy and Leslie, 1989; Hoffman, Moses, et al., 1989; Hoffman, Rabe, et al., 1989). Electrophysiological studies performed in vivo (Frohlich et al., 1994) have provided additional evidence that low-to-moderate concentrations of ethanol antagonize NMDA-induced increases in firing rate. Rats trained to discriminate doses of ethanol (1.0, 1.5, and 2.0 g/kg) from water substituted the noncompetitive NMDA antagonists, phencyclidine (PCP) and MK-801 (dizocipline) for higher doses of ethanol (Grant and Colombo, 1993). In contrast, the competitive NMDA receptor antagonist, CPPene, did not substitute for ethanol in this paradigm (Grant et al., 1991). It was concluded that antagonism of NMDA receptor function by a channel-blocking NMDA antagonist is perceived by the animal as equivalent to the administration of ethanol (Grant and Colombo, 1993). This latter finding indicates that inhibition of NMDA receptors is an important mechanism by which ethanol affects brain function. Thus, strong evidence supports that moderate concentrations of ethanol antagonize NMDA responses and that this action of ethanol has functional consequences.

Differential Action of Ethanol on NMDA-Stimulated Responses

Following the seminal findings concerning ethanol antagonism of NMDA (Simson et al., 1993; Simson et al., 1991), using in vivo recording techniques in anesthetized rats, it was found that systemically administered ethanol antagonized the effect of NMDA on some, but not all, cells in the medial septum. Local application of ethanol onto neurons was later found to reduce NMDA stimulated responses, eliminating the possibility that systemic administration of ethanol was acting at distant brain sites to inhibit NMDA at the recording site (Criswell et al., 1993; Simson et al., 1993). Initial extracellular recordings that found sensitive and insensitive NMDA-stimulated responses in the medial septum and substantia nigra reticulata (SNR) (Breese et al., 1993; Criswell et al., 1993; Simson et al., 1993), have been extended to additional sites in the brain including the ventral tegmental area, the deep mesencephalic nucleus, and the red nucleus (Yang et al., 1996). In the hippocampus, ethanol inhibited NMDA responses from all neurons, but did not antagonize NMDA-stimulated responses in the lateral septum, suggesting a degree of brain regional specificity for ethanol's inhibition. Using calcium flux, Wilson et al. (1990) also found regional differences in ethanol inhibition of NMDA-stimulated responses that were consistent with earlier findings (Criswell et al., 1993; Simson et al., 1993; Simson et al., 1991). Regional differences in NMDA antagonism by ethanol support the hypothesis that these differences were due to regional differences in NMDA receptor isoform expression.

NMDA Receptor Isoforms and Differential Ethanol Sensitivity

The existence of a relationship between the ability of ifenprodil and ethanol to inhibit NMDA-stimulated responses is supported by recent studies. During a four-week period, neocortical neurons in culture showed a decreased sensitivity to both ethanol and ifenprodil inhibition of NMDA-stimulated responses as the neurons matured (Lovinger, 1995). Both ifenprodil and ethanol were found to inhibit recombinant NMDA receptors containing the NMDAR-2B subunit. The ability of ethanol to inhibit NMDA responses was recently compared to ifenprodil (Yang et al., 1996). Whenever ethanol antagonized an NMDA-stimulated response, ifenprodil also inhibited this response. However, neurons were identified to which ifenprodil antagonized NMDA-stimulated responses, but ethanol did not (Yang et al., 1996). Thus, the most likely mechanism of differential ethanol inhibition of NMDA-stimulated responses appears to be related to the expression of different NMDA receptor isoforms, i.e., different receptor isoforms are more or less sensitive to ethanol inhibition (Breese et al., 1993; Criswell et al., 1993; Simson et al., 1993; Yang et al., 1996).

Several studies support the hypothesis that ethanol has a differential action on NMDA receptor isoforms. As mentioned earlier, ifenprodil most potently inhibits a subset of NMDA receptors that contain the NMDAR-2B subunit (Williams et al., 1993) and inhibits NMDA receptors that are sensitive to ethanol inhibition in cultured neurons (Lovinger, 1995) and in vivo (Yang et al., 1996). Reconstitution studies also suggest that ethanol has selective actions on particular subtypes of NMDA receptors. Several investigators have combined the NMDAR-1A variant with the four NMDAR-2 subunits in *Xenopus* oocytes or HEK-293 cells and examined the action of ethanol on responses to NMDA (Buller et al., 1995; Chu et al., 1995; Lovinger, 1995; Masood et al., 1994; Mirshahi and Woodward, 1995). Consistent with neuronal studies that suggest NMDAR-2B and ifenprodil predict potent inhibitory actions of ethanol, the ε2 subunit (mouse NMDAR-2B subunit) when expressed with the ζ1 (mouse NMDAR-1A variant) in *Xenopus* oocytes is significantly inhibited by concentrations of ethanol less than 25 mM (Masood et al., 1994). Higher concentrations of ethanol also inhibited ε1 (mouse NMDAR-2A subunit) combined with the ζ1, but concentrations as high as 100 mM had little or no effect on ε3 (mouse NMDAR-2C subunit) and ε4 (mouse NMDAR-2D subunit) combined with ζ1 (mouse NMDAR-1A subunit). Similar studies done by Buller et al. (1995) found both NMDAR-2A and NMDAR-2B in combination with NMDAR-1A to be the NMDA receptor isoforms most sensitive to inhibition by ethanol. All studies agree that the recombinant NMDA receptors containing either the NMDAR-2C or the NMDAR-2D subunits with the NMDAR-1A subunit are not sensitive to ethanol inhibition (Buller et al., 1995; Lovinger, 1995; Masood et al., 1994). Lovinger (1995) found that the NMDA receptor formed from NMDAR-1A and NMDAR-2A was inhibited by ethanol, however, when NMDAR-2B was added, the recombinant NMDA receptor was considerably more sensitive to ethanol inhibition of NMDA than the recombinant receptor containing only the NMDAR-2A subunit. In vivo, NMDA receptors in the cerebral cortex likely contain combinations of NMDAR-1,

NMDAR-2A, and NMDAR-2B subunits (Sheng et al., 1994). Taken together, the findings suggest that NMDA receptors containing NMDAR-2B subunits, alone or in combination with NMDAR-2A subunits, are likely to make up the NMDA receptor isoforms most sensitive to ethanol inhibition whereas those containing NMDAR-2C or NMDAR-2D subunits are likely to be relatively insensitive to inhibition by ethanol.

The presence of specific NMDAR-1 subunit variants (Monyer et al., 1992) may also contribute to differential sensitivity of NMDA isoforms to inhibition by ethanol. Koltchine and colleagues (1993) provided evidence that four of the NMDAR-1 variants had differential sensitivity to ethanol, with the variant containing both the N terminal and another cassette being the most sensitive to inhibition by ethanol when expressed in oocytes as homomeric assemblies. When the NMDAR-1B subunit, which contains the N-terminal cassette, was combined with the NMDAR-2B or NMDAR-2A subunit, the resulting isoforms were more sensitive to ethanol inhibition of NMDA than isoforms with NMDAR-2C or -2D subunits (Chu et al., 1995). Since NMDAR-1A variants, which lack an N-terminal insert (Durand et al., 1993; Durand et al., 1992), are also sensitive to ethanol when combined with the NMDAR-2B subunit, it is possible that the NMDAR-1 variants in combination with the NMDAR-2 variants indicate that there is a wide spectrum of NMDA receptor isoforms with differential sensitivity to inhibition by ethanol. Thus, for the NMDAR-1 variants investigated, an interaction of both the R1 splice variant properties combined with the various NMDAR-2 subunits appears to modulate the sensitivity to ethanol, with NMDAR-1 variants containing inserts and NMDAR-2B subunits apparently being the most sensitive to inhibition by ethanol.

NMDA Receptor Modulatory Sites and Differential Sensitivity to Ethanol

Another aspect regarding differential inhibition of NMDA receptors by ethanol could involve an interaction with specific modulatory sites on the NMDA receptor (Johnson and Ascher, 1987; Peters et al., 1987; Reynolds and Miller, 1989). Glycine was reported to reverse ethanol inhibition of NMDA-induced calcium flux and cyclic guanosine monophosphate (cGMP) in cerebellar granule cells (Dildy and Leslie, 1989; Hoffman, Rabe, et al., 1989; Rabe and Tabakoff, 1990). However, glycine did not reverse ethanol inhibition of NMDA-stimulated excitotoxicity in cerebral cortical neurons (Chandler et al., 1993) or patch clamp responses in cultured hippocampal neurons (Peoples and Weight, 1992). Studies by Buller and colleagues (1995) may explain these contradictory results. Buller and colleagues demonstrated that NMDA-stimulated responses in *Xenopus* oocytes containing the recombinant NMDAR-1A/NMDAR-2B subunits were desensitized by the addition of ethanol when subsaturating concentrations of glycine were present (Buller et al., 1995). Increasing the concentration of glycine reversed this desensitization. However, other aspects of this study clearly demonstrate glycine-independent components. This work suggests that ethanol can have two distinct effects on NMDA-stimulated responses depending on the glycine concentration. Manipulations of various other modulatory sites (e.g., polyamines, Mg^{2+}, Zn^{2+}) or the presence of the drug dithiothreitol (i.e., oxidation and reduction) did not affect ethanol inhibition of NMDA in recombinant systems (Chu et al., 1995; Matsumoto et al., 1993).

NMDA Receptor Phosphorylation and Differential Sensitivity to Ethanol

Phosphorylation is important in direct and indirect modulation of NMDA receptors and several studies have demonstrated that phosphorylation may contribute to NMDA receptors' differential sensitivity to ethanol (Huganir and Greengard, 1990; Wright et al., 1993). The NMDA receptor subunits contain a site that allows for phosphorylation by protein kinase C (PKC) and other kinases (Lieberman and Mody, 1994; Monyer et al., 1992; Nakanishi et al., 1992). Snell and colleagues (1994) found that staurosporine or calphostin, PKC inhibitors, reversed the inhibitory effect of ethanol on NMDA-stimulated responses, suggesting that ethanol may facilitate phosphorylation of the NMDA receptor and thereby inhibit NMDA-stimulated responses. Consequently, the proper phosphorylation state of the NMDA receptor may be required for ethanol and ifenprodil inhibition of NMDA. However, Tabakoff (1995) noted that PKC does not appear to have the same role in all cell populations in determining the effect of ethanol on NMDA-stimulated responses, and stated that more investigation is needed to clearly define the role of NMDA receptor phosphorylation in differential sensitivity to ethanol.

Differential Action of Ethanol on AMPA/ Kainate-Stimulated Responses

Initial investigations with low-to-moderate concentrations of ethanol suggested that ethanol did not affect the function of non-NMDA glutamate receptors (Hoffman, Rabe, et al., 1989; Lovinger et al., 1989; Simson et al., 1993). These reports have given way to data indicating that ethanol can inhibit agonist-stimulated responses, but some controversy and uncertainty still exists about the concentration of ethanol required for this action to occur.

Lovinger et al. (1989) reported that only high concentrations of ethanol (~100 mM) can antagonize kainate-stimulated responses in cultured neurons from fetal rodent brains. Likewise, ethanol (>100 mM) was shown to inhibit responses from recombinant AMPA-type glutamate receptor subunits expressed in kidney 243 cells (Lovinger, 1993). Based on work with cultured neurons Weight and colleagues (1993) reported that only ethanol concentrations above 50 mM affected the non-NMDA receptors, suggesting that ethanol's ability to produce general anesthesia could be attributed to inhibition of kainate and AMPA receptor function. High concentrations of ethanol (100 mM) have also been found to inhibit kainate and AMPA responses in vivo in the rat locus coeruleus (Frohlich et al., 1994). Collectively, these data suggested that non-NMDA receptors are considerably less sensitive to ethanol than NMDA receptors, although some regional differences may exist in brain (Gonzales, 1990).

A particularly important observation made by Dildy-Mayfield and Harris (1992a,b) was that ethanol inhibition was potentiated at lower, rather than higher, concentrations of kainate. In fact, the inhibition of a low concentration of AMPA by ethanol was similar to that seen for NMDA. The region of the brain may also be a contributing factor as to whether ethanol affects non-NMDA receptors (Dildy-Mayfield and Harris, 1992a,b). Martin and colleagues (1995) found that ethanol inhibited agonist responses to the non-NMDA receptors in hippocampal slices, but as noted in earlier studies, this action depended greatly on the concentration of the agonist used. Similarly, Chandler and colleagues (1994) found that AMPA-stimulated nitrous oxide formation in cerebral cortical cultures was inhibited by ethanol. Thus, there is no question that ethanol can inhibit non-NMDA receptor stimulated responses. However, a complete understanding of the differences observed between the various studies as to the concentration of ethanol required to inhibit kainate- or AMPA-stimulated responses has yet to be resolved. It is possible that the variable effects of ethanol relate to the differing subunit composition of various non-NMDA receptor subtypes. Additionally, consensus sites are found on some subunits for protein kinase II and protein kinase C (Keinanen et al., 1990; Wright et al., 1993). Thus, phosphorylation could account for some of the differences observed. These potential reasons for the varying observations need to be critically tested.

Until recently there has been much controversy regarding the effect of ethanol on kainate receptors. This was mainly due to the inability of researchers to pharmacologically isolate kainate receptors from other glutamate receptors. The few studies mentioned previously found that ethanol inhibited kainate receptor function in recombinant receptor systems. But these findings only suggested such an effect was possible, as the characteristics of recombinant kainate receptors differ from endogenous receptors.

AMPA receptor antagonists recently became available allowing researchers to characterize endogenous kainate receptors and ethanol's effect upon them. Two groups have since investigated kainate receptors and their sensitivity to ethanol, one in cerebellar granule cells (Valenzuela, Cardoso, et al., 1998) and one in CA3 pyramidal neurons (Weiner et al., 1999). Both groups found that intoxicating concentrations of ethanol inhibited kainate currents and Weiner's group also found that ethanol in concentrations as low as 20 mM depressed kainate excitatory postsynaptic currents. Further studies are necessary to more fully characterize ethanol's inhibition of kainate receptors and any behavioral or cognitive consequences that may occur.

ETHANOL EFFECTS ON GABA$_A$/BENZODIAZEPINE RECEPTORS

γ-aminobutyric acid (GABA) is the most ubiquitous inhibitory neurotransmitter in the brain. GABA interacts with a family of receptors containing recognition sites for the anxiolytic and sedative benzodiazepines, barbiturates, and endogenous neurosteroids. These binding sites are linked allosterically to a GABA recognition site, and each site is involved directly or indirectly in the gating properties of integral chloride channels. GABA receptor-mediated activation of Cl^- conductance results in membrane hyperpolarization and decreased neuronal excitability (Skolnick and Paul, 1982). Ethanol alters the gating properties of this receptor complex; however, ethanol binds with little or no affinity to recognition sites for GABA, benzodiazepines, barbiturates, or cage convulsants (Davis and Ticku, 1981; Greenberg et al., 1984). GABA$_A$ receptor isoforms are heteromeric protein complexes consisting of five distinct, yet homologous, membrane-spanning glycoprotein subunits. These subunits exist in six major classes: α, β, γ, δ, and ρ (Levitan et al., 1988; Schofield, 1989; Schofield et al., 1987). Within each class of subunits, there are various isoforms that include α1-6, ß1-4, γ1-4, δ, and ρ1-2 (Cutting et al., 1992; Cutting et al., 1991). Additional variants are possible due to post-translational processing (see Macdonald and Olsen, 1994, for review; Seeburg et al., 1990). The structural features of GABA$_A$ receptor channels have been inferred to a large extent by analogy to nicotinic, cholinergic, and glycine receptors which are members of the superfamily of ligand-gated ion channels (Unwin, 1989). However, the pentameric structure of native GABA$_A$ receptors has been confirmed by electron microscopy and rotational spin analysis of isolated receptors (Nayeem et al., 1994).

The actual subunit composition of GABA$_A$ receptor isoforms in vivo is not yet known. However, it is clear that subunit composition determines the pharmacological and functional properties of GABA$_A$ receptor isoforms.

For example, the coexpression of different ß and γ subunits in recombinant expression systems results in $GABA_A$ receptors with different pharmacological properties, and may account for the functional heterogeneity of $GABA_A$ receptors (Levitan et al., 1988; Pritchett, Lüddens, et al., 1989; Pritchett, Sontheimer, et al., 1989; Puia et al., 1991; Wafford et al., 1990). In transient expression systems, benzodiazepine type I binding characteristics are observed with the expression of $\alpha2\beta x\gamma2$ subunits (where x indicates any ß subunit). In contrast, the expression of $\alpha2\beta x\gamma2$, $\alpha3\beta x\gamma2$, or $\alpha5\beta x\gamma2$ subunits results in benzodiazepine type II pharmacology (Pritchett, Lüddens, et al., 1989). Further diversity of γ2 subunits are created by an eight-amino-acid insertion site of the $GABA_A$ receptor γ2L subunit, which encodes a sequence that can be phosphorylated by protein kinase C (Whiting et al., 1990) and appears to confer ethanol sensitivity to recombinant $GABA_A$ receptors expressed in some circumstances (Wafford et al., 1991; Wafford and Whiting, 1992). There is increasing evidence that all $GABA_A$ receptor subunit combinations contribute to specific functional properties in assembled receptors. The expression of $\alpha1$, $\alpha2$, $\alpha3$, or $\alpha5$ subunits with $\beta1$, $\beta2$, or $\beta3$ subunits in conjunction with γ2L subunits in frog oocytes results in twelve receptors that exhibit unique pharmacological properties (White and Gurley, 1995). Understanding the heterogeneity of native $GABA_A$ receptors will provide additional insight into heterogeneous signaling in the brain.

The functional properties of $GABA_A$ receptors may also be influenced by posttranslational mechanisms that are presumed to alter receptor conformation. The potential role of phosphorylation in the regulation of GABA responses is controversial. Evidence suggests that GABA receptor phosphorylation is both associated with (Heuschneider and Schwartz, 1989; Leidenheimer et al., 1990; Porter et al., 1990) or prevents (Gyenes et al., 1988; Stelzer et al., 1988) $GABA_A$ receptor desensitization. Artifacts related to the actions of cAMP, which are independent of protein phosphorylation, have been described (Heuschneider and Schwartz, 1989; Leidenheimer et al., 1990) and complicate the interpretation of the results of these studies. In addition, the heterogeneity of $GABA_A$ receptors may explain some of the conflicting results. Another mechanism may involve $GABA_A$ receptor isoforms that are phosphorylated by maximal GABA stimulation, whereas other isoforms are not. $GABA_A$ receptors contain putative phosphorylation sites on ß1-3 and γ2L subunits (Wang and Burt, 1991; Ymer et al., 1989), but the expression of these subunits varies in different brain regions (Wang and Burt, 1991; Zhang et al., 1995). Thus, the potential role of phosphorylation and other posttranslational processes remains obscure.

Ethanol Interactions with GABA_A Receptors

Ethanol is believed to act at many sites in the brain, but $GABA_A$/benzodiazepine receptors may be the major targets responsible for many of its behavioral effects. GABA-mimetic drugs enhance and prolong the behavioral effects of ethanol, while antagonists shorten ethanol narcosis (Frye and Breese, 1982; Martz et al., 1983). Likewise, benzodiazepines and GABA-mimetics ameliorate the symptoms of ethanol withdrawal (Frye et al., 1983a; Sellers and Kalant, 1976), while GABA antagonists potentiate these symptoms (Goldstein, 1973). Furthermore, benzodiazepine receptor inverse agonists, such as Ro15-4513 and FG-7142, antagonize many ethanol-induced behaviors in the rat, including intoxication (Koob et al., 1989; Lister, 1988; Suzdak, Glowa, et al., 1986; Suzdak et al., 1988). The behavioral effects of various chain-length alcohols have also been used to establish a link between alcohol interactions with GABA receptors and the production of their behavioral effects. Recent studies have shown that while short-chain alcohols activate $GABA_A$ receptors (Suzdak et al., 1987), long-chain alcohols (greater than ten carbons) no longer activate $GABA_A$ receptors (Dildy-Mayfield et al., 1996). This loss of GABA activation correlates with the effects of various length alcohols on the loss of righting reflex in tadpoles (Dildy-Mayfield et al., 1996). Site-specific effects of ethanol on $GABA_A$ receptors that result in sedation have been demonstrated in the medial septum (Givens and Breese, 1990b).

Direct evidence that ethanol interacts with $GABA_A$ receptors at pharmacologically relevant concentrations has been demonstrated in studies using subcellular brain preparations and cultured embryonic neurons, wherein ethanol and other short-chain alcohols have been shown to stimulate (Suzdak et al., 1987; Suzdak, Schwartz, et al., 1986) or potentiate $GABA_A$ receptor-mediated $^{36}Cl^-$ uptake (Allan and Harris, 1986; Mehta and Ticku, 1988; Suzdak et al., 1987; Suzdak, Schwartz, et al., 1986; Ticku et al., 1986). Electrophysiological studies have confirmed that ethanol enhances $GABA_A$ receptor-mediated Cl^- conductance, but only in specific brain regions (Celentano et al., 1988; Givens and Breese, 1990a,b; Mereu and Gessa, 1985; Nestores, 1980) or cell populations (Aguayo, 1990; Reynolds and Prasad, 1991). The regional specificity of ethanol interactions with GABA was first observed by Givens and Breese (1990a,b), who demonstrated that ethanol enhances GABA responses in the medial septal nucleus, but not the lateral septal nucleus. Subsequent studies have defined several brain regions where electrophysiological responses to GABA are both sensitive and insensitive to ethanol (Criswell et al., 1993, 1995). Several researchers have suggested that the subunit composition of $GABA_A$ receptors determines the presence or absence of ethanol sensitivity (Breese et al., 1993; Criswell et al., 1993;

Givens and Breese, 1990a; Morrow et al., 1992; Wafford et al., 1990). This hypothesis has been supported by studies of mammalian brain regions in which ethanol sensitivity is highly correlated with the simultaneous presence of benzodiazepine type I ([^{3}H]zolpidem) binding sites (Breese et al., 1993; Criswell et al., 1993, 1995) and GABA$_A$ receptor α1, β2, and γ2 subunits (Criswell et al., 1993; Duncan et al., 1995). It is not clear from these studies whether the γ2 subunit splice variants influence ethanol sensitivity in the rat brain, since γ2L subunits were abundant in both ethanol-sensitive and ethanol-insensitive sites (Criswell et al., 1993; Duncan et al., 1995). However, it is clear that ethanol potentiation of GABA$_A$ receptors may be limited to very specific subtypes of GABA$_A$ receptors that have a unique regional distribution in the brain.

Additional evidence suggests that other GABA$_A$ receptor isoforms may exhibit ethanol sensitivity under certain circumstances. Several investigators have found that ethanol modulates GABA responses in cerebellar Purkinje cells if α-adrenergic receptors are coactivated (Knapp et al., 1995; Lin et al., 1991; Palmer et al., 1988). Cerebellar granule cells contain recognition sites for the benzodiazepine inverse agonist, Ro15-4513, which antagonizes the effects of ethanol on GABA-mediated responses such as the righting reflex. Since this site is not sensitive to zolpidem, it is assumed that it identifies a distinct GABA$_A$ receptor isoform that responds to ethanol. The subunit composition of this receptor is likely to include α6 subunits since this subunit appears to contain the Ro15-4513 recognition site (Lüddens et al., 1990). In the cerebral cortex, Ro15-4513 appears to label a GABA$_A$ receptor comprised of α4 subunits (Wisden et al., 1991). Chronic ethanol administration increases [$_3$H]Ro15-4513 binding in the cortex and cerebellum (Mhatre et al., 1988), as well as α4 (Devaud, Morrow, et al., 1995) and α6 subunits (Mhatre and Ticku, 1993; Morrow et al., 1992), respectively. Therefore, these GABA$_A$ receptor isoforms probably exhibit ethanol sensitivity in vivo.

The question of whether ethanol enhancement of GABA responses is dependent on receptor subunit composition has been directly addressed in various recombinant expression systems. In frog oocytes, the expression of the human γ2L subunit has been reported to be required for ethanol potentiation of GABA responses (Wafford et al., 1991; Wafford and Whiting, 1992), but other studies have not confirmed this effect (Mihic et al., 1994; Sigel et al., 1993). In mouse LTK cells, α1β1 γ2L and α1β1 γ2S recombinant receptors are sensitive to ethanol, though greater sensitivity was observed when the γ2L subunit was expressed (Ryan-Jastrow and Macdonald, 1993). Using the HEK293 expression system, the γ2 splice variant does not influence ethanol enhancement of GABA responses (Ryan-Jastrow and Macdonald, 1993). Conversely, stably transfected PA3 cells are only sensitive to ethanol when the γ2L variant is expressed with α1 and β1 subunits (Harris, Proctor, et al., 1995). The lack of consistent results in recombinant expression systems suggests that factors other than subunit composition can influence ethanol interactions with $GABA_A$ receptors. These factors could include differences in membrane properties, intracellular messengers, and/or receptor assembly that may exist among recombinant expression systems and mammalian brains. The extent to which these factors modulate the functional properties of $GABA_A$ receptors is a question of considerable importance in the interpretation of structure-function studies in recombinant expression systems.

Ethanol's Effects on $GABA_A$ Receptors Mediated by Posttranslational Modifications

Recent studies in recombinant receptor systems, where subunit expression is controlled by a dexamethasone-sensitive promoter, exhibit changes in receptor function that cannot be attributed to alterations in subunit expression (Klein et al., 1995). A possible explanation for these changes in receptor function may involve posttranslational modification of $GABA_A$ receptors and second messenger systems. Tyrosine phosphorylation of $GABA_A$ receptors has been shown to enhance $GABA_A$ receptor-gated currents (Valenzuela et al., 1995) and, as noted previously, tyrosine phosphorylation of NMDA receptors has been linked to the development of acute tolerance of NMDA receptors. PKC, PKA, and calmodulin kinase II have been reported to phosphorylate and/or alter the function of NMDA or $GABA_A$ receptors. Additionally, mouse mutants that lack a PKC isoform exhibit a loss of ethanol sensitivity both in vivo and at the cellular level (Harris, McQuilkin, et al., 1995). Thus, ethanol tolerance and dependence may also involve second messengers associated with $GABA_A$ receptors.

CHANGES IN NMDA AND $GABA_A$ RECEPTORS DURING CHRONIC ALCOHOL ABUSE AND WITHDRAWAL

Chronic Ethanol Alters NMDA Receptor Function and Expression

Hyperexcitability of the central nervous system (CNS) is a key component of ethanol withdrawal and a sign of alcohol dependence (Frye et al., 1983a,b; Grant et al., 1990). Both a reduction in GABA-mediated inhibition (Frye et al., 1983a,b) and a supersensitive NMDA response appear to be involved. One of the earliest findings suggesting glutamate involvement was the finding that [³H]glutamate binding is increased in the hippocampus of alcoholics (Michaelis et al., 1990). Although the isoform of glutamate receptor involved is not known, this is consistent with increased glutamate receptor density. Several studies of neuronal cells in culture have indicated that a few days of chronic ethanol treatment leads to supersensitive NMDA-stimulated calcium flux (Ahern et al., 1994; Iorio et al., 1992), as well as NMDA-stimulated excitotoxicity (Ahern et al., 1994; Chandler et al., 1993; Crews and Chandler, 1993; Crews et al., 1993; Iorio et al., 1993) and NMDA-stimulated nitric oxide formation (Chandler et al., 1995). Although the mechanisms are not totally resolved, it is clear that chronic ethanol can induce NMDA supersensitivity and likely contributes to the hyperexcitability and seizures associated with ethanol withdrawal. It may also cause neurotoxicity. Supersensitivity could occur through a number of mechanisms including increased density of the NMDA receptors, changes in subunit composition, and increased release of glutamate.

Nitric oxide has been implicated in toxicity due to the formation of highly oxidative metabolites (Crews and Chandler, 1993). Although both nitric oxide and excitotoxicity show supersensitivity as indicated by left shifts in the dose response curves, the finding that nitric oxide production is maximal at the minimum threshold concentration for NMDA-stimulated excitotoxicity suggests that nitric oxide may contribute to excitotoxicity, but is likely not the only factor involved. Although supersensitivity was found in both nitric oxide and excitotoxicity, changes in the amount of NMDAR1 immunoreactivity were not found, suggesting that changes in the NMDA receptor subunit composition, phosphorylation, or other posttranslational factors are most likely responsible for the super-sensitive NMDA response.

Ligand-binding studies support the hypothesis that changes in subunit composition are involved. Grant et al. (1990) reported that seven days of 7 percent ethanol diet increased [3H]MK-801 binding in hippocampal membranes by approximately 16 percent. Another autoradiographic study also reported increased [3H]MK-801 binding in the cortex, hippocampus, and striatum (Gulya et al., 1991). Well-controlled extensions of these experiments found changes in the hippocampus but not the cerebral cortex (Snell et al., 1993). These studies found that [3H]MK-801 and NMDA-specific [3H]glutamate binding slightly increased in the hippocampus during chronic ethanol treatment, but there were no changes in [3H] glycine or [3H] CGS19755, a competitive NMDA antagonist, in the hippocampus. No changes in any ligand binding were found in the cerebral cortex (Snell et al., 1993). Reconstitution studies using NMDAR-1A and NMDAR-2A subunits found receptors containing both glutamate antagonist and channel-blocking antagonist binding sites (Lynch et al., 1994). Further studies combining NMDAR-1A and NMDAR-2B subunits resulted in different receptor properties, particularly in the modulation of the channel by polyamines and high-affinity ifenprodil binding. Thus, subunit composition changes and not an increased density of channels may cause the changes in NMDA ligand-binding sites seen in these experiments.

Further supporting this theory, Trevisan and colleagues (1994) found that 12 weeks of ethanol liquid diet in rats increased the levels of NMDAR-1 immunoreactivity in the hippocampus, but not the cortex, striatum, or nucleus accumbens. Of interest, studies of levels of NMDAR-1 mRNA have indicated that chronic ethanol does not change NMDAR-1 mRNA but increases NMDAR-2A and NMDAR-2B mRNA levels in the hippocampus and cortex (Follesa and Ticku, 1995). Since Merck compound 801 (MK801) requires both an NMDAR-1 and NMDAR-2 subunit for binding, an increase in binding could be due to changes in receptor subunits without a concomitant increase in the density of channels. Other studies have not found increases in MK801 binding following chronic ethanol treatment of mice (Carter et al., 1995) or rats (Rudolph et al., 1997). These differences could be due to different ethanol treatment protocols or the responses of different animals. Long-term treatment of rats with ethanol (12 weeks) increased NMDAR-1 immunoreactivity in the ventral tegmental area, whereas one or six weeks of chronic 5 percent ethanol liquid diet did not (Oritz et al., 1995). Another factor that may relate to differences in ethanol treatment is that stress and treatment with glucocorticoids have been shown to increase NMDA receptor binding in a manner similar to ethanol (Yoneda et al., 1994). Since ethanol increases glucocorticoids and is a stressor, it is possible that increased glucocorticoid levels play a role in ethanol-induced increases in NMDA receptor binding in the brain. However, the supersensitivity observed in vitro by several groups cannot be related to stress-induced changes in NMDA receptor binding. Although the exact molecular processes require additional experimentation, a number of studies support the hypothesis that chronic ethanol consumption results in supersensitive NMDA receptors.

Chronic ethanol consumption also affects the functioning of NMDA receptors by altering the levels of extracellular glutamate through changes in glutamate release. While an acute dose of ethanol lowers extracellular glutamate levels in the CNS (Carboni et al., 1993; Moghaddam and Bolinao, 1994), ethanol-dependent rats show tolerance as their levels of extracellular glutamate return to normal levels. During withdrawal, however, levels of extracellular glutamate increased threefold, paralleling the time course of the withdrawal syndrome (Fadda and Rossetti, 1998; Gonzales et al., 1996; Rossetti and Carboni, 1995). It is therefore likely that the hyperexcitable state seen during ethanol withdrawal is caused not only by supersensitive NMDA receptor response, but also due to an increase in glutamate release.

Chronic Ethanol Consumption Alters GABA$_A$ Receptor Function and Receptor Subunit Assembly

Ethanol shares several pharmacologic actions with barbiturates and benzodiazepines including anxiolytic and sedative activity (Liljequist and Engel, 1984), cross-tolerance, and dependence (Boisse and Okamoto, 1980; Le et al., 1986). The similarities between the actions of ethanol, benzodiazepines, and barbiturates suggest that all three drugs share some mechanism(s) of action. Tolerance to the sedative and intoxicating effects of ethanol has been postulated to result from a compensatory decrease in GABA-mediated inhibition in the brain (Hunt, 1983). Other studies suggest that alterations in the function of GABA$_A$ receptor chloride channels also contribute to the signs and symptoms of ethanol withdrawal syndrome. Chronic exposure of rats to ethanol produces physical dependence and tolerance (Frye et al., 1981; Goldstein and Pal, 1971; Karanian et al., 1986; Morrow et al., 1988, 1992), which are associated with a decreased sensitivity of the GABA$_A$ receptor in the cerebral cortex (Sanna et al., 1993), when blood ethanol levels were greater than 0.15 percent (Morrow et al., 1988). In vitro studies have also shown that chronic ethanol decreases the sensitivity of GABA$_A$ receptors. Muscimol-stimulated $^{36}C^-$ uptake was decreased by 26 percent and pentobarbital-stimulated $^{36}C^-$ uptake was decreased by 25 percent following chronic ethanol treatment. Following chronic ethanol administration, the ability of ethanol (20 mM) to potentiate muscimol-stimulated $36C^-$ uptake was completely lost in rat cerebral cortical synaptoneurosomes (Morrow et al., 1988) and in mouse cerebellar microsacs (Allan and Harris, 1987). Cross-tolerance was also demonstrated as benzodiazepine enhancement of muscimol-stimulated chloride flux was reduced in the cerebral cortex of mouse microsacs, while the functional efficacy of inverse agonists was enhanced (Buck and Harris, 1990). This cross-tolerance was also seen in behavioral responses to injections of muscimol into the substantia nigra (Gonzalez and Czachura, 1989) and to subcutaneous THIP (a GABA agonist) injections (Martz et al., 1983) that were reduced following chronic ethanol administration. Following the completion of ethanol withdrawal, the decrease in muscimol-stimulated $^{36}Cl^-$ uptake in rat cerebral cortical synaptoneurosomes (Morrow et al., 1988) and flunitrazepam potentiation in mouse cortical microsacs (Buck and Harris, 1990) was completely reversed, as would be predicted if these neurochemical changes were related to the behavioral states of alcohol withdrawal.

Alterations in the density or affinity of brain GABA$_A$ receptors following chronic ethanol administration have yielded conflicting results and cannot explain the development of tolerance or withdrawal. For example, Ticku and colleagues (1986), Ticku and Burch (1980), and Unwin and Taberner (1980) have reported a decrease in the density of low-affinity [^{3}H]agonist binding sites in the brain following chronic ethanol exposure to rats or mice. deVries and colleagues (1987) have reported a reduction in the ability of GABA to enhance [^{3}H]flunitrazepam binding in brain membranes prepared from ethanol-treated mice. However, others have failed to find alterations in the number or affinity of GABA$_A$ receptors (Volicer, 1980; Volicer and Biagioni, 1982b). Chronic ethanol administration does not alter the density of [^{3}H] flunitrazepam (Karobath et al., 1980; Rastogi et al., 1986; Volicer and Biagioni, 1982a) or [^{35}S]t-butylbicyclophosphorothionate binding sites (Rastogi et al., 1986; Thyagarajan and Ticku, 1985) in brain. Mhatre et al. (1988) reported an increase in the density of specific binding sites for [^{3}H]Ro15-4513 in the rat cortex and cerebellum following chronic ethanol administration, as well as increased sensitivity to its behavioral effects (Mehta and Ticku, 1989). It has been proposed that the alterations in GABA$_A$ receptor function observed following chronic ethanol administration are the result of a change in the synthesis and expression of GABA$_A$ receptor isoforms. Chronic ethanol administration may have differential effects on the expression of individual GABA$_A$ receptor subunits, accounting for the diverse effects of ethanol on different radioligand binding sites. If ethanol alters the expression of specific populations of GABA$_A$ receptor isoforms, radioligands, which measure all GABA receptors, may lack the selectivity to detect changes in one or more receptor subunits or populations of GABA$_A$ receptor isoforms.

Chronic ethanol administration differentially alters the expression of GABA$_A$ receptor subunit mRNAs in the cerebral cortex (Devaud, Smith, et al., 1995; Montpied et al., 1991; Morrow et al., 1990) and cerebellum (Morrow et al., 1992). The levels of GABA$_A$ receptor $\alpha 1$ subunit mRNAs are reduced while $\alpha 4$ subunit mRNAs are increased by approximately equal amounts in the cerebral cortex (Devaud, Smith, et al., 1995). Likewise in the cerebellum, decreases in GABA$_A$ receptor $\alpha 1$ subunit mRNAs and increases in $\alpha 6$ subunit mRNA levels are found (Mhatre and Ticku, 1992; Morrow et al., 1992). These changes in mRNA levels suggest alterations in the expression of the corresponding proteins that could account for the alterations in receptor function and binding that have been observed. For example, the increases in $\alpha 4$ and $\alpha 6$ subunit expression probably explain the increases in [^{3}H]Ro-15-4513 (Mhatre et al., 1988) and sensitivity (Buck and Harris, 1990; Mehta and Ticku, 1989) following chronic ethanol administration. The increased expression of $\alpha 4$ subunits may also underlie the reduced sensitivity to GABA (Morrow et al., 1988) and benzodiazepine agonists (Buck and Harris, 1990), since recombinant GABA receptors with $\alpha 4$ $\beta 2\gamma 2$ subunits are less sensitive to GABA agonists and benzodiazepines than $\alpha 1$ $\beta 2\gamma 2$ receptors (Whittemore et al., 1995). Ethanol-dependent and withdrawn rats are also sensitized to the effects of the neurosteroid $3\alpha,5\alpha$-THP (Devaud et al., 1996; Devaud, Purdy, et al., 1995). This effect may be related to the increase in $\gamma 1$ subunit mRNAs following chronic ethanol exposure (Devaud et al., 1996; Devaud, Smith, et al., 1995), since $\gamma 1$ subunits convey greater neurosteroid sensitivity in recombinant expression studies (Puia et al., 1994).

As seen with chronic ethanol exposure, ethanol withdrawal is also associated with dynamic changes in $GABA_A$ receptor subunit mRNAs. During withdrawal, $GABA_A$ receptor $\alpha 1$ and $\alpha 4$ subunit mRNAs return to control levels, while $\beta 2$ and $\beta 3$ subunit mRNA levels increase compared to both control and dependent rats (Devaud et al., 1996). At this time, corresponding changes in protein expression are unlikely since the receptor turnover rate $(t_{1/2})$ is estimated to be one to two days. Therefore, while $GABA_A$ receptor polypeptide expression during withdrawal is probably similar to that found in ethanol-dependent rats, profound changes in $GABA_A$ receptor expression may occur shortly after withdrawal.

The observation that ethanol tolerance is associated with changes in subunit composition also supports the hypothesis that subunit composition influences ethanol sensitivity. As previously discussed, ethanol potentiation of $GABA_A$ receptor function is abolished at the cellular level in rats that are ethanol tolerant and dependent. The changes in subunit expression resulting from chronic exposure to ethanol may contribute to this reduction in ethanol sensitivity (Devaud, Smith, et al., 1995; Morrow et al., 1992).

Chronic Ethanol Alters Phosphorylation and Localization of NMDA and GABA_A Receptors

Whether the phosphorylation state of NMDA and $GABA_A$ receptors is altered by chronic ethanol exposure is not yet known. Chronic ethanol can increase PKC levels and activity (Coe, Yao, et al., 1996; DePetrillo and Liou, 1993; Gordon et al., 1997; Messing et al., 1991; Roivainen et al., 1993) and induce heterologous desensitization of cAMP signaling with decreased PKA activity (Coe, Dohrman, et al., 1996; Gordon et al., 1986; Rabin et al., 1992). Some of these effects of ethanol could relate to changes in subcellular translocation and localization. Ethanol has been shown to stimulate translocation to the nucleus of the catalytic subunit of PKA where it remains sequestered for as long as ethanol is present (Dohrman et al., 1996), and to stimulate translocation of PKC-δ and PKC-ϵ to new intracellular sites (Gordon et al., 1997). Translocation of PKC and PKA isozymes to subcellular anchoring proteins is thought to be important in targeting specific signaling events. Furthermore, PKA and calcineurin (protein phosphatase

2B) are concentrated in postsynaptic densities via a common A-kinase anchoring protein (AKAP79), putting them in a position to regulate phosphorylation and/or dephosphorylation of key postsynaptic proteins (Coghlan et al., 1995). Clearly, changes in PKA and/or PKC activity and subcellular targeting could play an important role in ethanol-induced changes in synaptic function, including modulation of NMDA and GABA$_A$ receptors.

Another potentially important process in NMDA and GABA$_A$ receptor adaptation during ethanol exposure is receptor-cytoskeletal interaction (Chandler et al., 1998). NMDA receptors are required for activity-dependent synaptic remodeling during development, and studies in hippocampal cultures have shown that the subcellular distribution of NMDA receptors is modulated by receptor activity. Chronic treatment with an NMDA receptor antagonist leads to increased NMDA receptor clustering at synaptic sites and, conversely, spontaneous activity leads to decreased synaptic NMDA receptor clustering (Rao and Craig, 1997). Because studies in primary neuronal cell cultures might more closely model developmental processes, an important question to be addressed is whether this activity-dependent redistribution of NMDA receptors also occurs in mature neurons. Furthermore, it is not known whether the functional property of the NMDA receptor itself is altered by clustering and redistribution (i.e., synaptic versus non-synaptic). However, receptor redistribution could represent a novel form of activity-dependent synaptic modification (plasticity), and prolonged inhibition of the NMDA receptor during chronic ethanol exposure might also lead to an increase in NMDA receptor clustering at synaptic sites.

BRAIN DAMAGE IN ALCOHOLICS

Morphological Changes Caused by Chronic Alcohol Abuse

Alcohol-induced changes in brain structure have been studied in both humans and rodents. A variety of postmortem histological analyses, as well as supporting imaging analysis, suggest that chronic alcohol intoxication changes brain structure (Crews, 2000; Sullivan, Rosenbloom, and Pfefferbaum, 2000). Computerized tomography (CT) and magnetic resonance imaging (MRI) studies have repeatedly shown enlargement of the cerebral ventricles and sulci in most alcoholics. The enlargement of the ventricles and sulci reflect a shrinking of brain mass. This is consistent with studies on postmortem brain tissue, wherein alcoholics have a reduction in total brain weight. Particularly severe alcoholics also have reductions in global cerebral hemisphere and cerebellar brain weights compared to controls and moderate drinkers (Harper and Kril, 1993). Some of this loss of brain mass is likely due to loss of neurons (gray matter) and myelin sheaths (white matter). However, a portion of the loss in brain mass is also likely to be due to a reduction in the brain parenchyma, i.e., the size of the cells and their processes, during chronic alcohol abuse. Recent studies have indicated that within one to five months of sustained abstinence, the size of the brain returns to normal levels. It is likely that this return involves an increase in neuronal cell size, arborization, and density of the neuronal processes that make up cellular brain mass, as well as increases in the number and size of glial cells (Franke et al., 1997). Although it is not exactly clear how alcoholism leads to a reduction in brain weight and volume, it is clear that this occurs during active alcohol abuse, and that some recovery of brain mass occurs during abstinence. More research is needed to clearly understand how chronic alcohol abuse leads to a reduction in brain mass and how recovery of brain mass occurs during abstinence.

The frontal lobes appear to be particularly affected in persons with chronic alcoholism as first observed in neuropathological studies (Courville, 1955) and confirmed more recently with neuropathological (Harper and Kril, 1990) and in vivo neuroradiological studies (Nicolas et al., 1997; Pfefferbaum et al., 1997; Ron et al., 1982). Quantitative morphometry suggests that the frontal lobes of the human brain show the greatest loss, and account for much of the associated ventricular enlargement (Jernigan et al., 1991). Studies have found that neuronal density in the superior frontal cortex is reduced by 22 percent in alcoholics compared to nonalcoholic controls, in contrast to other areas of the cortex, which were not different between the groups (Harper et al., 1987). Further, the complexity of the basal dendritic arborization of layer III pyramidal cells in both superior frontal and motor cortices were significantly reduced in alcoholics compared to controls. Decreases in the amounts of N-acetyl aspartate in the frontal lobe, a measure of neuron levels, also illustrates frontal lobe degeneration in alcoholics (Jagannathan et al., 1996). One reason these frontal lobe changes are more evident is the greater proportion of white matter to cortical gray matter in the frontal regions.

Other brain regions are also affected by chronic alcohol abuse. A reduction in dendritic arborization of Purkinje cells in the anterior superior vermis of the cerebellum is also found in alcoholics. Temporal lobe shrinkage occurs particularly in individuals with alcohol-withdrawal seizure history (Sullivan et al., 1996). Taken together, the data demonstrate a selective neuronal loss, dendritic simplification, and reduction of synaptic complexity in specific brain regions of alcoholics.

In addition to the global shrinkage of brain regions, certain key neuronal nuclei that have broad-ranging functions on brain activity are selectively lost with chronic alcohol abuse. One important nucleus altered in alcoholism is the cholinergic basal forebrain nuclei, which is also lost in Alzheimer's disease, causing loss of memory formation. Arendt (1993) found a significant loss of neurons in this region in alcoholic Korsakoff psychosis patients. Cholinergic blockade has been shown to cause the anterograde amnesia seen in both Korsakoff and Alzheimer patients (Kopelman and Corn, 1988).

Additional brain nuclei such as the locus coeruleus and raphe nuclei appear to be particularly sensitive. These two nuclei contain many of the noradrenergic and serotonergic neurons within the brain, respectively. Although these nuclei are small in size, they are particularly important because their neuronal processes project throughout the brain and modulate global aspects of brain activity. Chemical studies have shown abnormally low levels of serotonergic metabolites in the cerebral spinal fluid of alcoholics with Wernike-Korsakoff syndrome, and more recent morphological studies have found a 50 percent reduction in the number of serotonergic neurons from the raphe nuclei of all alcoholic cases studied compared to controls. Thus the serotonergic system appears to be disrupted in alcoholics, especially in severe alcoholics (Baker et al., 1996; Halliday et al., 1995). Several studies have also reported significant noradrenergic cell loss in the locus coeruleus (Arango et al., 1996; Arendt et al., 1995; Lu et al., 1997), although not all studies have found this loss (Harper and Kril, 1993). Studies have also indicated that certain neurons that contain the peptide vasopressin may be sensitive to chronic ethanol-induced neurotoxicity in both rats and humans (Harding et al., 1996; Madeira et al., 1997). Damage to hypothalamic vasopressin and other peptide-containing neurons could disrupt a variety of hormone functions as well as daily rhythms that are important for healthy living. Thus, studies have suggested that cholinergic and biogenic amine brain nuclei appear particularly sensitive to ethanol neurotoxicity.

Although human alcoholic neuropathology is associated with years of alcohol abuse, studies have found that long-term ethanol intoxication is not necessary to cause brain damage. Just a few days of intoxication can lead to neuronal loss in several brain areas including temporal dentate gyrus, entorhinal, piriform, and perirhinal cortices, and in the olfactory bulb (Collins et al., 1998; Crews et al., 2000). These structures are involved in integrating cortical inputs through the limbic system. These findings are consistent with recent human studies that report damage to the entorhinal cortex (Ibanez et al., 1995) and significant hippocampal shrinkage in alcoholics (Harding et al., 1997). Hippocampal damage during chronic ethanol treatment has been correlated with deficits in spatial learning and memory (Franke et al., 1997). Thus, cortical and hippocampal damage occur with chronic ethanol treatment and relatively short durations of alcohol abuse may cause some form of damage.

Cognitive Dysfunction Caused by Chronic Alcohol Abuse

Alcoholics who do not have Korsakoff's syndrome show decreased neuropsychological performance on tests of learning, memory, abstracting, problem solving, visuospatial and perceptual motor functioning, and information processing when compared to peer nonalcoholics (Parsons, 1993). Alcoholics are not only less accurate, they take considerably longer to complete tasks. Alcoholics are differentially vulnerable to these deficits. Further, many of the deficits appear to recover to age-appropriate levels of performance over a four-to-five-year period of abstinence (Parsons, 1993). Although global cerebral atrophy rebounds to normal levels with extended abstinence, not all cognitive functions return. Some abstinent alcoholics appear to have permanent cognitive impairments, particularly in memory and visual-spatial-motor skills (Di Sclafani et al., 1995). Other studies support a loss of logical memory and paired association learning tasks in alcoholics that may be long lasting (Eckardt et al., 1996; see Chapter 3 for further discussion). Thus, various psychological tests suggest long-term changes in brain function following chronic alcohol abuse.

Exciting studies have begun to address the effects of gender on brain damage. Interestingly, alcoholic women appear to have an increased sensitivity for brain damage when compared to alcoholic men (Hommer et al., 1996). This appears to be true for liver disease as well. Although more men than women are diagnosed as alcoholic, the number of female alcoholics is increasing. The increased susceptibility of women to alcoholic pathology is an area that needs further investigation.

Mechanisms of Alcohol-Induced Brain Damage

Although the neurotoxicity of alcohol is well established, the mechanisms of alcohol-induced brain damage are not clear. Human studies indicate loss of both white matter and gray matter, e.g., myelinated nerve track areas and primarily neuronal areas, respectively. It is generally thought that the loss of neurons leads to a loss of myelinated tracks. However, there is little or no evidence to support this hypothesis in humans. Although their methodologies are different, basic studies report neuronal toxicity with no clear loss of myelin or the oligodendroglia that form myelin. A number of mechanisms have been proposed for alcohol-induced brain damage with strong evidence for NMDA-mediated excitotoxicity and losses of trophic factors with less evidence for osmotic and oxidative stress mechanisms. These mechanisms, in combination with diet and other factors, such as genetics, cause alcohol-induced brain damage. Understanding the mechanisms of alcohol-induced brain damage will improve prevention, intervention, treatment, and recovery efforts as well as increase our understanding of neurodegeneration and neurobiological health.

Excitotoxicity

One of the leading theories that explains ethanol-induced neurotoxicity is excitotoxicity. Hyperexcitability of the central nervous system is a key component of ethanol withdrawal and a supersensitive NMDA response appears to be involved. Early research showing that [³H] glutamate binding was increased in the hippocampus of alcoholics (Michaelis et al., 1990) reinforced the hypothesis that a supersensitive NMDA response was responsible, either through an increase in NMDA receptor density or a change in subunit composition. NMDA receptors have a unique property, in that excessive stimulation of these receptors triggers a process in neurons that leads to neuronal death. This process is referred to as excitotoxicity. Glutamate can be excitotoxic in vivo through NMDA in combination with kainate and other glutamate receptors. Excitotoxicity plays a key role in neurodegenerative diseases in general, as well as stroke, brain trauma, and other types of brain damage (Crews and Chandler, 1993).

In vitro studies of excitotoxicity have indicated that long-term exposure to ethanol is not necessary to induce NMDA excitotoxic supersensitivity. Several studies of isolated neuronal cells have indicated that only a few days of ethanol treatment leads to supersensitive NMDA-stimulated calcium flux (Ahern et al., 1994; Iorio et al., 1992), as well as NMDA-stimulated excitotoxicity (Crews and Chandler, 1993; Crews et al., 1993; Iorio et al., 1993). This led researchers to investigate the role of excitotoxicity in an in vivo rat-binge model of ethanol exposure which found extensive mesocorticolimbic neuronal damage. Attempts to block binge ethanol-induced brain damage with NMDA antagonists were not successful (Table 4.1). Thus, general agreement exists among laboratories that chronic alcohol consumption leads to NMDA receptor supersensitivity. This finding predicts that NMDA antagonists would block alcohol withdrawal and alcohol-induced brain damage. Although alcohol withdrawal is blocked, brain damage is not.

Although thiamin deficiency is thought to play a key role in Wernicke's syndrome, the mechanism of the neurodegeneration in this model appears to involve excitotoxicity from glutamate (Langlais and Zhang, 1993). An animal model of Wernicke's syndrome which used pyrithiamine to create thiamin-deficient animals found extracellular concentrations of glutamate increased several fold during ethanol withdrawal seizures (Langlais and Zhang, 1993). Furthermore, MK-801, an NMDA antagonist, reduced experimental

TABLE 4.1. Drugs Tested for Effects on Neurodegeneration Caused by Binge Ethanol Exposure

Drug	Class	Hypothesis	Effect	Reference
Nimodipine	Voltage-gated Ca^{2+} channel blocker	Chronic Etoh increases Ca^{2+} channels in brain	Reduced damage in dentate gyrus Increased damage in piriform cortex	Corso et al., 1998
Nimodipine	L-type Ca^{2+} channel blocker	Chronic Etoh increases Ca^{2+} channels in brain	No neuroprotection	Hamelink, 1998, 2000
DNQX	AMPA antagonist NMDA antagonist at glycine site	High densities of AMPA receptors in the dentate gyrus, Ca fields, entorhinal cortex, piriform, frontal cortex	No effect	Corso et al., 1998
MK-801	NMDA antagonist	Chronic Etoh causes excitotoxicity	Increased damage in entorhinal cortex, orbital cortex, and periamygdala	Corso et al., 1998
MK-801	NMDA antagonist	Chronic Etoh causes excitotoxicity	No effect	Collins et al., 1998
MK-801	NMDA antagonist	Chronic Etoh causes excitotoxicity	No neuroprotection	Hamelink, 1998, 2000
Memantine	NMDA antagonist	Chronic Etoh causes excitotoxicity	No neuroprotection	Hamelink, 1998, 2000
Olfactory bulbectomies	Surgical procedure	Chronic Etoh causes excitotoxic cascade	No neuroprotection	Hamelink, 1998, 2000
L-NAME	Nitric oxide synthase inhibitor	Chronic Etoh increases NO production	No change/increased damage	Zou et al., 1996

Note: Shown are the results of experiments which tested hypotheses regarding mechanisms of alcohol-induced brain damage, particularly those regarding glutamate NMDA receptor supersensitivity to excitotoxicity (see Crews and Chandler, 1993). Each of the hypotheses has a basis in the basic brain studies that are referenced. Specific antagonists were used as tests. Binge treatment with ethanol differs slightly among studies, but in general involves very high alcohol consumption for several days. Although NMDA supersensitivity appears to be involved in ethanol dependence and withdrawal, it does not appear to be central to ethanol-induced neurotoxicity in these binge-drinking models.

neurological symptoms and decreased neural lessening in models of thiamin deficiency in rats (Langlais and Mair, 1990). In any case, there is strong evidence that ethanol withdrawal hyperexcitability is related at least in part to NMDA supersensitivity and that this supersensitivity could underlie ethanol-induced brain damage.

Osmotic Changes and Increased Intracranial Pressure

Another possible mechanism of ethanol-induced brain damage involves osmotic changes and increases in intracranial pressure. Although difficult to test, some studies have hypothesized that cerebral edema occurs with moderate doses of ethanol (McQueen and Posey, 1975; Weiss and Craig, 1978) and that this may cause alcoholic brain damage (Lambie, 1985). Recent investigations have tested the edema mechanisms of binge-drinking-induced brain damage using furosemide, which could reduce vasogenic and cytotoxic edema, and mannitol, a commonly used agent to reduce intracerebral pressure. Mannitol is an inert molecule that increases the osmolarity of the blood and decreases water content and brain volume (Paczynski et al., 1997). No protective effects have been found with binge-drinking models (see Figure 4.1). However, Collins and colleagues (1998) treated rats once daily with ethanol, much less than binge-drinking models, for ten days and found that furosemide reduced brain hydration and neurodegeneration in the entorhinal cortex and dentate gyrus, though no attenuation of olfactory bulb degeneration was found. Neurodegeneration mechanisms may differ depending upon the extent and duration of alcohol consumption.

Oxidative Stress

Another possible mechanism of ethanol-induced brain damage involves increased oxidative stress of neurons. Cells use oxygen for energy metabolism and normally have mechanisms that protect against oxidative damage. Studies that have examined the effects of both acute and chronic ethanol administration upon cellular oxidation have primarily focused either on ethanol's effects upon intracellular antioxidant mechanisms such as α-tocopherol, ascorbate, glutathione, catalase, and superoxide dismutase (SOD) activity (Ledig et al., 1981; Montoliu et al., 1994; Nordmann, 1987; Rouach et al., 1987) or potential sources of oxidative radicals such as CYP2E1 (Montoliu et al., 1994, 1995). Chronic ethanol-induced increases in CYP2E1 and other oxidases have been related to increased lipid peroxidation and reactive oxygen radicals in the brain (Montoliu et al., 1994). Because it is rich in polyunsaturated fatty acids, which are especially prone to reactive oxygen injury,

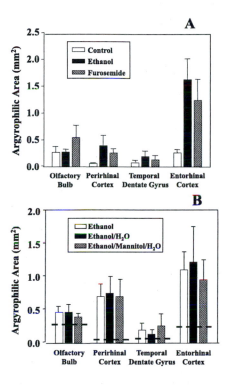

FIGURE 4.1. Edema and Binge Ethanol-Induced Brain Damage. To determine whether cerebral edema was involved in binge ethanol-induced brain damage, furosemide (a loop diuretic) was concomitantly administered to binge ethanol-exposed rats (A). Sprague-Dawley rats were treated using a four-day binge ethanol episode as previously described (Knapp and Crews, 1999). Furosemide, 6.7 mg/kg, was administered three times daily i.p. Immediately after the last dose of ethanol was administered, the rats were euthanized and their brains sectioned at 40 μm. Every eighth section was stained by the amino curpric silver method of de Olmos (1994). Shown is the mean total argyrophilia per rat ± SE. There was a main effect of drug treatment ($F_{(2,17)}$ = 5.481; p < .05). To determine whether vasogenic edema or hydration state was involved in binge ethanol-induced brain damage, the experiment in panel B was performed. Mannitol is an inert molecule that increases the osmolarity of the blood and decreases brain water content (Paczynski et al., 1997). The rats were hydrated to 25.9 ml/kg water per day and/or 0.75 g/kg mannitol was administered three times daily. After the final dose of ethanol, the rats were euthanized and treated as in panel A. Shown is the mean total argyrophilia per rat ± SE. The broken lines represent the average level of argyrophilic area in control-treated animals. There was no significant effect of hydration or mannitol ($F_{(2,13)}$ = .032; p > .05) on binge ethanol-induced brain damage as measured by argyrophilic area.

the brain is particularly susceptible to lipid peroxidation. It has been demonstrated that a single dose of ethanol elevates lipid hydroperoxide levels and decreases glutathione levels in rat brain homogenates (Nordmann et al., 1990, 1992; Uysal et al., 1986, 1989). However, it is not clear how this increased oxidation translates to increased brain damage or whether it does at all. Oxidative stress has been implicated in a variety of conditions, particularly aging, Alzheimer's disease, Parkinson's disease, stroke, and other neurodegenerative diseases. More research is needed to completely understand how oxidation damages neurons, and how other brain cells respond to increased oxidative stress. Ethanol-induced neurodegeneration may be related to an induction of oxidative enzymes, and alcohol research provides an opportunity to clearly address this aspect of neurodegeneration which could impact a broad range of mental diseases.

Hepatic Encephalopathy

Hepatic encephalopathy (HE) is caused by liver cirrhosis and other hepatotoxic syndromes that start with subtle personality changes and disturbances of sleep patterns and progress to muscle incoordination, flapping tremors, coma, and death. HE is caused by several factors, including increased levels of neurotoxic substances in the brain, in particular ammonia and manganese, and is often associated with alcohol cirrhosis (Hazell and Butterworth, 1999). HE causes severe alterations in astrocytes, including changes in expression of peripheral-type benzodiazepine receptors (Lavoie et al., 1990), monoamine oxidase B (Rao et al., 1993) and glutamine synthetase (Lavoie et al., 1987), and the glutamate transporter GLT-1 (Knecht et al., 1997; Norenberg et al., 1997). These changes during acute liver failure cause accumulation of glutamine (an ammonia metabolite) in the brain and cytotoxic edema (Levin et al., 1989; Takahashi et al., 1991), and in chronic liver failure result in Alzheimer type II astrocytosis (Hazell and Butterworth, 1999). Neurotransmitter systems such as glutamate, serotonin, GABA, and opioids are also disturbed in HE, although the causes and effects of these alterations are not as well understood (Bergeron et al., 1989; Layrargues and Butterworth, 1992; Thorton and Losowsky, 1988; Young et al., 1975). This suggests that the neurodegeneration associated with chronic alcoholism may be caused in part by changes in hepatic function.

Brain Damage, Alcohol Dependence, and Recovery

Alcoholism is a progressive disease that begins with experimentation and progresses to addiction, usually over the course of 10 to 15 years (Vaillant,

1996). Progressive increases in abuse often develop into complete fixation on obtaining and consuming alcohol. Addiction involves the loss of control over the ability to abstain from alcohol or other drugs, even in the face of adverse consequences, and perseverative preoccupation with obtaining and using the drugs desired. Perseveration refers to continued repetitive behaviors of a previous appropriate or correct response, even though the repeated response has since become inappropriate and incorrect. Perseveration is associated with cortical damage. One hypothesis regarding the development of alcoholism is that an initial state of disinhibition/hyperexcitability, perhaps due to low frontal-cortical impulse inhibition, predisposes a person to developing alcoholism (Begleiter and Porjesz, 1999). Both clinical and experimental studies support frontal-cortical involvement in neuropsychological dysfunction in alcoholics, particularly those with Korsakoff's syndrome (Oscar-Berman and Hutner, 1993). Studies have found that the ventromedial prefrontal cortex mediates goal-oriented actions that are guided by motivational and emotional factors (Gallagher et al., 1999). Damage to this area results in a loss of the ability to associate incentive values with stimuli. Thus the effects of negative stimuli on behavior are blunted by ventromedial prefrontal damage and result in maladaptive behaviors (Bechara et al., 2000; Gallagher et al., 1999). Humans with ventromedial prefrontal cortical lesions are insensitive to future consequences and are primarily guided by immediate prospects (Bechara et al., 2000). As mentioned earlier, a variety of evidence has focused attention on the prefrontal cortex as an area of brain that is particularly sensitive to alcohol-induced brain damage. Various regions of the frontal and prefrontal cortex are involved in learned associations, emotional decision making, and executive cognitive functions. Executive cognitive function (ECF) is the ability to utilize higher mental abilities such as attention, planning, organization, sequencing, and abstract reasoning, to adaptively modulate future behavior based on external and internal feedback (Foster et al., 1994). Executive cognitive function is disrupted in alcoholics and other patients who exhibit prefrontal damage (Boller et al., 1995), and this disruption has been implicated in aggression associated with alcohol and drug abuse (Hoaken et al., 1998). ECF/prefrontal disruption is associated with decreased regulation of human social behavior, including disinhibition syndrome (characterized by impulsivity, socially inappropriate behavior, and aggression) (Giancola and Zeichner, 1995). These studies suggest that some of the greatest sociopathic problems of alcoholism, e.g., violence and loss of control over the drug, may be directly related to the neurotoxic effects of ethanol on prefrontal cortical function. The prefrontal cortex is closely linked to the amygdala and temporal lobes which also show damage in cases of alcoholism. These structures are known to play a role in automatic or nonconscious decision making (Kubota et al., 2000). Emotional factors are often subconscious processes that are below the level of aware-ness. Addiction involves continued behaviors out of conscious control. The progression from experimentation with alcohol to alcohol addiction gener-ally occurs over an extended period of many years with increased consump-tion of alcohol, increased neurotoxicity, increased distortions of thinking, and preoccupation with the drug. A hypothetical scheme of the progression to alcoholism is depicted in the Spiral of Distress (Figure 4.2; see Koob et al., 1997 for additional discussions). Figure 4.2 attempts to relate the neurochemical changes in the brain induced by alcohol to the progression to addiction. Addiction is presented as an end point reached when cortical damage results in perseverative drinking behavior without conscious recog-nition of negative consequences and the inability to consciously control behavior. Each of these characteristics occurs with frontal and temporal lobe cortical lesions suggesting that progressive neurotoxicity may underlie the progression to addiction. Future studies are needed to directly determine the relationship of prefrontal cortical function to alcohol-induced brain damage and addiction.

Treatment and Recovery for Alcoholism

The principal approach to treatment for alcoholism is abstinence from drinking alcohol. A variety of treatments including elements of supportive therapy, cognitive behavioral therapy, and Alcoholics Anonymous and other group therapies and recovery programs in various forms and combina-tions have helped millions of people. In general, treatments are effective for many, but not all, individuals. During recovery, behavioral and neuroana-tomical changes persist long after the end of the physical alcohol with-drawal syndrome, which typically lasts less than one week. Human studies have shown that within the first month of recovery alcoholics show a signifi-cant decrease in ventricular and sulci size (i.e., the brain mass actually in-creases and returns to normal values) (Pfefferbaum et al., 1995). Over the following months regrowth of brain mass continues. In abstinent alcoholics a significant increase in brain volume occurs over a period of months. Re-lapsing alcoholics do not show increased gains in brain mass (Pfefferbaum et al., 1995). It is possible that changes in behavior essential for successful recovery from addiction require neurophysiological and perhaps anatomi-cal changes in the brain to sustain the recovery. The findings that those who are successful at recovery have brain regrowth whereas those who relapse have no regrowth could be due to continued ethanol neurotoxicity in relaps-ing addicts (Pfefferbaum et al., 1998) or due to the need for brain regrowth and return of key brain functions to sustain abstinence. Those individuals

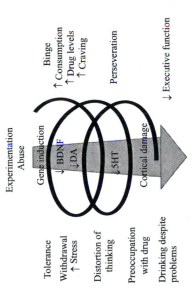

Experimentation
Abuse

Gene induction

Tolerance

Withdrawal
↑ Stress

Distortion of
thinking

Preoccupation
with drug

Drinking despite
problems

↓ BDNF
↓ DA

↓ 5HT

Cortical damage

Binge
↑ Consumption
↑ Drug levels
↑ Craving

Perseveration

↓ Executive function

ADDICTION

FIGURE 4.2. The Spiral of Distress. This model depicts the progression from experimentation to addiction. On the left are criteria for the diagnosis of alcohol dependence. Included are increasing tolerance; alcohol withdrawal due to physical dependence, which increases stress; increasing preoccupation with the drug; spending large amounts of time obtaining and consuming alcohol; and continued use despite negative consequences and problems associated with the use of alcohol. In the middle are known changes in the brain that occur during chronic alcohol use. Changes in gene expression are well documented as occurring during the development of dependence. Studies have shown changes in biogenic amines, particularly serotonin (5 hydroxytryptamine, 5HT) and dopamine, key neurotransmitters involved in dependence (see Crews et al., 1999, for more details). Cortical damage and shrinkage occurs in alcoholics, particularly in frontal and temporal regions. Binge drinking, on the right, is indicative of the behavior most likely to induce tolerance, dependence, and changes in brain structure and function. Loss of biogenic amines could increase craving and drinking. Cortical damage can cause perseveration—the persistence of behavior once the reward is removed—and could be analogous to preoccupation with alcohol. Frontal cortical damage is associated with loss of executive functions and could be related to failure to associate negative consequences with drinking, inability to set goals, and inability to inhibit behaviors, ultimately leading to addiction. *Source:* Adapted from Koob and Le Moal, 1997.

without regrowth and return of functions (e.g., executive functions that include setting and maintaining goals) may be more prone to relapse. Behavioral counseling and other therapies may activate and train cortical regions, strengthening and stimulating neuronal function and neuronal regrowth. Thus, successful recovery may involve brain regrowth due to abstinence and the removal of ethanol neurotoxicity, as well as exercising emotional-association cortical areas to regain functions needed for appropriate emotional decision making, executive function, and appropriate responses to environmental stimuli (Figure 4.3).

SUMMARY

Alcohol dependence is one of the most common maladies in our society, touching most families and communities. At least a portion of the acute actions of alcohol are due to its effects at glutamate and GABA receptors. Glutamate NMDA receptors are abundant excitatory receptors in the brain and are among the most sensitive receptors to inhibition by ethanol. NMDA receptors are heterogeneous and the effects of alcohol on NMDA receptors differ among brain regions, likely due to differences in subunit composition, phosphorylation state, and other factors. Kainate and AMPA glutamate excitatory receptors are also inhibited in certain circumstances. In contrast, the major inhibitory receptor in the brain, the $GABA_A$ receptor, is potentiated by ethanol. $GABA_A$ receptor potentiation also varies across brain regions due to subunit composition, phosphorylation state, and other possible heterogeneous modulators. $GABA_A$ receptor potentiation is shared by ethanol with barbiturates and benzodiazepines as well as many sedative, anticonvulsant, and anxiolytic behavioral actions. Chronic ethanol abuse leads to adaptive changes in both NMDA glutamate and $GABA_A$ receptor responses. NMDA receptor supersensitivity likely contributes to the hyperexcitability of ethanol withdrawal syndrome and may contribute to alcoholic brain damage, although other mechanisms appear to contribute as well. The mechanism of supersensitivity appears to be more complicated than a simple increased number of receptors and requires additional studies to elucidate the mechanisms of NMDA supersensitivity in alcohol dependence. $GABA_A$ receptor responses are altered during chronic ethanol consumption as well in a complex manner consistent with tolerance and dependence. It is clear that many of ethanol's acute and chronic pharmacological effects are due to actions at glutamate NMDA and $GABA_A$ receptors.

Alcohol abuse and dependence clearly result in neurodegeneration. Alcoholics have lesions in specific cholinergic, biogenic amine, and other brain nuclei as well as cortical shrinkage and ventricular enlargement. The

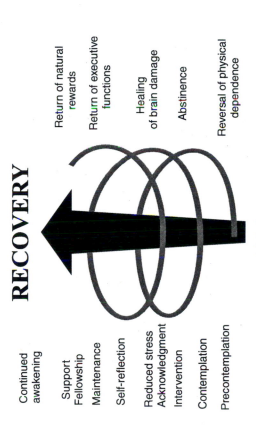

FIGURE 4.3. The Path to Recovery. This model illustrates the stages of change, including reversal of brain damage and return of executive function involved in recovery from addiction (Prochasta and DiClemente, 1992). These stages begin with precontemplation, in which individuals are unaware of the problem, have no intention of changing, and possibly have difficulty associating negative consequences of drug taking due to cortical dysfunction. Contemplation refers to the point at which individuals are aware of the problem and interventions to make the patient aware help motivate change. Abstinence allows the return of cortical functions and regrowth of the cortex. Self-reflection strengthens associations of negative consequences with drug taking, perhaps invigorating cortical regions involved in these associations. Return of executive functions, including impulse inhibition and goal setting, support the maintenance of abstinence. Increased fellowship with other abstainers reduces craving and helps with motivation, leading to continued awakening and return of natural rewards. Models of this type can be used to test associations between recovery and changes in brain function.

117

frontal, prefrontal, associative, and temporal lobe cortexes appear to be particularly sensitive to alcohol neurotoxicity. The mechanisms of neurotoxicity appear to be multifaceted, including NMDA supersensitivity and other toxic factors that lead to neuronal loss and degeneration. The progressive nature of addiction may be related to a progressive loss of brain tissue associated with chronic alcohol abuse neurotoxicity. Recovery from alcoholism is associated with a return of cerebral mass that could play a role in the success of the recovery process. Additional studies are needed to fully understand the process of addiction and how it relates to the effects of chronic alcohol abuse on brain function.

REFERENCES

Aguayo, L.G. (1990). Ethanol potentiates the $GABA_A$-activated Cl^- current in mouse hippocampal and cortical neurons. *Eur J Pharmacol* 187:127-130.

Ahern, K.B.; Lustig, H.S.; Greenberg, D.A. (1994). Enhancement of NMDA toxicity and calcium responses by chronic exposure of cultured cortical neurons to ethanol. *Neurosci Lett* 165:211-214.

Allan, A.M.; Harris, R.A. (1986). Gamma-aminobutyric acid and alcohol actions: Neurochemical studies of long sleep and short sleep mice. *Life Sci* 39:2005-2015.

Allan, A.M.; Harris, R.A. (1987). Acute and chronic ethanol treatments alter GABA receptor-operated chloride channels. *Pharmacol Biochem Behav* 27:665-670.

Arango, V.; Underwood, M.D.; Pauler, D.K.; Kass, R.E.; Mann, J.J. (1996). Differential age-related loss of pigmented locus coeruleus neurons in suicides, alcoholics, and alcoholic suicides. *Alcohol Clin Exp Res* 20:1141-1147.

Arendt, T. (1993). The cholinergic differentiation of the cerebral cortex induced by chronic consumption of alcohol: Reversal by cholinergic drugs and transplantation. In Hunt, W.A.; Nixon, S.J. (Eds.), *Alcohol-Induced Brain Damage,* Vol 22, pp. 431-460. Rockville, MD: NIAAA/NIH.

Arendt, T.; Bruckner, M.K.; Magliusi, S.; Krell, T. (1995). Degeneration of rat cholinergic basal forebrain neurons and reactive changes in nerve growth factor expression after chronic neurotoxic injury-I. Degeneration and plastic response of basal forebrain neurons. *Neuroscience* 65:633-645.

Baker, K.G.; Halliday, G.M.; Kril, J.J.; Harper, C.G. (1996). Chronic alcoholism in the absence of Wernicke-Korsakoff syndrome and cirrhosis does not result in the loss of serotonergic neurons from the median raphe nucleus. *Metab Brain Dis* 11:217-227.

Bechara, A.; Tranel, D.; Damasio, H. (2000). Characterization of the decision-making deficit of patients with ventromedial prefrontal cortex lesions. *Brain* 123: 2189-2202.

Begleiter, H.; Porjesz, B. (1999). What is inherited in the predisposition toward alcoholism? A proposed model. *Alcohol Clin Exp Res* 23:1125-1135.

Bergeron, M.; Reader, T.A.; Layrargues, G.P.; Butterworth, R.F. (1989). Mono-amines and metabolites in autopsied brain tissue from cirrhotic patients with hepatic encephalopathy. *Neurochem Res* 14:853-859.

Bettler, B.; Mulle, C. (1995). Neurotransmitter receptors II AMPA and kainate receptors. *Neuropharmacology* 34:123-139.

Boisse, N.N.; Okamoto, M. (1980). Ethanol as a sedative-hypnotic: Comparison with barbiturate and non-barbiturate sedative-hypnotics. In Rigter, H.; Crabbe, J.C. (Eds.), *Alcohol Tolerance and Dependence,* pp. 265-292. Amsterdam: Elsevier.

Boller, F.; Traykov, L.; Dao-Castellana, M.H.; Fontaine-Dabernard, A. (1995). Cognitive functioning in "diffuse pathology": Role of prefrontal and limbic structures. *Ann NY Acad Sci* 769:23-39.

Bowe, M.A.; Nadler, J.V. (1995). Polyamines antagonize *N*-methyl-D-aspartate-evoked depolarizations, but reduce Mg^{2+} block. *Eur J Pharmacol* 278:55-65.

Breese, G.R.; Morrow, A.L.; Simson, P.E.; Criswell, H.E.; McCown, T.J.; Duncan, G.E.; Keir, W.J. (1993). The neuroanatomical specificity of ethanol action with ligand-gated ion channels: A hypothesis. *Alcohol Alcohol Suppl* 2:309-313.

Buck, K.J.; Harris, R.A. (1990). Benzodiazepine agonist and inverse agonist actions on $GABA_A$ receptor-operated chloride channels. II. Chronic effects of ethanol. *J Pharmacol Exp Ther* 253:713-719.

Buller, A.L.; Larson, H.C.; Morrisett, R.A.; Monaghan, D.T. (1995). Glycine modulates ethanol inhibition of heteromeric *N*-methyl-D-aspartate receptors expressed in *Xenopus* oocytes. *Mol Pharmacol* 48:717-723.

Buller, A.L.; Larson, H.C.; Schneider, B.E.; Beaton, J.A.; Morrisett, R.A.; Monoghan, D.T. (1994). The molecular basis of NMDA receptor subtypes: Native receptor diversity is predicted by subunit composition. *J Neurosci* 14:5471-5484.

Butterworth, R.F. (1995). Pathophysiology of alcoholic brain damage: Synergistic effects of ethanol, thiamine deficiency and alcoholic liver disease. *Metab Brain Dis* 10:1-8.

Carboni, S.; Isola, R.; Gessa, G.L.; Rossetti, Z.L. (1993). Ethanol prevents the glutamate release induced by *N*-methyl-D-aspartate in the rat striatum. *Neurosci Lett* 152:133-136.

Carter, L.A.; Belknap, J.K.; Crabbe, J.C.; Janowsky, A. (1995). Allosteric regulation of the *N*-methyl-D-aspartate receptor-linked ion channel complex and effects of ethanol in ethanol-withdrawal seizure-prone and -resistant mice. *J Neurochem* 64:213-219.

Celentano, J.J.; Gibbs, T.T.; Farb, D.H. (1988). Ethanol potentiates GABA- and glycine-induced chloride currents in chick spinal cord neurons. *Brain Res* 455: 377-380.

Chandler, L.J.; Guzman, N.; Sumners, C.; Crews, F.T. (1994). Induction of nitric oxide synthase in brain glial cells: Possible interaction with ethanol in reactive neuronal injury. In Lancaster, F.E. (Ed.), *Alcohol and Glial Cells,* Vol 27, pp. 195-214. Rockville, MD: NIAAA.

Chandler, L.J.; Harris, R.A.; Crews, F.T. (1998). Ethanol tolerance and synaptic plasticity. *Trends Pharmacol Sci* 19:491-495.

Chandler, L.J.; Newson, H.; Sumners, C.; Crews, F.T. (1993). Chronic ethanol exposure potentiates NMDA excitotoxicity in cerebral cortical neurons. *J Neurochem* 60:1578-1581.

Chandler, L.J.; Sumners, C.; Crews, F.T. (1995). Chronic ethanol increases NMDA-stimulated NO formation but not MK-801 binding or NMDAR1 subunits in primary neuronal cultures. *Mol Pharmacol* 19:6A-14.

Chu, B.; Anantharam, V.; Treistman, S.N. (1995). Ethanol inhibition of recombinant heteromeric NMDA channels in the presence and absence of modulators. *J Neurochem* 65:140-148.

Coe, I.R.; Dohrman, D.P.; Constantinescu, A.; Diamond, I.; Gordon, A.S. (1996). Activation of cyclic AMP-dependent protein kinase reverses tolerance of a nucleoside transporter to ethanol. *J Pharmacol Exp Ther* 276:365-369.

Coe, I.R.; Yao, L.; Diamond, I.; Gordon, A.S. (1996). The role of protein kinase C in cellular tolerance to ethanol. *J Biol Chem* 271:29468-29472.

Coghlan, V.M.; Perrino, B.A.; Howard, M.; Langeberg, L.K.; Hicks, J.B.; Gallatin, W.M.; Scott, J.D. (1995). Association of protein kinase A and protein phosphatase 2B with a common anchoring protein. *Science* 267:108-111.

Collins, M.A.; Zou, J-Y.; Neafsey, E.J. (1998). Brain damage due to episodic alcohol exposure in vivo and in vitro: Furosemide neuroprotection implicates edema-based mechanism. *FASEB J* 12:221-230.

Corso, T.D.; Mostafa, H.M.; Collins, M.A.; Neafsey, E.J. (1998). Brain neuronal degeneration caused by episodic alcohol intoxication in rats: Effects of nimodipine, 6,7-dinitro-quinoxalne-2,3-dione, and MK-801. *Alcohol Clin Exp Res* 22(1):217-224.

Courville, C.B. (1955). *Effects of Alcohol on the Nervous System in Man.* Los Angeles: San Lucas Press.

Crews, F.T. (1999). Alcohol and neurodegeneration. *CNS Drug Reviews* 5:379-394.

Crews, F.T. (2000). Neurotoxicity of alcohol: Excitotoxicity, oxidative stress, neurotrophic factors, apoptosis, and cell adhesion molecules. In Noronha, M.; Eckardt, M.; Warren, K. (Eds.), *Review of NIAAA's Neuroscience and Behavioral Research Portfolio,* Monograph No. 34, pp. 189-206. Bethesda, MD: National Institutes of Health.

Crews, F.T.; Braun, C.J.; Hoplight, B.; Switzer, R.C.; Knapp, D.J. (2000). Binge ethanol consumption causes differential brain damage in young-adolescent compared to adult rats. *Alcohol Clin Exp Res* 24:1712-1723.

Crews, F.T.; Chandler, L.J. (1993). Excitotoxicity and the neuropathology of ethanol. In Hunt, W.A.; Nixon, S.J. (Eds.), *Alcohol-Induced Brain Damage,* Vol. 22, pp. 355-371. Rockville, MD: NIAAA Monograph.

Crews, F.T.; Newsom, H.; Gerber, M.; Sumners, C.; Chandler, L.J.; Freund, G. (1993). Molecular mechanisms of alcohol neurotoxicity. In Alling, C.; Sun, G. (Eds.), *Alcohol, Cell Membranes, and Signal Transduction in Brain,* pp. 123-138. Lund, Sweden: Plenum Press.

Crews, F.T.; Waage, H.G.; Wilkie, M.B.; Lauder, J.M. (1999). Ethanol pretreatment enhances NMDA excitotoxicity in biogenic amine neurons: protection by brain derived neurotrophic factor. *Alcohol Clin Exp Res* 23:1834-1842.

Criswell, H.E.; Simson, P.E.; Duncan, G.E.; McCown, T.J.; Herbert, J.S.; Morrow, A.L.; Breese, G.R. (1993). Molecular basis for regionally specific action of ethanol on γ-aminobutyric acid A receptors: Generalization to other ligand-gated ion channels. *J Pharmacol Exp Ther* 267:522-537.

Criswell, H.E.; Simson, P.E.; Knapp, D.J.; Devaud, L.L.; McCown, T.J.; Duncan, G.E.; Morrow, A.L.; Breese, G.R. (1995). Effect of zolpidem on γ-aminobutyric acid (GABA)-induced inhibition predicts the interaction of ethanol with GABA on individual neurons in several rat brain regions. *J Pharmacol Exp Ther* 273: 526-536.

Cutting, G.R.; Curristin, S.; Zoghbi, H.; O'Hara, B.; Seldin, M.F.; Uhl, G.R. (1992). Identification of a putative gamma-aminobutyric acid (GABA) receptor subunit rho2 cDNA and colocalization of the genes encoding rho2 (GABRR2) and rho1 (GABRR1) to human chromosome 6q14-q21 and mouse chromosome 4. *Genomics* 12:801-806.

Cutting, G.R.; Lu, L.; O'Hara, B.F.; Kasch, L.M.; Montrose-Rafizadeh, C.; Donovan, D.M.; Shimada, S.; Antonarakis, S.E.; Guggino, W.B.; Uhl, G.R.; Kazazian, H.H. Jr. (1991). Cloning of the gamma-aminobutyric acid (GABA) rho1 cDNA: A GABA receptor subunit highly expressed in the retina. *Proc Natl Acad Sci USA* 88:2673-2677.

Davies, J.; Francis, A.A.; Jones, A.W.; Watkins, J.C. (1981). 2-Amino-5-phosphonovalerate (2APV), a potent and selective antagonist of amino acid-induced and synaptic excitation. *Neurosci Lett* 21:77-81.

Davis, W.C.; Ticku, M.K. (1981). Ethanol enhances [3H]diazepan binding at the benzodiazepine-GABA receptor ionophore complex. *Mol Pharmacol* 20:287.

de Olmos, J.S.; Beltramino, C.A.; de Olmos de Lorenzo, S. (1994). Use of an amino-cupric-silver technique for the detection of early and semiacute neuronal degeneration caused by neurotoxicants, hypoxia and physical trauma. *Neurotoxicol Teratol* 16(6): 545-561.

de Vries, D.J.; Johnston, G.A.R.; Ward, L.C.; Wilce, P.A.; Shanley, B.C. (1987). Effects of chronic ethanol inhalation on the enhancement of benzodiazepine binding to mouse brain membranes by GABA. *Neurochem Int* 10:231-235.

DePetrillo, P.B.; Liou, C.S. (1993). Ethanol exposure increases total protein kinase C activity in human lymphocytes. *Alcohol Clin Exp Res* 17:351-354.

Devaud, L.L.; Morrow, A.L.; Criswell, H.E.; Breese, G.R.; Duncan, G.E. (1995). Regional differences in the effects of chronic ethanol administration on [3H]zolpidem binding in rat brain. *Alcohol Clin Exp Res* 19:910-914.

Devaud, L.L.; Purdy, R.H.; Finn, D.A.; Morrow, A.L. (1996). Sensitization of γ-aminobutyric acid$_A$ receptors to neuroactive steroids in rats during ethanol withdrawal. *J Pharmacol Exp Ther* 278:510-517.

Devaud, L.L.; Purdy, R.H.; Morrow, A.L. (1995). The neurosteroid 3α-hydroxy-5α-pregnan-20-one protects against bicuculline-induced seizures during ethanol withdrawal in rats. *Alcohol Clin Exp Res* 19:350-355.

Devaud, L.L.; Smith, F.D.; Grayson, D.R.; Morrow, A.L. (1995). Chronic ethanol consumption differentially alters the expression of g-aminobutyric acidA receptor subunit mRNAs in rat cerebral cortex: Competitive, quantitative reverse transcriptase-polymerase chain reaction analysis. *Mol Pharmacol* 48:861-868.

Di Sclafani, V.; Ezekiel, F.; Meyerhoff, D.J.; MacKay, S.; Dillon, W.P.; Weiner, M.W. (1995). Brain atrophy and cognitive function in older abstinent alcoholic men. *Alcohol Clin Exp Res* 19:1121-1126.

Dildy, J.E.; Leslie, S.W. (1989). Ethanol inhibits NMDA-induced increases in free intracellular Ca+2 in dissociated brain cells. *Brain Res* 499:383-387.

Dildy-Mayfield, J.E.; Harris, R.A. (1992a). Acute and chronic ethanol exposure alters the function of hippocampal kainate receptors expressed in *Xenopus* oocytes. *J Neurochem* 58:1569-1572.

Dildy-Mayfield, J.E.; Harris, R.A. (1992b). Comparison of ethanol sensitivity of rat brain kainate, DL-a-amino-3-hydroxy-5-methyl-4-isoxalone proprionic acid and *N*-methyl-D-aspartate receptors expressed in *Xenopus* oocytes. *J Pharmacol Exp Ther* 262:487-494.

Dildy-Mayfield, J.E.; Mihic, S.J.; Liu, Y.; Deitrich, R.A.; Harris, R.A. (1996). Actions of long chain alcohols on GABA$_A$ and glutamate receptors: Relation to in vivo effects. *Br J Pharmacol* 118:378-384.

Dohrman, D.P.; Diamond, I.; Gordon, A.S. (1996). Ethanol causes translocation of cAMP-dependent protein kinase catalytic subunit to the nucleus. *Proc Natl Acad Sci USA* 93:10217-10221.

Duncan, G.E.; Breese, G.R.; Criswell, H.E.; McCown, T.J.; Herbert, J.S.; Devaud, L.L.; Morrow, A.L. (1995). Distribution of [3H]zolpidem binding sites in relation to mRNA encoding the α1, β2 and γ2 subunits of GABA$_A$ receptors in rat brain. *Neuroscience* 64:1113-1128.

Durand, G.M.; Bennett, M.V.; Zukin, R.S. (1993). Splice variants of the *N*-methyl-D-aspartate receptor NR1 identify domains involved in regulation by polyamines and protein kinase C. *Proc Natl Acad Sci USA* 90:6731-6735.

Durand, G.M.; Gregor, P.; Zheng, X.; Bennett, M.L.V.; Uhl, G.R.; Zukin, R.S. (1992). Cloning of an apparent splice variant of the rat *N*-methyl-D-aspartate receptor NMDAR1 with altered sensitivity to polyamines and activators of protein kinase C. *Proc Natl Acad Sci USA* 89(19):9359-9363.

Eckardt, M.J.; Rohrbaugh, J.W.; Stapleton, J.M.; Davis, E.Z.; Martin, P.R.; Weingartner, H.J. (1996). Attention-related brain potential and cognition in alcoholism-associated organic brain disorders. *Biol Psychiatry* 39:143-146.

Fadda, F.; Rossetti, Z. (1998). Chronic ethanol consumption: From neuroadaptation to neurodegeneration. *Prog Neurobiol* 56:385-431.

Follesa, P.; Ticku, M. (1995). Chronic ethanol treatment differentially regulates NMDA receptor subunit mRNA expression in rat brain. *Mol Brain Res* 29:99-106.

Foster, J.; Eskes, G.; Stuss, D. (1994). The cognitive neuropsychology of attention: A frontal lobe perspective. *Cognitive Neuropsychology* 11:133-147.

Franke, H.; Kittner, H.; Berger, P.; Wirkner, K.; Schramek, J. (1997). The reaction of astrocytes and neurons in the hippocampus of adult rats during chronic ethanol treatment and correlations to behavioral impairments. *Alcohol* 14:445-454.

Frohlich, R.; Patzelt, C.; Illes, P. (1994). Inhibition by ethanol of excitatory amino acid receptors and nicotinic acetylcholine receptors at rat locus coeruleus neurons. *Naunyn Schmiedebergs Arch Pharmacol* 350(6):626-631.

Frye, G.D.; Breese, G.R. (1982). GABAergic modulation of ethanol-induced motor impairment. *J Pharmacol Exp Ther* 223:752-756.

Frye, G.; Chapin, R.; Vogel, R.; Mailman, R.; Kilts, C.; Mueller, R.; Breese, G. (1981). Effects of acute and chronic 1,3-butanediol treatment on central nervous system function: A comparison with ethanol. *J Pharmacol Exp Ther* 216:306-314.

Frye, G.D.; McCown, T.J.; Breese, G.R. (1983a). Characterization of susceptibility to audiogenic seizures in ethanol-dependent rats after microinjections of gamma-aminobutyric acid (GABA) agonists into the inferior coliculus, substantia nigra or medial septum. *J Pharmacol Exp Ther* 227:663-670.

Frye, G.D.; McCown, T.J.; Breese, G.R. (1983b). Differential sensitivity of ethanol withdrawal signs in the rat to gamma-aminobutyric acid (GABA) mimetics: Blockade of audiogenic seizures but not forelimb tremors. *J Pharmacol Exp Ther* 226:720-725.

Gallagher, M.; McMahan, R.W.; Schoenbaum, G. (1999). Orbitofrontal cortex and representation of incentive value in associative learning. *J Neurosci* 19:6610-6614.

Giancola, P.R.; Zeichner, A. (1995). Alcohol-related aggression in males and females: Effects of blood alcohol concentration, subjective intoxication, personality, and provocation. *Alcohol Clin Exp Res* 19:130-134.

Givens, B.S.; Breese, G.R. (1990a). Electrophysiological evidence for an involvement of the medial septal area in the acute sedative effects of ethanol. *J Pharmacol Exp Ther* 253:95-103.

Givens, B.S.; Breese, G.R. (1990b). Site-specific enhancement of γ-aminobutyric acid-mediated inhibition of neural activity by ethanol in the rat medial septum. *J Pharmacol Exp Ther* 254:528-538.

Goldstein, D.B. (1973). Alcohol withdrawal reactions in mice: Effects of drugs that modify neurotransmission. *J Pharmacol Exp Ther* 186:1-9.

Goldstein, D.B.; Pal, N. (1971). Alcohol dependence produced in mice by inhalation of ethanol: Grading the withdrawal reaction. *Science* 172:288-290.

Gonzales, R.A. (1990). NMDA receptors excite alcohol research. *Trends Pharmacol Sci* 11:137-139.

Gonzales, R.; Bungay, P.M.; Kiianmaa, K.; Samson, H.H.; Rossetti, Z.L. (1996). In vivo links between neurochemistry and behavioral effects of ethanol. *Alcohol Clin Exp Res* 20(suppl):203A-205A.

Gonzalez, L.P.; Czachura, J.F. (1989). Reduced behavioral responses to intranigral muscimol following chronic ethanol. *Physiol Behav* 46:473-477.

Gordon, A.S.; Collier, K.; Diamond, I. (1986). Ethanol regulation of adenosine receptor-stimulated cAMP levels in a clonal neural cell line: An in vitro model of cellular tolerance to ethanol. *Proc Natl Acad Sci USA* 83:2105-2108.

Gordon, A.S.; Yao, L.; Wu, Z.L.; Coe, I.R.; Diamond, I. (1997). Ethanol alters the subcellular localization of delta- and epsilon protein kinase C in NG 108-15 cells. *Mol Pharmacol* 52:554-559.

Grant, B.F.; Dawson, D.A. (1997). Age of onset of alcohol use and its association with DSM-IV alcohol abuse and dependence: Results from the National Longitudinal Alcohol Epidemiologic Survey. *J Substance Abuse* 9:103-110.

Grant, K.A.; Colombo, G. (1993). Discriminative stimulus effects of ethanol: Effect of training dose on the substitution of *N*-methyl-D-aspartate antagonists. *J Pharmacol Exp Ther* 264:1261-1247.

Grant, K.A.; Knisely, J.S.; Tabakoff, B.; Barrett, J.E.; Balster, R.L. (1991). Ethanol-like discriminative stimulus effects of noncompetitive *N*-methyl-D-aspartate antagonists. *Behavioral Pharmacology* 2:87-95.

Grant, K.A.; Valverius, P.; Hudspith, M.; Tabakoff, B. (1990). Ethanol withdrawal seizures and the NMDA receptor complex. *Eur J Pharmacol* 176:289-296.

Greenberg, D.A.; Cooper, E.C.; Gordon, A.; Diamond, I. (1984). Ethanol and the γ–aminobutyric acid receptor complex. *J Neurochem* 42:1062-1068.

Gulya, K.; Grant, K.A.; Valverius, P.; Hoffman, P.L.; Tabakoff, B. (1991). Brain regional specificity and time-course of changes in the NMDA receptor-ionophore complex during ethanol withdrawal. *Brain Res* 547:129-134.

Gyenes, M.; Farrant, M.; Farb, D.H. (1988). "Run-down" of γ-aminobutyric acid$_A$ receptor function during whole cell recording: A possible role for phosphorylation. *Mol Pharmacol* 34:719-723.

Halliday, G.; Baker, K.; Harper, C. (1995). Serotonin and alcohol-related brain damage. *Metab Brain Dis* 10:25-30.

Hamelink, C.R.; Carpenter-Hylana, E.P.; Meiri, N.; Ondo, J.G.; Castronguay, T.W.; Eskay, R.L. (1998). Short-term binge alcohol exposure lesions hippocampal-entorhinal cortex and impairs spatial memory. *Society for Neuroscience Abstracts* 24:1239.

Hamelink, C.R.; Hampson, A.J.; Axelrod, J.; Eskay, R.L. (2000). Antioxidants prevent neurotoxicity in a binge-drinking model of alcoholism. *Society for Neuroscience Abstracts* 26:582.3.

Harding, A.J.; Halliday, G.M.; Ng, J.L.; Harper, C.G.; Kril, J.J. (1996). Loss of vasopressin-immunoreactive neurons in alcoholics is dose-related and time-dependent. *Neuroscience* 72:699-708.

Harding, A.J.; Wong, A.; Svoboda, M.; Kril, J.J.; Halliday, G.M. (1997). Chronic alcohol consumption does not cause hippocampal neuron loss in humans. *Hippocampus* 7:78-87.

Harper, C.G.; Kril, J.J. (1990). Neuropathology of alcoholism. *Alcohol* 25:207-216.

Harper, C.G.; Kril, J.J. (1993) Neuropathological changes in alcoholics. In Hunt, W.A.; Nixon, S.J. (Eds.), *Alcohol-Induced Brain Damage,* Vol 22, pp. 39-70. Rockville, MD: NIAAA/NIH.

Harper, C.G.; Kril, J.J.; Daly, J. (1987). Are we drinking our neurons away? *Br Med J* 294:534-536.

Harris, R.A.; McQuilkin, S.J.; Paylor, R.; Abeliovich, A.; Tonegawa, S.; Wehner, J.M. (1995). Mutant mice lacking the gamma isoform of protein kinase C show decreased behavioral actions of ethanol and altered function of gamma-aminobutyrate type A receptors. *Proc Natl Acad Sci USA* 92:3658-3662.

Harris, R.A.; Proctor, W.R.; McQuilkin, S.J.; Klein, R.L.; Mascia, M.P.; Whatley, V.; Whiting, P.J.; Dunwiddie, T.V. (1995). Ethanol increases GABA$_A$ responses in cells stably transfected with receptor subunits. *Alcohol Clin Exp Res* 19:226-232.

Hazell, A.S.; Butterworth, R.F. (1999). Hepatic encephalopathy: An update of pathophysiologic mechanisms. *Proc Soc Exp Biol Med* 222:99-112.

Heuschneider, G.; Schwartz, R.D. (1989). cAMP and forskolin decrease γ-aminobutyric acid-gated chloride flux in rat brain synaptoneurosomes. *Proc Natl Acad Sci USA* 86:2938-2942.

Hoaken, P.N.S.; Giancola, P.R.; Pihl, R.O. (1998). Executive cognitive functions as mediators of alcohol-related aggression. *Alcohol Alcohol* 33:47-54.

Hoffman, P.L.; Moses, F.; Tabakoff, B. (1989). Selective inhibition by ethanol of glutamate-stimulated cyclic GMP production in primary cultures of cerebellar granule cells. *Neuropharmacology* 28:1239-1243.

Hoffman, P.L.; Rabe, C.S.; Moses, F.; Tabakoff, B. (1989). N-methyl-D-aspartate receptors and ethanol: Inhibition of calcium flux and cyclic GMP production. *J Neurochem* 52:1937-1940.

Hollmann, M.; Boulter, J.; Maron, C.; Beasley, L.; Sullivan, J.; Pecht, G.; Heinemann, S. (1993). Zinc potentiates agonist-induced currents at certain splice variants of the NMDA receptor. *Neuron* 10:943-954.

Hollmann, M.; Heineman, S. (1994). Cloned glutamate receptors. *Annu Rev Neurosci* 17:31-108.

Hollmann, M.; O'Shea-Greenfield, A.; Rogers, S.W.; Heinemann, S. (1989). Cloning by functional expression of a member of the glutamate receptor family. *Nature* 342:643-648.

Hommer, D.; Momenan, R.; Rawlings, R.; Ragan, P.; Williams, W.; Rio, D.; Eckardt, M. (1996). Decreased corpus callosum size among alcoholic women. *Arch Neurol* 53:359-363.

Huganir, R.L.; Greengard, P. (1990). Regulation of neurotransmitter receptor desensitization by protein phosphorylation. *Neuron* 5:555-567.

Hunt, W.A. (1983). The effect of ethanol on GABAergic transmission. *Neurosci Biobehav Rev* 7:87-95.

Ibanez, J.; Herrero, M.T.; Insausti, R.; Balzunegui, T.; Tunon, T.; Garcia-Bragado, F.; Gonzalo, L.M. (1995). Chronic alcoholism decreases neuronal nuclear size in the human entorhinal cortex. *Neurosci Lett* 183:71-74.

Igarashi, K.; Williams, K. (1995). Antagonist properties of polyamines and bis(ethyl)polyamines at N-methyl-D-aspartate receptors. *J Pharmacol Exp Ther* 272:1101-1109.

Iorio, K.R.; Reinlib, L.; Tabakoff, B.; Hoffman, P.L. (1992). Chronic exposure of cerebellar granule cells to ethanol results in increased N-methyl-D-aspartate receptor function. *Mol Pharmacol* 41:1142-1148.

Iorio, K.R.; Tabakoff, B.; Hoffman, P.L. (1993). Glutamate-induced neurotoxicity is increased in cerebellar granule cells exposed chronically to ethanol. *Eur J Pharmacol* 248:209-212.

Ishii, T.; Moriyoshi, K.; Sugihara, H.; Sakurada, K.; Kadotani, H.; Tokoi, M.; Akazawa, C.; Shigemoto, R.; Mizuno, N.; Masu, M.; Nakanishi, S. (1993). Molecular characterization of the family of the NMDA receptor subunits. *J Biol Chem* 286:2636-2643.

Jagannathan, M.R.; Desai, M.G.; Raghunathan, P. (1996). Brain metabolite changes in alcoholism: An in vivo proton magnetic resonance spectroscopy. *Magn Reson Imaging* 14:553-557.

Jernigan, T.L.; Butters, N.; DiTraglia, G.; Schafer, K.; Smith, T.; Irwin, M.; Grant, I.; Schuckit, M.; Cermak, L.S. (1991). Reduced cerebral grey matter observed in alcoholics using magnetic resonance imaging. *Alcohol Clin Exp Res* 15:418-427.

Johnson, J.W.; Ascher, P. (1987). Glycine potentiates the NMDA response in cultured mouse brain neurons. *Nature* 325:529-531.

Karanian, J.W.; Yergey, J.; Lister, R.; D'Souza, N.; Linnoila, M.; Salem, N. (1986). Characterization of an automated apparatus for precise control of inhalation chamber ethanol vapor and blood ethanol concentrations. *Alcohol Clin Exp Res* 10:443-447.

Karobath, M.; Rogers, J.; Bloom, F.E. (1980). Benzodiazepine receptors remain unchanged after chronic ethanol administration. *Neuropharmacology* 19:125-128.

Keinanen, K.; Wisden, W.; Sommer, B.; Werner, P.; Herb, A.; Verdoorn, T.A.; Sakmann, B.; Seeburg, P.H. (1990). A family of AMPA-selective glutamate receptors. *Science* 249:556-560.

Kleckner, N.W.; Dingledine, R. (1988). Requirement for glycine in activation of NMDA-receptors expressed in *Xenopus* oocytes. *Science* 241:835-837.

Klein, R.L.; Mascia, M.P.; Whiting, P.J.; Harris, R.A. (1995). GABA$_A$ receptor function and binding in stably transfected cells: Chronic ethanol treatment. *Alcohol Clin Exp Res* 19:1338-1344.

Knapp, D.J.; Crews, F.T. (1999). Induction of cyclooxygenase-2 in brain during acute and chronic ethanol treatment and ethanol withdrawal. *Alcohol Clin Exp Res* 23:1-11.

Knapp, D.J.; Criswell, H.E.; Breese, G.R. (1995). Regional effects of isoproterenol on ethanol enhancement of GABA responses in vivo. *Soc Neurosci Abstr* 21:354.

Knecht, K.; Michalak, A.; Rose, C.; Rothstein, J.D.; Butterworth, R.F. (1997). Decreased glutamate transporters (GLT-1) expression in frontal cortex of rats with acute liver failure. *Neurosci Lett* 229:201-203.

Koltchine, V.; Anantharam, V.; Wilson, A.; Bayley, H.; Treistman, S.N. (1993). Homomeric assemblies of NMDAR1 splice variants are sensitive to ethanol. *Neurosci Lett* 152:13-16.

Koob, G.F.; Le Moal, M. (1997). Drug abuse: Hedonic homeostatic dysregulation. *Science* 278:52-58.

Koob, G.F.; Percy, L.; Britton, K.T. (1989). The effects of Ro15-4513 on the behavioral actions of ethanol in an operant reaction time test and a conflict test. *Pharmacol Biochem Behav* 31:757-760.

Kopelman, M.D.; Corn, T.H. (1988). Cholinergic "blockade" as a model for cholinergic depletion. A comparison of the memory deficits with those of Alzheimer-type dementia and the alcoholic Korsakoff syndrome. *Brain* 111: 1079-1110.

Kubota, Y.; Sato, W.; Murai, T.; Toichi, M.; Ikeda, A.; Sengoku, A. (2000). Emotional cognition without awareness after unilateral temporal lobectomy in humans. *J Neurosci* 20:1-5.

Kumar, K.N.; Tilakaratne, N.; Johnson, P.S.; Allen, A.E.; Michaelis, E.K. (1991). Cloning of cDNA for the glutamate-binding subunit of an NMDA receptor complex. *Nature* 354:70-73.

Kutsuwada, T.; Kashiwabuchi, N.; Mori, H.; Sakimura, K.; Kushiya, E.; Araki, K.; Meguro, H.; Masaki, H.; Kumanishi, T.; Arakawa, M.; Mishina, M. (1992). Molecular diversity of the NMDA receptor channel. *Nature* 358:36-41.

Lambie, D.G. (1985). Alcoholic brain damage and neurological symptoms of alcohol withdrawal—manifestations of overhydration. *Med Hypotheses* 16:377-388.

Langlais, P.J.; Mair, R.G. (1990). Protective effects of the glutamate antagonist MK-801 on pyrithiamine-induced lesions and amino acid changes in rat brain. *J Neurosci* 10:1664-1674.

Langlais, P.J.; Zhang, S.X. (1993). Extracellular glutamate is increased in thalamus during thiamine deficiency-induced lesions and is blocked by MK-801. *J Neurochem* 61:2175-2182.

Laurie, D.J.; Seeburg, P.H. (1994). Regional and developmental heterogeneity in splicing of the rat brain NMDAR1 mRNA. *J Neurosci* 14:335-345.

Lavoie, J.; Giguere, J.F.; Layrargues, G.P.; Butterworth, R.F. (1987). Activities of neuronal and astrocytic marker enzymes in autopsied brain tissue from patients with hepatic encephalopathy. *Metab Brain Dis* 2:283-290.

Lavoie, J.; Layrargues, G.P.; Butterworth, R.F. (1990). Increased densities of peripheral-type benzodiazepine receptors in brain autopsy samples from cirrhotic patients with hepatic encephalopathy. *Hepatology* 11:874-878.

Layrargues, G.P.; Butterworth, R.F. (1992). Efficacy of Ro15-1788 in cirrhotic patients with hepatic coma: Results of a randomized, double-blind placebo-controlled crossover trial. *Hepatology* 16:311-319.

Le, A.D.; Khanna, J.M.; Kalant, H.; Grossi, F. (1986). Tolerance to and cross-tolerance among ethanol, pentobarbital and chlordiazepoxide. *Pharmacol Biochem Behav* 24:93-98.

Ledig, M.; M'Paria, J.; Mandel, P. (1981). Superoxide dismutase activity in rat brain during acute and chronic alcohol intoxication. *Neurochem Res* 6:385-390.

Leidenheimer, N.J.; Browning, M.D.; Dunwiddie, T.V.; Hahner, L.D.; Harris, R.A. (1990). Phosphorylation-independent effects of second messenger system modulators on gamma-aminobutyric acidA receptor complex function. *Mol Pharmacol* 38:823-828.

Levin, L.H.; Koehler, R.C.; Brusilow, S.W.; Jones, J.; Traystman, R.J. (1989). Elevated brain water during urease-induced hyperammonemia in dogs. In Hoff, J.T.; Betz, A.L. (Eds.), *Intracranial Pressure,* pp. 1032-1088. Berlin: Springer-Verlag.

Levitan, E.S.; Schofield, P.R.; Burt, D.R.; Rhee, L.M.; Wisden, W.; Kohler, M.; Fujita, N.; Rodriguez, H.F.; Stephenson, F.A.; Darlison, M.G.; Barnard, E.A.; Seeburg, P.H. (1988). Structural and functional basis for GABA$_A$ receptor heterogeneity. *Nature* 335:76-79.

Lieberman, D.N.; Mody, I. (1994). Regulation of NMDA channel function by endogenous Ca^{2+}-dependent phosphatase. *Nature* 369:235-239.

Liljequist, S.; Engel, J.A. (1984). The effects of GABA and benzodiazepine receptor antagonists on the anti-conflict action of diazepam or ethanol. *Pharmacol Biochem Behav* 21:521-526.

Lima-Landman, M.T.; Albuquerque, E.X. (1989). Ethanol potentiates and blocks NMDA-activated single-channel currents in rat hippocampal pyramidal cells. *FEBS Lett* 247:61-67.

Lin, A.M-Y.; Freund, R.K.; Palmer, M.R. (1991). Ethanol potentiation of GABA-induced electrophysiological responses in cerebellum: Requirement for catecholamine modulation. *Neurosci Lett* 122:154-158.

Lister, R.G. (1988). Partial reversal of ethanol-induced reductions in exploration by two benzodiazepine antagonists (flumazenil and ZK 93426). *Brain Res Bull* 21:765-770.

Lovinger, D.M. (1993). High ethanol sensitivity of recombinant AMPA-type glutamate receptors expressed in mammalian cells. *Neurosci Lett* 159:83-87.

Lovinger, D.M. (1995). Developmental decrease in ethanol inhibition of N-methyl-D-aspartate receptors in rat neocortical neurons: Relation to the actions of ifenprodil. *J Pharmacol Exp Ther* 274:164-172.

Lovinger, D.M.; White, G.; Weight, F.F. (1989). Ethanol inhibits NMDA-activated ion current in hippocampal neurons. *Science* 243:1721-1724.

Lovinger, D.M.; White, G.; Weight, F.F. (1990). NMDA receptor-mediated synaptic excitation selectively inhibited by ethanol in hippocampal slice from adult rat. *J Neurosci* 10:1372-1379.

Lu, W.; Jaatinen, P.; Rintala, J.; Sarviharju, M.; Kiianmaa, K.; Hervonen, A. (1997). Effects of life-long ethanol consumption on rat locus coeruleus. *Alcohol Alcohol* 32:463-470.

Lüddens, H.; Pritchett, D.B.; Kohler, M.; Killisch, I.; Keinanen, K.; Monyer, H.; Sprengel, R.; Seeburg, P.H. (1990). Cerebellar $GABA_A$ receptor selective for a behavioral alcohol antagonist. *Nature* 346:648-651.

Lynch, D.R.; Anegawa, N.J.; Verdoorn, T.; Pritchett, D.B. (1994). N-methyl-D-aspartate receptors: Different subunit requirements for binding of glutamate antagonists, glycine antagonists, and channel-blocking agents. *Mol Pharmacol* 45:540-545.

Lynch, D.R.; Lawrence, J.J.; Lenz, S.; Anegawa, N.J.; Dichter, M.; Pritchett, D.B. (1995). Pharmacological characterization of heterodimeric NMDA receptors composed of NR 1a and 2B subunits: Differences with receptors formed from NR 1a and 2A. *J Neurochem* 64:1462-1468.

Macdonald, R.L.; Olsen, R.W. (1994). GABA A receptor channels. *Annu Rev Neurosci* 17:569-602.

Madeira, M.D.; Andrade, J.P.; Lieberman, A.R.; Sousa, N.; Almeida, O.F.; Paula-Barbosa, M.M. (1997). Chronic alcohol consumption and withdrawal do not induce cell death in the suprachiasmatic nucleus, but lead to irreversible depression of peptide immunoreactivity and mRNA levels. *J Neurosci* 17:1302-1319.

Martin, D.; Tayyeb, M.I.; Swartzwelder, H.S. (1995). Ethanol inhibition of AMPA and kainate receptor-mediated depolarizations of hippocampal area CA1. *Alcohol Clin Exp Res* 19:1312-1316.

Martin, P.R.; Adinoff, B.; Weingartner, H.; Mukherjee, A.B.; Edhardt, M.J. (1986). Alcoholic organic brain disease: Nosology and pathophysiologic mechanisms. *Prog Neuropsychopharmacol Biol Psychiatry* 10:147-164.

Martz, A.; Dietrich, R.A.; Harris, R.A. (1983). Behavioral evidence for the involvement of γ-aminobutyric acid in the actions of ethanol. *Eur J Pharmacol* 89:53-62.

Masood, K.; Wu, C.; Brauneis, U.; Weight, F.F. (1994). Differential ethanol sensitivity of recombinant N-methyl-D-aspartate receptor subunits. *Mol Pharmacol* 45:324-329.

Massey, J.T.; Moore, T.F.; Parsons, V.L.; and Tadros, W. (1989). Design and estimation for the National Health Interview Survey, 1985-1994. *Vital and Health Statistics,* 2(110):1-33. Hyattsville, MD: National Center for Health Statistics.

Matsumoto, I.; Leah, J.; Shanley, B.; Wilce, P. (1993). Immediate early gene expression in the rat brain during ethanol withdrawal. *Mol Cell Neurosci* 4:485-491.

Mayer, M.L.; Westbrook, G.L.; Guthrie, P.B. (1984). Voltage-dependent block by Mg^{2+} of NMDA responses in spinal cord neurons. *Nature* 309:261-263.

McQueen, J.D.; Posey, J.B. (1975). Changes in intracranial pressure and brain hydration during acute ethanolism. *Surgical Neurology* 4(4):375-379.

Meguro, H.H.; Mori, K.; Araki, E.; Kushiya, T.; Kutsuwada, M.; Yamazaki, T.; Kumanishi, M.; Arakawa, T.; Sakimura, S.; Mishina, M. (1992). Functional characterization of a heteromeric NMDA receptor channel expressed from cloned cDNAs. *Nature* 357:70-74.

Mehta, A.K.; Ticku, M.K. (1988). Ethanol potentiation of GABAergic transmission in cultured spinal cord neurons involves γ-aminobutyric acid-gated chloride channels. *J Pharmacol Exp Ther* 246:558-564.

Mehta, A.K.; Ticku, M.K. (1989). Chronic ethanol treatment alters the behavioral effects of Ro 15-4513, a partially negative ligand for benzodiazepine binding sites. *Brain Res* 489:93-100.

Mereu, G.; Gessa, G.L. (1985). Low doses of ethanol inhibit the firing of neurons in the substantia nigra pars reticulata: A GABAergic effect? *Brain Res* 360:325-330.

Messing, R.O.; Petersen, P.J.; Henrich, C.J. (1991). Chronic ethanol exposure increases levels of protein kinase C delta and epsilon and protein kinase C-mediated phosphorylation in cultured neural cells. *J Biol Chem* 266:23428-23432.

Mhatre, M.; Mehta, A.K.; Ticku, M.K. (1988). Chronic ethanol administration increases the binding of the benzodiazepine inverse agonist and alcohol antagonist [3H]Ro15-4513 in rat brain. *Eur J Pharmacol* 153:141-145.

Mhatre, M.C.; Ticku, M.K. (1992). Chronic ethanol administration alters gamma-aminobutyric acidA receptor gene expression. *Mol Pharmacol* 42:415-422.

Mhatre, M.C.; Ticku, M.K. (1993). Alcohol: Effects on GABA$_A$ receptor function and gene expression. *Alcohol Alcohol* Suppl 2:331-335.

Michaelis, E.K.; Freed, W.J.; Galton, N.; Foye, J.; Michaelis, M.L.; Phillips, I.; Kleinmann, J.E. (1990). Glutamate receptor changes in brain synaptic membranes from human alcoholics. *Neurochemical Research* 15:1055-1063.

Mihic, S.J.; McQuilkin, S.J.; Eger, E.I. II; Ionescu, P.; Harris, R.A. (1994). Potentiation of gamma-aminobutyric acid type A receptor-mediated chloride currents by novel halogenated compounds correlates with their abilities to induce general anesthesia. *Mol Pharmacol* 46:851-857.

Mirshahi, T.; Woodward, J.J. (1995). Ethanol sensitivity of heteromeric NMDA receptors: Effects of subunit assembly, glycine and NMDAR1 Mg^{2+}-insensitive mutants. *Neuropharmacology* 34:347-355.

Moghaddam, B.; Bolinao, M.L. (1994). Biphasic effect of ethanol on extracellular accumulation of glutamate in the hippocampus and the nucleus accumbens. *Neurosci Lett* 178:99-102.

Molinoff, P.B.; Williams, K.; Pritchett, D.B.; Zhong, J. (1994). Molecular pharmacology of NMDA receptors: Modulatory role of NR2 subunits. *Prog Brain Res* 100:39-45.

Monaghan, D.T. (1991). Differential stimulation of [3H]-MK-801 binding to subpopulations of NMDA receptors. *Neurosci Lett* 122:21-24.

Montoliu, C.; Sancho-Tello, M.; Azorin, I.; Burgal, M.; Valles, S.; Renau-Piqueras, J.; Guerri, C. (1995). Ethanol increases cytochrome P4502E1 and induces oxidative stress in astrocytes. *J Neurochem* 65:2561-2570.

Montoliu, C.; Valles, S.; Renau-Piqueras, J.; Guerri, C. (1994). Ethanol-induced oxygen radical formation and lipid peroxidation in rat brain: Effect of chronic alcohol consumption. *J Neurochem* 63:1855-1862.

Montpied, P.; Morrow, A.L.; Karanian, J.W.; Ginns, E.I.; Martin, B.M.; Paul, S.M. (1991). Prolonged ethanol inhalation decreases gamma-aminobutyric acid A receptor alpha subunit mRNAs in the rat cerebral cortex. *Mol Pharmacol* 39: 157-163.

Monyer, H.; Burnashev, N.; Laurie, D.J.; Sakmann, B.; Seeburg, P.H. (1994). Developmental and regional expression in rat brain and functional properties of four NMDA receptors. *Neuron* 12:529-540.

Monyer, H.; Sprengel, R.; Schoepfer, R.; Herb, A.; Higuchi, M.; Lomeli, H.; Burnashev, N.; Sakmann, B.; Seeburg, P.H. (1992). Heteromeric NMDA receptors: Molecular and functional distinction of subtypes. *Science* 258:597-603.

Moriyoshi, K.; Masu, M.; Ishii, T.; Shigemoto, R.; Mizuno, N.; Nakanishi, S. (1991). Molecular cloning and characterization of the rat NMDA receptor. *Nature* 354:31-37.

Morrow, A.L.; Herbert, J.S.; Montpied, P. (1992). Differential effects of chronic ethanol administration on $GABA_A$ receptor $\alpha 1$ and $\alpha 6$ subunit mRNA levels in rat cerebellum. *Mol Cell Neurosci* 3:251-258.

Morrow, A.L.; Pace, J.R.; Purdy, R.H.; Paul, S.M. (1990). Characterization of steroid interactions with gamma-aminobutyric acid receptor-gated chloride ion channels: Evidence for multiple steroid recognition sites. *Mol Pharmacol* 37: 263-270.

Morrow, A.L.; Suzdak, P.D.; Paul, S.M. (1988). Chronic ethanol administration alters GABA, pentobarbital and ethanol-mediated $^{36}Cl^-$ uptake in cerebral cortical synaptoneurosomes. *J Pharmacol Exp Ther* 246:158-164.

Nakanishi, N.; Axel, R.; Shneider, N.A. (1992). Alternative splicing generates functionally distinct *N*-methyl-D-aspartate receptors. *Proc Nat Acad Sci USA* 89:8552-8556.

Nayeem, N.; Green, T.P.; Martin, I.L.; Barnard, E.A. (1994). Quarternary structure of the native $GABA_A$ receptor determined by electron microscopic image analysis. *J Neurochem* 62:815-818.

Nestores, J.N. (1980). Ethanol specifically potentiates GABA-mediated neurotransmission in the feline cerebral cortex. *Science* 209:708-710.

Nicolas, C.; Carter, C. (1994). Autoradiographic distribution and characteristics of high- and low-affinity polyamine-sensitive [^{3}H]ifenprodil sites in the rat brain: Possible relationship to NMDAR2B receptors and calmodulin. *J Neurochem* 63:2248-2258.

Nicolas, J.M.; Estruch, R.; Salamero, M.; Orteu, N.; Fernandez-Sola, J.; Sacanella, E.; Urbano-Marquez, A. (1997). Brain impairment in well-nourished chronic alcoholics is related to ethanol intake. *Ann Neurol* 41:590-598.

Nordmann, R. (1987). Oxidative stress from alcohol in the brain. *Alcohol Alcohol* Suppl 1:75-82.

Nordmann, R.; Ribiere, C.; Rouach, H. (1990). Ethanol-induced lipid peroxidation and oxidative stress in extrahepatic tissues. *Alcohol Alcohol* 25:231-237.

Nordmann, R.; Ribiere, C.; Rouach, H. (1992). Implication of free radical mechanisms in ethanol induced cellular injury. *Free Radic Biol* 12:219-240.

Norenberg, M.D.; Huo, Z.; Neary, J.T.; Roig-Cantesano, A. (1997). The glial glutamate transporter in hyperammonemia and hepatic encephalopathy: Relation to energy metabolism and glutamatergic neurotransmission. *Glia* 21:124-133.

Nowak, L.; Bregestovski, P.; Ascher, A.; Herbert, A.; Prochiantz, A. (1984). Magnesium gates glutamate-activated channels in mouse central neurons. *Nature* 307:462-465.

Ortiz, J.; Fitzgerald, L.W.; Charlton, M.; Lane, S.; Trevisan, L.; Guitart, X.; Shoemaker, W.; Duman, R.S.; Nestler, E.J. (1995). Biochemical actions of chronic ethanol exposure in the mesolimbic dopamine system. *Synapse* 21:289-298.

Oscar-Berman, M.; Hutner, N. (1993). Frontal lobe changes after chronic alcohol ingestion. In Hunt, W.A.; Nixon, S.J. (Eds.), *Alcohol-Induced Brain Damage,* Vol 22, pp. 121-156. Rockville, MA: NIAAA/NIH.

Paczynski, R.P.; He, Y.Y.; Diringer, M.N.; Hsu, C.Y. (1997). Multiple-dose mannitol reduces brain water content in a rat model of cortical infarction. *Stroke* 28:1437-1444.

Palmer, M.R.; van Horne, C.G.; Harlan, J.T.; Moore, E.A. (1988). Antagonism of ethanol effects on cerebellar Purkinje neurons by the benzodiazepine inverse agonists Ro15-4513 and FG 7142: Electrophysiological studies. *J Pharmacol Exp Ther* 247:1018-1024.

Parsons, O.A. (1993). Impaired neuropsychological cognitive functioning in sober alcoholics. In Hunt, W.A.; Nixon, S.J. (Eds.), *Alcohol-Induced Brain Damage,* Vol 22, pp. 173-194. Rockville, MD: NIAAA/NIH.

Peoples, R.W.; Weight, F.F. (1992). Ethanol inhibition of *N*-methyl-D-aspartate-activated ion current in rat hippocampal neurons is not competitive with glycine. *Brain Res* 571:342-344.

Peters, S.; Koh, J.; Choi, D.W. (1987). Zinc selectively blocks the action of *N*-methyl-D-aspartate on cortical neurons. *Science* 236:589-593.

Pfefferbaum, A.; Lim, K.O.; Desmond, J.E.; Sullivan, E.V. (1996). Thinning of the corpus callosum in older alcoholic men: A magnetic resonance imaging study. *Alcohol Clin Exp Res* 20:752-757.

Pfefferbaum, A.; Sullivan, E.V.; Mathalon, D.H.; Lim, K.O. (1997). Frontal lobe volume loss observed with magnetic resonance imaging in older chronic alcoholics. *Alcohol Clin Exp Res* 21:521-529.

Pfefferbaum, A.; Sullivan, E.V.; Mathalon, D.H.; Shear, P.K.; Rosenbloom, M.J.; Lim, K.O. (1995). Longitudinal changes in magnetic resonance imaging brain volumes in abstinent and relapsed alcoholics. *Alcohol Clin Exp Res* 19:1177-1191.

Pfefferbaum, A.; Sullivan, E.V.; Rosenbloom, M.J.; Mathalon, D.H.; Lim, K.O. (1998). A controlled study of cortical gray matter and ventricular changes in alcoholic men over a 5-year interval. *Arch Gen Psychiatry* 55:905-912.

Porter, N.M.; Twyman, R.E.; Uhler, M.D.; Macdonald, R.L. (1990). Cyclic AMP-dependent protein kinase decreases $GABA_A$ receptor current in mouse spinal neurons. *Neuron* 5:789-796.

Pritchett, D.B.; Lüddens, H.; Seeburg, P.H. (1989). Type I and type II $GABA_A$-benzodiazepine receptors produced in transfected cells. *Science* 245:1389-1392.

Pritchett, D.B.; Sontheimer, H.; Shivers, B.D.; Ymer, S.; Kettenmann, H.; Schofield, P.R.; Seeburg, P.H. (1989). Importance of a novel $GABA_A$ receptor subunit for benzodiazepine pharmacology. *Nature* 338:582-585.

Prochasta, J.O.; DiClemente, C.D. (1992). Stages of change in the modification of problem behaviors. *Prog Behav Modif* 28:183-218.

Puia, G.; Ducic, I.; Vicini, S.; Costa, E. (1994). Does neurosteroid modulatory efficacy depend on $GABA_A$ receptor subunit composition? *Receptors Channels* 1:135-142.

Puia, G.; Vicini, S.; Seeburg, P.H.; Costa, E. (1991). Influence of recombinant gamma-aminobutyric acid-A receptor subunit composition on the action of allosteric modulators of gamma-aminobutyric acid-gated Cl⁻ currents. *Mol Pharmacol* 39:691-696.

Rabe, C.S.; Tabakoff, B. (1990). Glycine site-directed agonists reverse the actions of ethanol at the *N*-methyl-D-aspartate receptor. *Mol Pharmacol* 38:753-757.

Rabin, R.A.; Edelman, A.M.; Wagner, J.A. (1992). Activation of protein kinase A is necessary but not sufficient for ethanol-induced desensitization of cyclic AMP production. *J Pharmacol Exp Ther* 262:257-262.

Ransom, R.W.; Stec, N.L. (1988). Cooperative modulation of [³H]MK-801 binding to the *N*-methyl-D-aspartate receptor ion channel complex by L-glutamate, glycine, and polyamines. *J Neurochem* 51:830-836.

Rao, A.; Craig, A.M. (1997). Activity regulates the synaptic localization of the NMDA receptor in hippocampal neurons. *Neuron* 19:801-812.

Rao, V.L.; Giguere, J.F.; Layrargues, G.P.; Butterworth, R.F. (1993). Increased activities of MAO_A and MAO_B in autopsied brain tissue from cirrhotic patients with hepatic encephalopathy. *Brain Res* 621:349-352.

Rastogi, S.K.; Thyagarajan, R.; Clothier, J.; Ticku, M.K. (1986). Effect of chronic treatment of ethanol on benzodiazepine and picrotoxin sites on the GABA receptor complex in regions of the brain of the rat. *Neuropharmacology* 25:1179-1184.

Reynolds, I.J. (1990). Arcaine uncovers dual interactions of polyamines with the *N*-methyl-D-aspartate receptor. *J Pharmacol Exp Ther* 255:1001-1007.

Reynolds, I.J.; Miller, R.J. (1989). Ifenprodil is a novel type of *N*-methyl-D-aspartate receptor antagonist: Interaction with polyamines. *Mol Pharmacol* 36:758-765.

Reynolds, I.J.; Murphy, S.N.; Miller, R.J. (1987). 3H-labeled MK-801 binding to the excitatory amino acid receptor complex from rat brain is enhanced by glycine. *Proc Natl Acad Sci USA* 84:7744-7748.

Reynolds, J.N.; Prasad, A. (1991). Ethanol enhances $GABA_A$ receptor-activated chloride currents in chick cerebral cortical neurons. *Brain Res* 564:138-142.

Rock, D.M.; Macdonald, R.L. (1995). Polyamine regulation of *N*-methyl-D-aspartate receptor channels. *Annu Rev Pharmacol Toxicol* 35:463-482.

Roivainen, R.; McMahon, T.; Messing, R.O. (1993). Protein kinase C isozymes that mediate enhancement of neurite outgrowth by ethanol and phorbol esters in PC12 cells. *Brain Res* 624:85-93.

Ron, M.A.; Acker, R.W.; Shaw, G.K.; Lishman, W.A. (1982). Computerized tomography of the brain in chronic alcoholism: A survey and follow-up study. *Brain* 105:497-514.

Rossetti, Z.L.; Carboni, S. (1995). Ethanol withdrawal is associated with increased extracellular glutamate in the rat striatum. *Eur J Pharmacol* 283:177-183.

Rouach, H.; Park, M.K.; Orfanelli, M.T.; Janvier, B.; Nordmann, R. (1987). Ethanol-induced oxidative stress in the rat cerebellum. *Alcohol Alcohol* 22:207-211.

Rudolph, J.G.; Walker, D.W.; Iimuro, Y.; Thurman, R.G.; Crews, F.T. (1997). NMDA receptor binding in adult rat brain after several chronic ethanol treatment protocols. *Alcohol Clin Exp Res* 21:1508-1519.

Ryan-Jastrow, T.; Macdonald, R.L. (1993). Ethanol sensitivity of recombinant $\alpha 1\beta 1\gamma 2$ $GABA_A$ receptors expressed in mammalian cells do not require the $\gamma 2L$ splice variant. *Soc Neurosci Abstr* 19:852.

Sanna, E.; Serra, M.; Cossu, A.; Colombo, G.; Follesa, P.; Cuccheddu, T.; Concas, A.; Biggio, G. (1993). Chronic ethanol intoxication induces differential effects on $GABA_A$ and NMDA receptor function in the rat brain. *Alcohol Clin Exp Res* 17:115-123.

Schofield, P.R. (1989). The $GABA_A$ receptor: Molecular biology reveals a complex picture. *Trends Pharmacol Sci* 10:476-478.

Schofield, P.R.; Darlison, M.G.; Fujita, N.; Burt, D.R.; Stephenson, F.A.; Rodriguez, H.; Rhee, L.M.; Ramachandran, J.; Reale, V.; Glencorse, T.A.; et al. (1987). Sequence and functional expression of the $GABA_A$ receptor shows a ligand-gated super-family. *Nature* 328:221-227.

Seeburg, P.H.; Wisden, W.; Verdoorn, T.A.; Pritchett, D.B.; Werner, P.; Herb, A.; Lüddens, H.; Sprengel, R.; Sakmann, B. (1990). The GABA$_A$ receptor family: Molecular and functional diversity. *Cold Spring Harbor Sym Quant Biol* 55:29-38.

Sellers, E.M.; Kalant, H. (1976). Alcohol intoxication and withdrawal. *New Eng J Med* 294:757-762.

Sheng, M.; Cummings, J.; Roldan, L.A.; Jan, Y.N.; Jan, L.Y. (1994). Changing subunit composition of heteromeric NMDA receptors during development of rat cortex. *Nature* 368:144-147.

Sigel, E.; Baur, R.; Malherbe, P. (1993). Recombinant GABA$_A$ receptor function and ethanol. *FEBS Lett* 324:140-142.

Simson, P.E.; Criswell, H.E.; Breese, G.R. (1993). Inhibition of NMDA-evoked electrophysiological activity by ethanol in selected brain regions: Evidence for ethanol-sensitive and ethanol-insensitive NMDA responses. *Brain Res* 607:9-16.

Simson, P.E.; Criswell, H.E.; Johnson, K.B.; Breese, G.R. (1991). Ethanol inhibits NMDA-evoked electrophysiological activity in vivo. *J Pharmacol Exp Ther* 257:225-231.

Skolnick, P.; Paul, S.M. (1982). Molecular pharmacology of the benzodiazepines. *Int Rev Neurobiol* 23:103-140.

Snell, L.D.; Tabakoff, B.; Hoffman, P.L. (1993). Radioligand binding to the *N*-methyl-D-aspartate receptor/ionophore complex: Alterations by ethanol in vitro and by chronic in vivo ethanol ingestion. *Brain Res* 602:91-98.

Snell, L.D.; Tabakoff, B.; Hoffman, P.L. (1994). Involvement of protein kinase C in ethanol-induced inhibition of NMDA receptor function in cerebellar granule cells. *Alcohol Clin Exp Res* 18:81-85.

Sommer, B.; Seeburg, P.H. (1992). Glutamate receptor channels: Novel properties and new clones. *Trends Pharmacol Sci* 13:291-296.

Sprengel, R.; Seeburg, P.H. (1993). The unique properties of glutamate receptor channels. *FEBS Lett* 325:90-94.

Standaert, D.G.; Testa, C.M.; Penney, J.B.; Young, A.B. (1993). Alternatively spliced isoforms of the NMDAR1 receptor subunit: Differential expression in the basal ganglia of the rat. *Neurosci Lett* 152:161-164.

Stelzer, A.; Kay, A.R.; Wong, R.K.S. (1988). GABA$_A$ receptor function in hippocampal cells is maintained by phosphorylation factors. *Science* 241:339-341.

Sugihara, H.; Moriyoshi, K.; Ishii, T.; Masu, M.; Nakanishi, S. (1992). Structures and properties of seven isoforms of the NMDA receptor generated by alternative splicing. *Biochem Biophys Res Commun* 185:826-832.

Sullivan, E.V.; Marsh, L.; Mathalon, D.H.; Lim, K.O.; Pfefferbaum, A. (1996). Relationship between alcohol withdrawal seizures and temporal lobe white matter volume deficits. *Alcohol Clin Exp Res* 20:348-354.

Sullivan, E.V.; Rosenbloom, M.J.; Lim, K.O.; Pfefferbaum, A. (2000). Longitudinal changes in cognition, gait, and balance in abstinent and relapsed alcoholic men: Relationships to changes in brain structure. *Neuropsychology* 14:178-188.

Sullivan, E.V.; Rosenbloom, M.J.; Pfefferbaum, A. (2000). Pattern of motor and cognitive deficits in detoxified alcoholic men. *Alcohol Clin Exp Res* 24:611-621.

Sullivan, J.M.; Traynelis, S.F.; Hen, H-S.V.; Escobar, W.; Heinemann, S.F.; Lipton, S.A. (1994). Identification of two cystine residues that are required for redox modulation of NMDA subtype of glutamate receptor. *Neuron* 13:929-936.

Suzdak, P.D.; Glowa, J.R.; Crawley, J.N.; Schwartz, R.D.; Skolnick, P.; Paul, S.M. (1986). A selective imidazobenzodiazepine antagonist of ethanol in the rat. *Science* 234:1243-1247.

Suzdak, P.D.; Glowa, J.R.; Crawley, J.N.; Skolnick, P.; Paul, S.M. (1988). Is ethanol antagonist Ro15-4513 selective for ethanol? Response to K.T. Britton et al. *Science* 239:649-650.

Suzdak, P.D.; Schwartz, R.D.; Paul, S.M. (1987). Alcohols stimulate GABA receptor-mediated chloride uptake in brain vesicles: Correlation with intoxication potency. *Brain Res* 444:340-344.

Suzdak, P.D.; Schwartz, R.D.; Skolnick, P.; Paul, S.M. (1986). Ethanol stimulates γ-aminobutyric acid receptor-mediated chloride transport in rat brain synaptoneurosomes. *Proc Natl Acad Sci USA* 83:4071-4075.

Tabakoff, B. (1995). Ethanol's action on the $GABA_A$ receptor: Is there a requirement for parsimony? *Alcohol Clin Exp Res* 24:810-821.

Takahashi, H.; Koehler, R.C.; Brusilow, S.W.; Traystman, R.J. (1991). Inhibition of brain glutamine accumulation prevents cerebral edema in hyperammonemia in rats. *Am J Physiol* 281:H826-H829.

Thornton, J.R.; Losowsky, M.S. (1988). Plasma methionine enkephalin concentration and prognosis in primary biliary cirrhosis. *Br Med J* 297:1241-1242.

Thyagarajan, R.; Ticku, M.K. (1985). The effect of in vitro and in vivo ethanol administration on [35S]t-butylbicyclophosphorothionate binding in C57 mice. *Brain Res Bull* 15:343-345.

Ticku, M.K.; Burch, T. (1980). Alterations in gamma-aminobutyric acid receptor sensitivity following acute and chronic ethanol treatments. *J Neurochem* 34: 417-423.

Ticku, M.K.; Lowrimore, P.; Lehoullier, P. (1986). Ethanol enhances GABA-induced $^{36}Cl^-$ influx in primary spinal cord cultured neurons. *Brain Res Bull* 17:123-126.

Trevisan, L.; Fitzgerald, L.W.; Brose, N.; Gasic, G.P.; Heinemann, S.F.; Duman, R.S.; Nestler, E.J. (1994). Chronic ingestion of ethanol up-regulates NMDAR1 receptor subunit immunoreactivity in rat hippocampus. *J Neurochem* 62:1635-1638.

Unwin, J.W.; Taberner, P.V. (1980). Sex and strain differences in GABA receptor binding after chronic ethanol drinking in mice. *Neuropharmacology* 19:1257-1259.

Unwin, N. (1989). The structure of ion channels in membranes of excitable cells. *Neuron* 3:665-676.

Uysal, M.; Keyer-Uysal, M.; Kocak-Toker, N.; Aykac, G. (1986). Effect of chronic ethanol ingestion on brain lipid peroxide and glutathione levels in rats. *Drug Alcohol Depend* 18:73-75.

Uysal, M.; Kutalp, G.; Ozdemirler, G.; Aykac, G. (1989). Ethanol-induced changes in lipid peroxidation and glutathione content in rat brain. *Drug Alcohol Depend* 23:227-230.

Vaillant, G.E. (1996). A long-term follow-up of male alcohol abuse. *Arch Gen Psychiatry* 53:243-249.

Valenzuela, C.F.; Bhave, S.; Hoffman, A.; Harris, R.A. (1998). Acute effects of ethanol on pharmacologically isolated kainate receptors in cerebellar granule neurons: Comparison with NMDA and AMPA receptors. *J Neurochem* 71:1777-1780.

Valenzuela, C.F.; Cardoso, R.A.; Lickteig, R.; Browning, M.D.; Nixon, K.M. (1998). Acute effects of ethanol on recombinant kainate receptors: Lack of role of protein phosphorylation. *Alcohol Clin Exp Res* 22:1292-1299.

Valenzuela, C.F.; Machu, T.K.; McKernan, R.M.; Whiting, P.; VanRenterghem, B.B.; McManaman, J.L.; Brozowski, S.J.; Smith, G.B.; Olsen, R.W.; Harris, R.A. (1995). Tyrosine kinase phosphorylation of $GABA_A$ receptors. *Brain Res Mol Brain Res* 31:165-172.

Volicer, L. (1980). GABA levels and receptor binding after acute and chronic ethanol administration. *Brain Res Bull* 5:809-813.

Volicer, L.; Biagioni, T.M. (1982a). Effect of ethanol administration and withdrawal on benzodiazepine receptor binding in the rat brain. *Neuropharmacology* 21:283-286.

Volicer, L.; Biagioni, T.M. (1982b). Effect of ethanol administration and withdrawal on GABA receptor binding in rat cerebral cortex. *Subst Alcohol Actions Misuse* 3:31-39.

Wafford, K.A.; Burnett, D.M.; Dunwiddie, T.V.; Harris, R.A. (1990). Genetic differences in the ethanol sensitivity of $GABA_A$ receptors expressed in *Xenopus* oocytes. *Science* 249:291-293.

Wafford, K.A.; Burnett, D.M.; Leidenheimer, N.J.; Burt, D.R.; Wang, J.B.; Kofuji, P.; Dunwiddie, T.V.; Harris, R.A.; Sikela, J.M. (1991). Ethanol sensitivity of the $GABA_A$ receptor expressed in *Xenopus* oocytes requires 8 amino acids contained in the gamma 2L subunit. *Neuron* 7:27-33.

Wafford, K.A.; Whiting, P.J. (1992). Ethanol potentiation of $GABA_A$ receptors requires phosphorylation of the alternatively spliced variant of the gamma2 subunit. *FEBS Lett* 313:113-117.

Wang, J.B.; Burt, D.R. (1991). Differential expression of two forms of $GABA_A$ receptor gamma2-subunit in mice. *Brain Res Bull* 27:731-735.

Watkins, J.C. (1962). The synthesis of some acidic amino acids possessing neuropharmacological activity. *J Med Pharm Chem* 5:1187-1199.

Weight, F.F. (1992). Cellular and molecular physiology of alcohol actions in the nervous system. *Int Rev of Neurobiol* 33:289-348.

Weight, F.F.; Peoples, R.W.; Wright, J.M.; Li, C.; Aguayo, L.G.; Lovinger, D.M.; White, G. (1993). Neurotransmitter-gated ion channels as molecular sites of alcohol action. In Alling, C. (Ed.), *Alcohol, Cell Membranes, and Signal Transduction in Brain,* pp. 107-122. New York: Plenum Press.

Weiner, J.L.; Dunwiddie, T.V.; Valenzuela, C.F. (1999). Ethanol inhibition of synaptically evoked kainate responses in rat hippocampal CA3 pyramidal neurons. *Mol Pharmacol* 56:85-90.

Weiss, M.H.; Craig, J.R. (1978). The influence of acute ethanol intoxication on intracranial physical dynamics. *Bull Los Angeles Neurol Soc* 43:1-5.

Westbrook, G.L.; Mayer, M.L. (1987). Micromolar concentration of Zn^{2+} antagonize NMDA and GABA responses of hippocampal neurons. *Nature* 328:640-643.

White, G.; Gurley, D.A. (1995). Primate-derived $GABA_A$ α1, α2, α3, α5 subunits in combination with either ß1γ2L, ß2g2L, form twelve pharmacologically distinct receptor subtypes in *Xenopus* oocytes. *Soc Neurosci Abstr* 21:850.

Whiting, P.; McKernan, R.M.; Iversen, L.L. (1990). Another mechanism for creating diversity in γ-aminobutyrate type A receptors: RNA splicing directs expression of two forms of gamma 2 phosphorylation site. *Proc Natl Acad Sci USA* 87:9966-9970.

Whittemore, E.R.; Yang, W.; Drewe, J.A.; Woodward, R.M. (1995). Functional and pharmacological characterization of the human $GABA_A$ receptor α4 subunit expressed in *Xenopus* oocytes. *Soc Neurosci Abstr* 21:850.

Williams, K.; Russel, S.L.; Shen, Y.M.; Molinoff, P.B. (1993). Developmental switch in the expression of NMDA receptors occurs in vivo and in vitro. *Neuron* 10:267-278.

Williams, K.; Zappia, A.M.; Pritchett, D.B.; Shen, Y.M.; Molinoff, P.B. (1994). Sensitivity of the *N*-methyl-D-aspartate receptor to polyamines is controlled by NR2 subunits. *Mol Pharmacol* 45:803-809.

Wilson, W.R.; Bosy, T.Z.; Ruth, J.A. (1990). NMDA agonists and antagonists alter the hypnotic response to ethanol in LS and SS mice. *Alcohol* 7:389-395.

Wisden, W.; Herb, A.; Wieland, H.; Keinänen, K.; Lüddens, H.; Seeburg, P.H. (1991). Cloning, pharmacological characteristics, and expression pattern of the rat $GABA_A$ receptor α4 subunit. *FEBS Lett* 289:227-230.

Wright, M.S.; Sefland, I.; Walaas, S.I. (1993). Cloning of the long intracellular loop of the AMPA-selective glutamate receptor for phosphorylation studies. *J Receptor Res* 13:653-665.

Yamazaki, M.; Araki, K.; Shibata, A.; Mishina, M. (1992). Molecular cloning of a cDNA encoding a novel member of the mouse glutamate receptor channel family. *Biochem Biophys Res Commun* 183:886-892.

Yang, X.; Criswell, H.E.; Simson, P.; Moy, S.S.; Breese, G.R. (1996). Evidence for a selective effect of ethanol on NMDA responses: Ethanol affects a subtype of the ifenprodil-sensitive NMDA receptor. *J Pharmacol Exp Ther* 278:782-786.

Ymer, S.; Schofield, P.R.; Draguhn, A.; Werner, P.; Kohler, M.; Seeburg, P.H. (1989). $GABA_A$ receptor ß subunit heterogeneity: Functional expression of cloned cDNAs. *EMBO J* 8:1665-1670.

Yoneda, Y.; Enomoto, R.; Kiyokazu, O. (1994). Supporting evidence for negative modulation by protons of an ion channel associated with the *N*-methyl-D-aspartate receptor complex in rat brain using ligand binding techniques. *Brain Res* 636:298-307.

Young, S.N.; Lal, S.; Feldmuller, F.; Aranoff, A.; Martin, J.B. (1975). Relationships between tryptophan in serum and CSF and 5-hydroxyindoleacetic acid in CSF of man: Effects of cirrhosis of the liver and probenecid administration. *J Neurol Neurosurg Psychiatry* 38:322-330.

Zhang, J-H.; Gong, Z.H.; Hellstrom-Lindahl, E.; Nordberg, A. (1995). Regulation of α4 and ß2 nicotinic acetylcholine receptors in M10 cells following treatment with nicotinic agents. *NeuroReport* 6:313-317.

Zhong, J.; Russell, S.L.; Pritchett, D.B.; Molinoff, P.B.; Williams, K. (1994). Expression of mRNAs encoding subunits of the N-methyl-D-aspartate receptor in cultured cortical neurons. *Mol Pharmacol* 45:846-853.

Zou, J.Y.; Martinez, D.B.; Neafsey, E.J.; Collins, M.D. (1996). Binge ethanol-induced brain damage in rats: Effect of inhibitors of nitric oxide synthase. *Alcohol Clin Exp Res* 20(8)1406-1411.

Chapter 5

Neuroanatomical and Neurobehavioral Effects of Heavy Prenatal Alcohol Exposure

Tara S. Wass
Sarah N. Mattson
Edward P. Riley

OVERVIEW

Suspicions about the harmful effects of prenatal alcohol exposure have surfaced throughout history (Streissguth, 1997). However, these suspicions were for the most part unsubstantiated until researchers in France (Lemoine et al., 1968) and the United States (Jones et al., 1973; Jones and Smith, 1973) identified a cluster of abnormalities in the children of female alcohol abusers, which came to be referred to as fetal alcohol syndrome (FAS). Three criteria provide the basis for the FAS diagnosis: a characteristic pattern of craniofacial anomalies, growth retardation, and central nervous system (CNS) dysfunction (Jones et al., 1973). Although the diagnostic criteria for FAS have been scrutinized and even criticized because many children thought to be affected by prenatal alcohol exposure do not meet criteria for the diagnosis, FAS continues to be diagnosed on the basis of the triad of features delineated in those original articles (Institute of Medicine [IOM], 1996).

The effects of prenatal alcohol exposure may be viewed as a continuum with FAS and fetal death at the extreme end of the spectrum. At the opposite end of the spectrum, there may be no observable effect on the fetus following minimal exposure. A wide range of effects has been observed between these extremes, including attention deficits, learning disabilities, and physical birth defects (IOM, 1996). The term fetal alcohol effects (FAE) has been used to refer to alcohol-exposed children who do not meet the diagnostic criteria for FAS but exhibit one or more of these effects. However, this term has repeatedly been criticized because of its lack of diagnostic specificity

This research was funded by grants AA10417 and AA07456 from NIAAA.

139

(Aase et al., 1995; IOM, 1996). In response to these criticisms, the Institute of Medicine (1996) proposed several diagnostic categories for alcohol-exposed children who did not meet the criteria for an FAS diagnosis. Two of these diagnoses, alcohol-related neurodevelopmental disorder (ARND) and alcohol-related birth defects (ARBD), are particularly important because they enable the classification of alcohol-affected children who do not present with craniofacial anomalies characteristic of FAS. These children may be particularly at risk for the development of secondary disabilities because they are not identified early in life and frequently do not qualify for services, although they display neurobehavioral deficits that are comparable to those observed in children with FAS (Streissguth et al., 1997; Mattson et al., 1997; Mattson et al., 1999).

Estimating the number of children affected by prenatal alcohol exposure can be difficult, in part due to the diagnostic issues just mentioned. Several studies have provided incidence estimates of FAS in the United States and around the world. One study estimated the worldwide incidence of FAS at 0.97 cases per 1,000 live births (Abel and Sokol, 1991). However, this may be an underestimate as others have argued that the true incidence of FAS is between 2.8 and 4.6 cases per 1,000 live births in the United States and Western European countries (Sampson et al., 1997). Sampson et al. (1997) further estimated the combined prevalence rate of FAS and ARND to be at least 9.1 cases per 1,000 live births. The Centers for Disease Control (CDC, 1995) estimated that the incidence of alcohol-affected births has increased from 1.0 affected child per 1,000 live births in 1979 to 6.7 affected children per 1,000 live births in 1993. Overall, these statistics suggest that alcohol may be a bigger public health threat than previously realized.

Since the identification of FAS, a multitude of animal and human studies have examined the impact of prenatal alcohol exposure on the developing organism. The most obvious and debilitating effects of heavy prenatal alcohol exposure are the persistent and pervasive neurobehavioral deficits which may include reductions in IQ, deficits in learning and memory, attention deficits, and increased behavioral problems (Mattson et al., 1998). These neurobehavioral changes are presumed to reflect alcohol-induced changes in the structure and/or function of the brain. To date, numerous studies have begun to characterize the neuropathological changes present in the brains of children with FAS or heavy prenatal exposure to alcohol (PEA) as a means of understanding the neurological underpinnings of the disorder and providing direction for further refining the behavioral phenotype of FAS. The current chapter reviews findings from autopsy, structural imaging, and functional imaging studies on children with FAS and PEA. In addition, research on cognitive and psychosocial functioning is briefly reviewed.

AUTOPSY STUDIES

Evidence that prenatal alcohol exposure affects human brain development first came from autopsy studies. Clarren (1986) summarized the findings from the first 16 autopsy reports that were available for infants with FAS who died within a year of birth. Since that time, a total of 25 autopsies have been reported and reviewed (Mattson and Riley, 1996).

The first autopsy was conducted on the child of a chronic alcoholic mother (Jones and Smith, 1973). The child, who was delivered at 32-weeks gestation and died at five days of age, had an abnormally small brain (microcephaly). Further, the child's left cerebral hemisphere was covered by a leptomeningeal neuroglial heterotopia, an abnormal sheet of neural and glial tissue. Below the leptomeningeal neuroglial heterotopia there was evidence of extensive neuronal disorganization, which ranged from cortical thinning to an absence of the normative laminar structure of the cortex. Abnormalities were not localized solely in the cerebral cortex. Agenesis (absence) of the corpus callosum and the anterior commissure were noted, as were abnormalities in both the cerebellum and the brainstem. The cerebellum was small and poorly shaped, while the medulla was covered by another small leptomeningeal neuroglial heterotopia. Thus, in this first autopsy case, damage to the brain was extensive and widespread.

Later autopsies have similarly reported widespread damage to cortical and subcortical structures following heavy prenatal exposure to alcohol. By far, the most consistent and common neuropathological change is a reduction in the size of the cranium, also referred to as microcephaly. Samson (1986) reported that microcephaly is present in more than 80 percent of children with FAS. In a review of autopsies done on children with FAS who died within one year of birth, Clarren (1986) reported that 56 percent of cases had microcephaly. In a later review, Mattson and Riley (1996) found that 73 percent of the 22 autopsy or MRI cases had microcephaly. Microcephaly could be caused by a variety of different mechanisms including disruptions in neuronal generation, neuronal differentiation, the establishment and maintenance of synaptic connections between neurons, and increased cell death. Many of these effects have been observed in animal models of FAS (Guerri, 1998; Bonthius and West, 1990; Miller, 1988).

Porencephaly and hydrocephaly have also been reported (Clarren et al., 1978; Peiffer et al., 1979). Hydrocephaly is characterized by an overabundance of cerebrospinal fluid (CSF), which results in enlargement of the ventricles. Enlargement of the ventricles causes the cerebral gray matter to be displaced and compressed, ultimately resulting in neuronal damage if the pressure is not released. In contrast, porencephaly is characterized by one or more fluid-filled cysts in the cerebral cortex, which are typically caused by a brain hemorrhage, trauma, or partial to complete occlusion of blood vessels.

Another neuropathological finding is holoprosencephaly (Jellinger et al., 1981; Coulter et al., 1993), a condition in which the forebrain fails to completely develop into two hemispheres. In the most severe cases, referred to as alobar holoprosencephaly, there is a complete fusion of all forebrain structures. Ronen and Andrews (1991) presented one case of alobar holoprosencephaly and two less-severe cases of semilobar holoprosencephaly. In all three cases there was only a single "square-shaped ventricle" and midline fusion of the basal ganglia and thalamic nuclei (p. 152). Holoprosencephaly has been induced in nonhuman primate and mouse models of FAS (Siebert et al., 1991; Sulik and Johnston, 1982), further strengthening the suggestion that alcohol exposure is one possible cause of this disorder. Finally, it is interesting to note that infants with FAS or holoprosencephaly both exhibit midline facial anomalies (Ronen and Andrews, 1991), although the anomalies observed in the two disorders are not identical. In both disorders, the severity of these craniofacial anomalies may covary with the severity of the underlying neuropathological abnormalities (Swayze et al., 1997).

In addition to these macroscopic cortical anomalies, microscopic changes and abnormalities resulting from abnormal neuronal and glial cell migration have frequently been reported. These include ectopic neurons scattered throughout the cortex, nonspecific cerebral disorganization or dysgenesis, incompletely developed sulci, and polymicrogyria (Clarren et al., 1978; Coulter et al., 1993; Wisniewski et al., 1983; Peiffer et al., 1979; Konovalov et al., 1997).

Abnormalities are not limited to the cerebral cortex. Both cerebellar and brainstem anomalies have been documented. For example, brainstem abnormalities have included absence of the pons and medulla, leptomeningeal neuroglial heterotopias, and brainstem dysgenesis (Clarren et al., 1978; Peiffer et al., 1979). Cerebellar abnormalities have been more widely reported and include underdevelopment of the cerebellum or the cerebellar vermis, hyperplastic folds of the cerebellum, and agenesis of the cerebellar vermis (Clarren et al., 1978; Wisniewski et al., 1983; Peiffer et al., 1979; Konovalav et al., 1997). In all, 10 of the 16 autopsy cases reviewed by Clarren (1986) displayed evidence of cerebellar abnormalities.

Agenesis of the corpus callosum and the anterior commissure was noted in Clarren and colleagues' original autopsy case (Jones and Smith, 1973). Two additional autopsy cases have presented with agenesis of the corpus callosum and one also presented with agenesis of the anterior commissure (Peiffer et al., 1979; Wisniewski et al., 1983). When the corpus callosum is present significant thinning has been reported (Clarren et al., 1978; Coulter et al., 1993).

A variety of other abnormalities have been found in numerous autopsy cases. These include fusion of the thalami or basal ganglia nuclei, absence of the olfactory bulbs, and hypoplasia of the optic nerves and hippocampus (Peiffer et al., 1979; Wisniewski, 1983; Coulter et al., 1993).

Even a cursory examination of the autopsy findings suggests that the damage caused by prenatal exposure to alcohol is widespread. On the basis of these autopsy findings, Clarren (1986) argued that due to the variability in the neuropathological findings in children with FAS, future research would be unable to document a pattern of behavioral or neuropsychological deficits that is representative of all children with FAS. While others have agreed with this position (Peiffer et al., 1979), it may be premature to presume that no commonalities in the neurological underpinnings or phenotypic expression of FAS will emerge across children. The cases evaluated in the autopsy studies represent the extreme for children with FAS. Primate studies suggest that prenatal alcohol exposure may not be lethal in the majority of cases. Two nonhuman primate studies have demonstrated that although exposure does decrease viability, 68 to 70 percent of exposed cases were live born (Clarren et al., 1987; Clarren and Astley, 1992). Further, only 6 percent (3 out of 47) of the live-born alcohol-exposed infants died within the first six months of life. Thus, in the vast majority of cases, prenatal alcohol exposure is not lethal, which suggests that the cases reviewed in the autopsy studies may be more severely affected than the average child with FAS. Consequently, it is possible that an examination of the brains of children with FAS who have survived will yield a more consistent pattern of neuropathological findings. Rapid advances in structural and functional imaging techniques have enabled researchers to examine living children with FAS or PEA and a much more consistent pattern of neuropathological findings is beginning to emerge.

MAGNETIC RESONANCE IMAGING STUDIES

Brain imaging techniques, such as magnetic resonance imaging (MRI) have become increasingly popular tools for documenting structural changes in the brain associated with various developmental disorders. These techniques have the potential to advance our understanding of the neurological changes associated with disorders such as FAS. Some MRI studies have provided clinical assessments and descriptions of MRI scans, indicating whether the images are normal or abnormal, while others have gone a step further and assessed the size of structures. Both techniques are important, although the latter techniques have proved more useful in the investigation of disorders caused by an insult to the brain in utero.

Clinical assessments of MRI data are sensitive to gross structural malformations of the brain that can be detected by the human eye. However, subtle changes such as small reductions in volume may not be observable. Further, clinical assessments negate the possibility of controlling for alcohol's global effect on the brain when examining individual brain structures. Since we already know that prenatal alcohol exposure frequently results in a reduction in overall brain size, it may be more informative to determine whether this reduction is uniform across the brain or whether certain structures appear to be more susceptible to alcohol's teratogenic effects. Certainly, isolated reductions in discrete brain structures would have important implications for the behavioral phenotype of FAS.

Cerebral Cortex

The most consistent and common neuropathological change associated with heavy prenatal alcohol exposure is a reduction in overall head or brain size (Roebuck et al., 1998). In a series of structural MRI studies, a significant reduction in cranial vault volume of children with FAS or PEA has been documented (Mattson et al., 1992; Mattson et al., 1994; Mattson, Riley, Sowell, et al., 1996; Archibald et al., 2001). PEA children are those with known histories of exposure to large amounts of alcohol in utero, but without the features of FAS. In one study, these reductions were accompanied by increases in cortical and subcortical fluid, which is further suggestive of brain atrophy (Mattson et al., 1992). Studies from other laboratories have noted cortical atrophy, enlargement of the lateral ventricles, and enlargement of the subarachnoid space, which are consistent with brain atrophy and reductions in overall brain size (Riikonen et al., 1999; Robin and Zachai, 1994; Swayze et al., 1997; Johnson et al., 1996; Goldstein and Arulanantham, 1978). In addition to microcephaly, imaging studies have documented other changes to the cortex, including a large infarct in the left hemisphere, delayed myelination, multifocal encephalopathy, and an abnormal configuration of the occipital lobes (Riikonen et al., 1999; Gabrielli et al., 1990; Clark et al., 2000).

Until recently, studies had not addressed whether the impact of prenatal alcohol exposure is consistent across all cortical areas. Archibald et al. (2001) used morphometric MRI analyses to examine whether the proportional cortical volume comprised by the frontal, parietal, temporal, and occipital lobes differed between children with FAS and normally developing children. After adjusting for overall brain size, only the parietal lobe was disproportionately reduced in children with FAS, indicating that all areas of the cortex were not equally affected.

Two studies have examined the effect of prenatal alcohol exposure on cerebral white and gray matter (Sowell et al., 2001; Archibald et al., 2001). Using the same pool of participants two distinct types of analyses were conducted, assessing relative density and volume, respectively, of these tissue types. Both studies revealed that prenatal alcohol exposure is related to disproportionate reductions in cerebral white matter with relative sparing of cerebral gray matter. When overall microcephaly in these individuals is taken into account, it appears that the parietal regions are particularly affected, with marked white matter volume reductions occurring in this area along with reductions in white matter density and increases in gray matter density. The parietal cortex is involved in a variety of functions including the representation of spatial relations, mathematical processing, attention, and processing of somatosensory information (Kolb and Whishaw, 1996). The data from Archibald and colleagues (2001) and Sowell and colleagues (2001) suggest that attention should be focused on these areas of neurobehavioral functioning as we attempt to determine whether a common neurobehavioral profile can be identified in alcohol-exposed children.

Cerebellum

Historically, studies of the cerebellum have focused on its role in the control of motor functions. This focus was driven in part by the knowledge that the cerebellum has reciprocal connections with multiple motor areas of the CNS including the spinal cord, the vestibular system, and the motor cortex, among others. Further, a number of studies have detailed the performance of individuals with cerebellar lesions on motor tasks. From the accumulated data, it is clear that the cerebellum is involved in a variety of motor skills, including postural control, gait, balance, and the coordination of bilateral movements (Diener et al., 1993).

Although largely overlooked, the idea that the cerebellum also plays a role in cognition is not new. For example, classical conditioning of the eyeblink response is known to be dependent upon the cerebellum and research on this phenomenon dates as far back as the early part of the twentieth century (Woodruff-Pak, 1997). Recently, there has been a surge of interest in the nonmotor functions of the cerebellum with researchers focusing on the role that the cerebellum plays in learning and memory (Ivry and Baldo, 1992; Schmahmann, 1997). The idea that the cerebellum could play a role in cognition is reinforced by neuroanatomical research that has demonstrated afferents from the association areas of the cortex via the pontine nucleus and efferents to the cortex via the thalamus (Schmahmann and Pandya, 1997). Current theories suggest that in addition to influencing motor control, the cerebellum influences attention (Townsend et al., 1999), planning (Hallett and Grafman, 1997), and temporal computation and perception (Keele and Ivry, 1990; Ackermann et al., 1999). Interestingly, deficits in attention and planning have been reported in children with FAS (Mattson et al., 1999; Kodituwakku et al., 1995; Kopera-Frye et al., 1997).

Cerebellar abnormalities associated with heavy prenatal exposure to alcohol have received extensive attention in the animal and human literature. Both autopsy studies and animal studies have suggested that the cerebellum is one of several neural structures sensitive to prenatal alcohol exposure. For example, animal studies have demonstrated that prenatal alcohol exposure causes a reduction in the number of cerebellar neurons resulting in a reduction in overall cerebellar volume (Pierce et al., 1989; Cragg and Phillips, 1985; Bonthius and West, 1990).

MRI studies have also revealed changes in the cerebellum in children with FAS or PEA. In a series of three MRI studies, significant reductions in the volume of the cerebellar vault of children with FAS were documented (Mattson et al., 1992; Mattson, Riley, Sowell, et al., 1996), along with marginally significant volume reductions in children with PEA (Mattson et al., 1994). Overall, 80 percent of the children with FAS or PEA who received MRI scans in these studies had a cerebellar vault volume below the range observed in normal controls. In a recent study, the earlier finding of significant reductions in the cerebellar vault of children with FAS was confirmed, along with marginal reductions in the cerebellar vault of children with PEA (Archibald et al., 2001).

Archibald and colleagues (2001) also examined the proportion of the cerebellar cortex composed of white and gray matter, but failed to find a significant difference. Thus, in contrast to the cerebral cortex data presented previously, the white and gray matter appeared to be more similarly affected in the cerebellum than in the cerebrum. This appeared to be due to relatively more severe effects on cerebellar gray matter, as cerebellar hypoplasia overall was more severe than was cerebral hypoplasia.

A global analysis of the cerebellum may not be sufficient to understand the relation between cerebellar changes and behavior in this population. Animal studies have demonstrated regional differences in sensitivity to prenatal alcohol exposure within the cerebellum. For example, animal research indicated that earlier maturing regions of the cerebellar vermis (lobules I-V, IX, and X) were more susceptible to the effects of alcohol than later maturing regions (lobules VI and VII) (Goodlett et al., 1990). Using MRI analyses in humans, the cerebellar vermis was divided into the anterior vermis (lobules I-V), the posterior vermis (lobules VI and VII), and the remaining vermal area (VIII to X) to examine whether reductions in volume were widespread or limited to the anterior regions and remaining vermal area, as would be predicted from the animal studies (Sowell et al., 1996). Results indicated there was a significant reduction in the anterior vermis of children with FAS or PEA. In contrast, neither the posterior vermis nor the remaining vermal area differed from controls.

These results are particularly interesting for two reasons. First, they are consistent with the animal literature. Second, these findings are inconsistent with cerebellar abnormalities observed in other developmental disorders. Specifically, studies of attention-deficit hyperactivity disorder (ADHD) have reported reductions in the posterior vermis with sparing of the anterior vermis (Mostofsky et al., 1998; Berquin et al., 1998). Studies of autism (Townsend et al., 1999; Courchesne et al., 1994; Bauman et al., 1997) have reported subtypes of autism patients who display either hyperplasia or hypoplasia in the posterior vermis with sparing of the anterior vermis. This pattern is opposite to what was observed in children with FAS or PEA, demonstrating that while cerebellar abnormalities are not solely caused by alcohol, the pattern of damage caused by prenatal alcohol exposure differs. This raises the possibility that specific patterns of strengths and weaknesses reflective of cerebellum function and dysfunction could be observed across these disorders. This pattern, in conjunction with other neuropathological findings, could increase the specificity of the behavioral phenotype observed in children with FAS or PEA, thereby improving the accuracy of the diagnosis.

Corpus Callosum

The corpus callosum is a large bundle of axonal fibers that connects the left and right hemispheres of the brain and allows for the efficient transfer of information between them. It is comprised of about 300 million fibers (Heimer, 1995) and can be separated into four sections: the rostrum, genu, body, and splenium (Kolb and Whishaw, 1996). Corpus callosum abnormalities were initially seen in autopsy studies of FAS. In fact, as mentioned previously, the first autopsied brain of an infant with FAS displayed agenesis (absence) of the corpus callosum (Jones and Smith, 1973; Clarren et al., 1978).

Agenesis of the corpus callosum is estimated to occur in 0.3 percent of the general population and in 2.3 percent of the developmentally disabled population (Jeret et al., 1986). In a sample of children in San Diego with FAS or PEA, it has been estimated that the incidence of complete agenesis of the corpus callosum is 6.8 percent (3 out of 44 children) (Riley et al., 1995). In addition to complete agenesis of the corpus callosum, other abnormalities such as partial agenesis or hypoplasia of the corpus callosum have been observed (Clark et al., 2000; Swayze et al., 1997; Riikonen, 1999). Corpus callosum abnormalities, even complete agenesis, are not unique to FAS, but rather have been observed in multiple developmental and genetic disorders including ADHD (Hynd et al., 1991), mental retardation (Schaefer et al., 1991), and Down's syndrome (Wang et al., 1992).

Quantitative analyses of the corpus callosum in children with FAS or PEA have been conducted (Riley et al., 1995). During the MRI analyses, the corpus callosum was divided into five equiangular regions, with region 1 corresponding to the genu, region 5 corresponding to the splenium, and regions 2 to 4 corresponding to the body of the corpus callosum. In addition, the area of the midsagittal section was computed in order to control for reductions in overall brain size when examining group differences. The midsagittal area was reduced by 14 percent in the alcohol-exposed children. In addition, there were significant reductions in areas 1, 3, 4, and 5 of the corpus callosum. Even after controlling for the reduction in the midsagittal area, areas 1, 4, and 5 were still significantly reduced in the corpus callosum of children with FAS or PEA. Thus, it was the most anterior and posterior regions of the corpus callosum that were affected by prenatal exposure. The selective pattern of reductions can provide information regarding the types of deficits one would expect to observe in children with FAS. For example, the anterior region of the corpus callosum contains fibers for the prefrontal cortex, while the posterior region contains fibers for the visual cortex, as well as the superior and inferior temporal cortexes.

Basal Ganglia

The basal ganglia are a group of subcortical nuclei that can be subdivided into the caudate and lenticular nuclei. The lenticular nuclei can be further subdivided into the globus pallidus and the putamen (Heimer, 1995). The basal ganglia have traditionally been thought to participate in motor activity for several reasons. First, the basal ganglia are part of a corticostriatal loop in which information is projected from the somatosensory and motor cortices to basal ganglia and eventually back to the motor and premotor cortices. This motor loop enables the basal ganglia to participate in both the initiation and modulation of motor activity (Kolb and Whishaw, 1996). Further, two diseases with known pathology in the basal ganglia, Huntington's and Parkinson's diseases, result in prominent motor dysfunction such as akinesia and hyperkinesia.

Current perspectives suggest that the basal ganglia play a role not only in motor activity, but also in cognitive functioning (Middleton and Strick, 1994, 2000; Rao et al., 1997). Cognitive deficits have been observed in patients with either Huntington's disease or Parkinson's disease and the degree of cognitive deficits has in some cases been linked to the degree of basal ganglial pathology (Bäckman et al., 1997; Watkins et al., 2000). Further, there is a second corticostriatal loop (cognitive loop) in which frontal, parietal, and temporal cortical association areas send projections to the caudate nucleus of the basal ganglia, which in turn sends projections back to the cortex, providing a means for the basal ganglia to influence cognition (Heimer, 1995).

A series of MRI studies has examined the basal ganglia in alcohol-exposed children and remarkable consistency has emerged. A clinical examination of the MRI scans taken by these studies revealed no abnormalities in the basal ganglia of children with FAS compared to normally developing children or children with Down's syndrome (Mattson et al., 1992). However, differences were revealed when morphometric analyses were conducted. The volume of the basal ganglia in the alcohol-exposed children was reduced beyond what would be expected given their overall brain size. In contrast, the children with Down's syndrome had proportionally larger basal ganglia than would be expected. Subsequently, two children with PEA were evaluated. In these less affected children, the volume of the basal ganglia was still significantly reduced even after controlling for the overall reduction in head size. Thus, analyses indicated that the basal ganglia were disproportionately reduced in the children with FAS or PEA and that mental retardation, degree of dysmorphology, and overall reductions in head size were not sufficient to explain the finding.

In a later study, six children with FAS were compared to seven age-appropriate, normally developing control children (Mattson, Riley, Sowell, et al., 1996). The morphometric analysis was refined to differentiate the caudate nucleus from the lenticular nuclei, since the caudate nucleus is more involved in the "cognitive loop," whereas the lenticular nuclei are more involved in the "motor loop." Analyses revealed that the caudate nucleus and lenticular nuclei were reduced in children with FAS relative to control children. However, only the caudate nucleus displayed a disproportionate reduction in volume after controlling for brain size. This finding was replicated in a recent study which incorporated a larger sample of FAS (N = 14), PEA (N = 12), and normally developing control children (N = 14) (Archibald et al., 2001). Based upon their intellectual functioning (range of intelligence scores: 40 to 103), this new sample was also more representative of the FAS and PEA populations at large. Archibald and colleagues found that the caudate nucleus, but not the lenticular nuclei, was disproportionately reduced in FAS children. There was a trend for a similar reduction in children with PEA; however, this did not reach significance, suggesting that either the magnitude or consistency of basal ganglial damage is diminished in children who do not manifest the full FAS phenotype.

The presence of significant reductions in the basal ganglia are interesting in light of autopsy studies that indicate prenatal alcohol exposure can cause severe damage to midline structures resulting in disorders such as holoprosencephaly. One might speculate that the midline is a "weak seam" during development and therefore midline structures as a whole are more susceptible to alcohol-induced damage (Johnson et al., 1996). While midline anomalies (e.g., agenesis of the corpus callosum, neural tube defects, holoprosencephaly) appear to occur at a higher than expected rate, MRI studies suggest that all midline structures are not equally sensitive to or affected by heavy prenatal alcohol exposure. As mentioned previously, the lenticular nuclei were not disproportionately reduced in children with FAS or PEA (Mattson, Riley, Sowell, et al., 1996; Archibald et al., 2001). Further, studies indicate that the limbic cortex and diencephalon were not disproportionately reduced in children with FAS or PEA (Mattson et al., 1994; Mattson, Riley, Sowell, et al., 1996). So while heavy alcohol exposure appears to result in a high rate of midline anomalies and can result in holoprosencephaly in rare cases, the bulk of MRI studies suggest that all midline structures are not equally sensitive to the effects of alcohol. Rather, the caudate nucleus of the basal ganglia appears to be especially sensitive since it is disproportionately reduced, while the reduction in many other midline structures is consistent with reductions in overall brain size.

OTHER STUDIES

Electroencephalogram (EEG) and Event-Related Potential (ERP) Studies

The earliest studies examining brain activity in children utilized electroencephalogram (EEG) and evoked response potential (ERP) methodologies. Numerous case studies have appeared throughout the literature. These reports indicated abnormal brain-wave activity, which included reduced voltage in the left temporal lobe (Goldstein and Arulanantham, 1978), markedly abnormal brainstem-auditory-evoked-response potentials (Johnson et al., 1996), theta-wave activity (Riikonen et al., 1999), and occasional delta-wave activity in the posterior cortex (Mattson et al., 1992).

Two studies have systematically utilized EEG or ERP methodologies to evaluate neural activity in children with FAS. Kaneko, Phillips, et al. (1996) compared brain-wave activity in normally developing children to children with either FAS or Down's syndrome. The EEG records for the children with

FAS were distinguishable from both the normally developing children and those with Down's syndrome. Brain activity in the children with Down's syndrome was characterized by a generalized slowing and a predominance of delta and theta waves. In contrast, the FAS children did not present with a generalized slowing of neural activity. However, alpha-frequency activity was significantly affected. Specifically, FAS children had significantly lower mean power in the alpha-frequency range in the left fronto-central and left parietal-occipital leads. They also displayed lower peak frequencies in the alpha frequency. These findings suggest immaturity of the cerebral cortex, particularly in the left hemisphere.

In a second study, Kaneko, Ehlers, et al. (1996) examined the same group of children using an oddball-plus-noise paradigm and ERP technology. Again, children with FAS were distinguishable from normally developing controls or children with Down's syndrome. Both children with Down's syndrome and FAS displayed longer P300 latencies. However, this finding was widespread in the Down's syndrome children and occurred in the presence of both the noise burst and infrequent tones. In the FAS children, the longer P300 latencies were isolated to the parietal cortex and only occurred in response to the noise burst.

Positron Emission Tomography (PET) and Single-Photon Emission Computerized Tomography (SPECT) Studies

While EEG provides information about the pattern of neuronal activity, its specificity is limited since it is typically difficult to accurately localize the source of the activity. Recently two new studies have utilized newer neuroimaging techniques to examine brain function in children with FAS.

Riikonen and colleagues (1999) utilized single-photon emission computerized tomography (SPECT) to examine the changes in the brain structure and activity of 11 children with FAS. SPECT is a variant of the better-known positron emission tomography (PET) methodology, which enables researchers to examine the amount of glucose utilized by different brain regions. Glucose utilization reflects the activity level of the brain with greater utilization indicating greater activity. Results indicated an absence of the hemispheric asymmetry characteristic of normally developing brains. Specifically, in normally developing children there is greater glucose utilization and cerebral blood flow in the left hemisphere. This hemispheric difference was absent in FAS children. Further, this finding was most pronounced in the frontal and parietooccipital regions.

In a similar study, Clark and colleagues (2000) utilized PET to examine brain activity in high functioning children with FAS. Rather than focus on cerebral asymmetry, Clark et al. examined the glucose metabolism of various cortical and subcortical structures relative to age-appropriate controls. Standardized glucose metabolism in the thalamus, head of the caudate, and the caudate/putamen was significantly lower in individuals with FAS than in controls. There was a bilateral reduction in glucose metabolism in each structure, with the exception of the caudate/putamen where the reduction was limited to the right side.

These newer studies complement the findings from the structural imaging studies. First, Riikonen et al. (1999) demonstrated a disruption of the normal hemispheric asymmetry, which was predominantly localized to the frontal and parietooccipital regions. Likewise, Riley and colleagues (1995) found that corpus callosum abnormalities were predominantly located in the anterior and posterior portions, which carry fibers from the frontal and occipital cortical regions and allow for the efficient transfer of information across the hemispheres. Second, Clark and colleagues (2000) demonstrated decreased rates of glucose metabolism in the thalamus, caudate, and caudate/putamen. These data are consistent with the findings of a disproportionate reduction in the size of the caudate nucleus of the basal ganglia. Thus, it appears that both structure and activity of the basal ganglia are impaired.

NEUROBEHAVIORAL EFFECTS

Intelligence

The effect of prenatal alcohol exposure on intelligence has received considerable attention, perhaps because prenatal alcohol exposure is the most frequent and preventable cause of mental retardation (Pulsifer, 1996). However, not all children with FAS or PEA are mentally retarded. In fact, it is estimated that only 25 percent of children with FAS have IQ scores that fall within the mental retardation range (IQ < 70) (Streissguth, 1997).

IQ scores vary widely in children with FAS or PEA. For example, IQ scores ranging from a low of 20 (Streissguth et al., 1991) to a high of at least 120 have been reported for children with FAS (Olson et al., 1998). Mean IQ for children with FAS is estimated to be between 65 and 72 (Mattson and Riley, 1997). At least during childhood, IQ scores tend to be correlated with dysmorphology (Steinhausen et al., 1994). Children with more dysmorphic features tend to have lower IQ scores than children with fewer dysmorphic features. Consequently, IQ scores tend to be higher in children classified as PEA or FAE than in those with FAS (Streissguth et al., 1991). However, it should be noted that children with PEA or FAE have significantly lower IQ scores than normally developing, non-alcohol-exposed children (Mattson et al., 1997). Thus, they tend to be less impaired than children with FAS, but are impaired when compared to non-alcohol-exposed peers.

Research indicates that the IQ scores of children with FAS derived from standardized intelligence tests such as the Wechsler Intelligence Scale for Children (WISC) (Wechsler, 1991) are very stable over time (Steinhausen et al., 1993; Steinhausen and Spohr, 1998). For example, Streissguth et al. (1991) found that test-retest correlations over an average eight-year interval ranged from 0.78 to 0.88 for FAS and PEA children respectively, indicating a high degree of stability in intellectual functioning across time.

Language

Delays in language development have been reported in a variety of studies. For example, Iosub et al. (1981) reported that in a sample of 63 patients with FAS, 84 percent of patients displayed some evidence of delayed or disordered speech or language development. Shaywitz et al. (1981) described two preschool age children who had expressive and receptive language skills that were delayed by at least two years. Further, they noted that these children failed to use language as a tool for initiating social interactions. Thus, early reports suggested that language impairments were widespread within this population.

Several systematic studies have examined language functioning in this population using standardized measures. Carney and Chermak (1991) tested 10 children with FAS and 17 normally developing children using the Test of Language Development. They found widespread impairments in language functioning, which included impairments in vocabulary and sentence imitation, grammatical understanding, and word discrimination. Impairments were noted in both expressive and receptive language. However, impairments appeared to be more extensive in the younger children. Older children were primarily impaired in their understanding and use of syntax. Although this study did not use a longitudinal design, it does suggest that language development may be delayed but not deviant.

This possibility was addressed in a study by Becker et al. (1990). Children with FAS were compared to chronological age (CA) and mental age (MA) control groups. A deficit in comparison to the CA group would suggest that language development was delayed. In contrast, a deficit in comparison to the MA group would suggest a qualitative shift in language development that is not easily accounted for by general cognitive functioning. This study utilized tests of grammar, semantics, and short-term memory. Significant differences were found between the children with FAS and the CA control group on a variety of measures including grammar, semantics, and memory. Thus, the data suggested that language development was delayed. However, the FAS group never differed significantly from the MA control group, indicating that while language development is delayed the observed language skills are consistent with the general intellectual functioning of the FAS group.

Overall, the data strongly indicate that language development is delayed, although consistent with general intellectual functioning. A variety of issues are likely to impede language development in this population. For example, Church et al. (1997) found that while 82 percent of their patients had receptive language delays almost all of them also had a hearing disorder. In addition, both Church and colleagues and Becker and colleagues (1990) reported abnormalities in the structure and function of the speech apparatus including cleft palate, high or narrow arches, and functional movements of the tongue and larynx, among other things. Both hearing disorders and abnormalities in the structure and function of the speech apparatus are likely to hinder age-appropriate language development.

Learning and Memory

Both verbal and nonverbal learning and memory have been assessed in children with FAS and appear to be impaired. Mattson, Riley, Delis, et al. (1996) examined verbal learning and memory in children with FAS in relation to chronological- and mental-age-matched controls using the Children's Verbal Learning Test-Children's Version (CVLT-C). Across five learning trials, children learn a 15-word list, which must be recalled following each presentation as well as after a 20-minute delay. Results indicated that FAS children learned fewer words across the five learning trials relative to chronological, but not mental, age-matched controls. Likewise, after a 20-minute delay, children with FAS exhibited significantly poorer recall for the list relative to their chronological, but not mental, age-matched controls. Of interest, when the number of words recalled after the 20-minute delay was compared to the number of words learned by the fifth learning trial, the groups did not differ in the percentage of learned words that were retained across the delay period. Thus, information that was learned tended to be equally retained by all groups. Some differences emerged between children with FAS and the mental-age-matched controls. Specifically, children with FAS had more difficulty discriminating the list words from distracters during a yes/no recognition test, resulting in more false positive errors. Additionally, they tended to make more perseverative errors during free- and cued-recall conditions.

A later study expanded these findings by comparing implicit and explicit memory in children with FAS. Mattson and Riley (1999) used a word-stem completion task to assess priming, a type of implicit memory, and used free-recall and recognition memory tasks to assess explicit memory. Results indicated that the children with FAS performed comparable to normally developing control children and better than children with Down's syndrome on the priming task, strongly suggesting that implicit memory is spared following prenatal exposure to alcohol. In contrast, children with FAS were significantly impaired in their ability to recall a list of words relative to normal controls. Further, they tended to make more perseveration errors when recalling the list of words. Thus, these studies suggest that while memory is impaired it is not globally impaired. Both recognition and implicit (priming) memory appear to be spared while free recall is impaired.

A similar disassociation occurs when one examines memory for objects and spatial location (Uecker and Nadel, 1996, 1998). In two related studies, children with FAS exhibited deficits in spatial memory, but not object memory. Specifically, children were instructed to remember the identity and spatial location of various objects they either estimated the price of or named. Children with FAS recalled a comparable number of objects during an immediate delay condition, but were significantly worse at accurately determining the original location of the object. After a 24-hour delay, children with FAS were still impaired in their ability to remember where the objects were originally located. Overall, the data suggested that spatial memory was impaired while object memory was spared.

The observed memory dissociations have implications for the types of neuroanatomical changes one would expect to find in alcohol-exposed children. For example, Mattson and Riley (1999) argued that the pattern of spared implicit memory and impaired explicit memory is comparable to that observed in patients with Huntington's disease. As mentioned previously, Huntington's disease is associated with pathological changes in the basal ganglia, an area that is reduced in children with FAS. Thus, the emerging neurobehavioral data converge with the existing neuroanatomical data. The dissociation between object and spatial memory provides us with a new avenue for exploration. The deficit in spatial memory suggests damage to the right hemisphere, particularly the temporal lobe and hippocampus (Smith and Milner, 1981) as well as damage to the basal ganglia (Lawrence et al., 2000). Damage to the hippocampus has been repeatedly observed in animal models of FAS (Berman and Hannigan, 2000). However, Riikonen and colleagues (1999) found that the right hippocampus was significantly larger than the left in children with FAS. Archibald and colleagues (2001) also found that the hippocampus was larger than expected in children with FAS given the size of other subcortical structures. Reductions in the temporal cortex have not been observed either (Archibald et al., 2001). As more sensitive neuroimaging techniques become available, further research should examine whether neuroanatomical differences in the hippocampus and temporal cortex emerge.

Attention and Activity

Attention and activity levels have received considerable focus. The inattentiveness and hyperactive behavioral patterns of children with FAS are frequently compared to those of children with ADHD. High levels of ADHD-like symptoms in this population would not be particularly surprising, since the prevalence of ADHD in special education classrooms is conservatively estimated to be between 9 and 33 percent (Pearson et al., 2000).

Steinhausen and colleagues (1993, 1994; Steinhausen and Spohr, 1998) examined rates of psychopathology in a sample of children with FAS and found that 63 percent displayed one or more psychiatric disorder, with hyperkinetic disorders (e.g., ADHD) predominant within the sample. The prevalence of hyperkinetic disorders ranged from approximately 42 to 63 percent depending upon the time of the assessment and the subsample evaluated. Further, while the presence of many other disorders, such as enuresis and language disorders, appeared to be age related, hyperkinetic disorders were present from an early age and persisted through adolescence in the majority of affected cases. The prevalence of hyperactivity in this sample is higher than the estimates for special education populations, suggesting that prenatal alcohol exposure may be one of many potential etiologies for hyperactivity.

Neuropsychological measures of attention have been employed in a number of studies to determine whether children with FAS exhibit deficits in attention. Kerns et al. (1997) reported that adults with FAS performed within normal limits on tests of simple auditory attention. However, complex sustained and alternating attention were impaired. In a similar study, Connor et al. (1999) compared the visual and auditory attention abilities of adults with FAS or FAE to nonexposed adults. The adults with FAS/FAE performed more poorly than controls on most measures and the results suggested that adults with FAS/FAE have difficulty focusing, sustaining, and shifting auditory attention, as well as focusing and sustaining visual attention.

Although children with FAS are frequently compared to children with ADHD, and data indicate that multiple components of attention are impaired, it is unclear whether the behavioral phenotype expressed by FAS children is identical to that expressed by children with ADHD. Two studies have explicitly compared the performance of children with ADHD or FAS. Nanson and Hiscock (1990) used parental reports and laboratory measures of attention to compare the performance of children with FAS or FAE to children with ADD or normally developing children. The parental reports for children with FAS/FAE or ADD were indistinguishable, suggesting that the presence and severity of hyperactive and inattentive symptoms was perceived to be significant in both groups. Likewise, children with ADD or FAS exhibited increased rates of impulsive errors on a delayed reaction time task. While children with ADD appeared to make a speed accuracy trade-off, children with FAS/FAE responded slowly and made many errors, indicating an increased difficulty with the task as well as possible impulsive responding. The slower responses exhibited by the FAS/FAE children on delayed reaction time task and vigilance tasks were likely attributable in part to the differences in IQ observed between the FAS/FAE children and other groups.

In a similar study, Coles and colleagues (1997) used parental reports and an attention battery to examine the profile of FAS/FAE children and ADHD children on four components of attention: focus, sustain, encode, and shift. Unlike the previous study, Coles and colleagues found that parents rated children with FAS/FAE differently from children with ADHD. Ratings for children with ADHD indicated they displayed significantly more behaviors associated with the disorder than either children with FAS/FAE or control children. Likewise, the profile of children with FAS/FAE tended to differ from that of children with ADHD on the attention battery. Both groups had difficulty focusing attention as measured by the WISC-R coding subtest. In addition, children with FAS/FAE had some difficulty encoding information and shifting attention. Children with ADHD performed significantly worse on measures of sustained attention. However, more than 50 percent of children with FAS/FAE or ADHD were unable to complete the sustained attention tasks, so the findings are difficult to interpret. Overall, Coles and colleagues found that while children with FAS/FAE exhibit attention deficits, the profile of deficits varies from that observed in children with ADHD. These phenotypic differences suggest that prenatal alcohol exposure may not cause classic ADHD symptoms, but rather a variant, which potentially could require different pharmacological and behavioral treatment protocols from those employed with nonexposed children with ADHD.

Executive Functioning

Executive functioning (EF) is a complex psychological construct that has been broadly defined as "the ability to maintain an appropriate problem solving set for the attainment of a goal" (Welsh and Pennington, 1988,

p. 201). A variety of cognitive domains are subsumed under this general definition including inhibition, set shifting and set maintenance, planning, working memory, and the ability to integrate information across time and space (Pennington and Ozonoff, 1996). EF plays a large role in our day-to-day functioning, as it is utilized in such diverse activities as interpersonal relations, organizing and conducting a search for missing keys, or organizing the tools and skills necessary to achieve a job or school assignment. Deficits in EF would be consistent with MRI studies that documented a reduction in the size of the basal ganglia. Studies of Parkinson's disease and Huntington's disease have documented impaired performance on EF tasks in association with pathology of the basal ganglia (Bäckman et al., 1997; Watkins et al., 2000).

The first systematic study of executive functioning in children with FAS investigated deficits in the self-regulation of action (Kodituwakku et al., 1995). Specifically, they measured three constructs: planning, the regulation of behavior, and the ability to utilize feedback to adapt behavior. Children with FAS or FAE were compared to normally developing children. The FAS/FAE children performed significantly worse on the Standard Progressive Matrices, which was used as a measure of fluid intelligence, indicating that they were more impaired than control children. Results from the EF battery were mixed. Children with FAS/FAE performed significantly worse on the Progressive Planning Test that was used to measure planning but also has a strong inhibitory component (Goel and Grafman, 1995). However, there were no group differences on two of the three tests of behavioral regulation. Finally, the FAS/FAE group performed significantly worse on one utilization of feedback test, the Wisconsin Card Sorting Test (WCST), but not on the go/no-go task. Children with FAS/FAE made significantly more perserverative responses and consequently did not complete as many categories as control children in the WCST. These data are consistent with those reported by Olson et al. (1998), although Coles and colleagues (1997) found no significant difference between children with FAS and normally developing children on this measure. Thus, while there were some deficits in EF, they were not as consistent as might have been expected, particularly since the two groups differed significantly on fluid intelligence.

Another systematic examination of EF in this population was recently published by Mattson et al. (1999). This study utilized the new Delis-Kaplan Executive Function System (D-KEFS) battery (Delis et al., 2001) to assess four domains of EF: cognitive flexibility, response inhibition, planning, and concept formation and reasoning. FAS/ PEA children had significantly lower IQ scores than the normally developing control children and group differences emerged across all four domains.

Cognitive flexibility and response inhibition were assessed with the California Trail Making Test and California Stroop Test, respectively. Both tests incorporate control conditions, although no group differences emerged across any control tasks. In the California Trail Making Test, the critical test requires children to connect a series of letters and numbers, alternating between the two categories (e.g., 1-A-2-B). FAS/PEA children performed significantly worse on this test. The California Stroop Test contains two critical tests: interference and set shifting. During the interference condition, children were presented with a color name printed in a different color of ink and were directed to name the ink color. During the set-shifting condition, children were presented with the same stimuli but were directed to read the word or name the ink color depending on a cue. The FAS/PEA children were significantly impaired on the interference condition. Only children with FAS differed from control children on the set-shifting condition. Thus, the data suggest that both cognitive flexibility and response inhibition may be impaired in children with FAS/PEA.

Planning was assessed using the Tower of California Test, a variant of the progressive planning test used by Kodituwakku and colleagues (1995), while concept formation and reasoning was assessed with the California Word Context Test. Consistent with Kodituwakku et al., the FAS/PEA children violated more rules and passed fewer items on the Tower of California Test, suggesting that planning was impaired. In the California Word Context Test, children must guess a target word on the basis of a series of five sequentially presented sentences that provide clues about the target word. Likewise, children with FAS/PEA required significantly more sentence cues to guess the target word than normally developing children.

The data from Mattson and colleagues (1999) and Kodituwakku and colleagues' (1995) studies suggest there may be deficits in EF in alcohol-exposed children. However, future studies should continue to examine the extent to which these executive-functioning deficits are greater than would be expected given observed reductions in intelligence.

Psychosocial Functioning

The majority of the research on the neurobehavioral consequences of heavy prenatal alcohol exposure has focused on cognitive skills and capabilities. However, the behavioral consequences of prenatal alcohol exposure are not limited to the cognitive arena as emphasized by a study on secondary disabilities across the lifespan in individuals with FAS and FAE (Streissguth et al., 1997). Secondary disabilities are those problems that are not directly caused by alcohol, but emerge after birth, and presumably could be prevented or ameliorated with intervention efforts. This initial study provided some alarming statistics. For example, 90 percent of 415 patients had sought help for or experienced a mental health problem. Further, more than half of the individuals with FAS had been in trouble with the law, and either dropped out of school, or had been suspended or expelled. These data indicate that individuals with FAS have significant and pervasive adaptive functioning deficits that persist into adulthood.

New studies have been initiated to determine what types of problem behaviors and deficits in adaptive functioning these children display during childhood and adolescence. A few older studies have examined adaptive behaviors, problem behaviors, or social skills (Streissguth et al., 1991; Steinhausen and Spohr, 1998; Steinhausen et al., 1993) with results indicating a spectrum of attention and social problems among children with FAS. However, they usually compared FAS children to normally developing control children or national norms. Since behavioral and social problems are not uncommon in developmentally disabled populations, it is not clear whether the problems are similar to those in other disabled populations or whether the difficulties exhibited by children with FAS are in some way unique.

Children with FAS also have significant deficits in social skills. Even when compared to children with similar IQ scores, children with FAS were significantly impaired in their interpersonal relationships and their ability to make appropriate use of their play and leisure time (Thomas et al., 1998). Further, FAS children display more problematic behaviors than children with comparable IQ scores (Mattson and Riley, 2000). Parents reported that FAS children engaged in more externalizing behaviors and had more social, thought, and attention problems. Further, according to their parents, FAS children engaged in more aggressive and delinquent behavior. These problems were not limited to the most severely affected children. Children with PEA displayed the same pattern of social and behavioral problems as children with FAS, indicating that overall intellectual functioning and dysmorphology were not sufficient to explain the pattern of maladaptive behaviors.

In a related study, the Personality Inventory for Children (PIC) was utilized to further examine the behavioral and psychological problems present in this population (Roebuck et al., 1999). As expected, FAS and PEA children scored poorly on the three subtests that measured intelligence, cognitive development, and achievement. In addition, they were in the clinical range for the subscales measuring delinquency and psychosis, with PEA children showing a level of impairment comparable to the FAS children.

Across multiple studies it is becoming clear that alcohol-exposed children display a wide variety of maladaptive behaviors and have significant problems in their social interactions. These maladaptive behaviors tend to be directed toward others rather than themselves and do not appear to be commensurate with their level of cognitive disability. FAS and PEA children are more likely to engage in antisocial behaviors and to disregard or fail to comprehend the rights and feelings of others. These findings are consistent with the secondary disabilities documented by Streissguth and colleagues (1997).

These studies have not determined why these children engage in antisocial behavior. Are children with FAS deliberately misbehaving or do their misdeeds reflect an inability to understand the consequences of their behaviors and the potential effect of their behaviors on others? Currently, many believe the latter to be the case. As mentioned above, some have suggested that children with FAS/PEA have deficits in EF (Mattson et al., 1999; Kodituwakku et al., 1995). Although this hypothesis needs to be further validated, executive-functioning deficits could be expressed as an inability to plan and foresee the consequences of actions as well as the inability to inhibit actions that may be inappropriate. Thus, although children with FAS may be engaging in risky and aversive behaviors, these behaviors may not be intentionally mischievous or antisocial. Rather they may reflect core deficits in foresight, planning, and the ability to read and understand social cues. Further research needs to be directed at determining the cause of social deficits and increased behavioral problems in children with FAS.

SUMMARY AND DISCUSSION

In summary, understanding of the neuroanatomical and neurobehavioral consequences of prenatal alcohol exposure is increasing rapidly. Although autopsy studies have suggested that heavy prenatal exposure to alcohol resulted in a diffuse, nonspecific pattern of neuropathological abnormalities, newer neuroimaging techniques are revealing a consistent pattern of anomalies across alcohol-affected children. Microcephaly is still the most common outcome following heavy exposure. However, it is now clear that the entire brain is not equally sensitive to the teratogenic effects of alcohol. The basal ganglia, corpus callosum, cerebellum, and parietal cortex appear to have a heightened susceptibility relative to other brain structures. Further research on the neuroanatomical effects of prenatal alcohol exposure is still needed. Most notably, there is a need for more studies that use developmentally disabled, rather than normally developing, children as controls in order to determine whether the observed neuropathology is in any way unique from that observed in a variety of other developmental disorders. The information gained about patterns of preserved and impaired brain structure and function is likely to greatly enhance efforts to define a behavioral phenotype that is specific to children with FAS.

Intellectual deficits have received considerable attention and this is not surprising since prenatal alcohol exposure remains the leading preventable cause of mental retardation and results in significant impairments in academic functioning. A number of other cognitive domains have also been examined including attention, learning and memory, executive functioning, and language. Questions remain unanswered in each of these domains. Most pressing is the need to determine the extent to which deficits in cognitive domains are consistent general declines in intellectual functioning. New research clearly indicates that deficits are not isolated to the cognitive domain. Children with FAS exhibit a high level of problem behaviors as well as impairments in their interpersonal relationships. It is critical that more research be directed toward exploring and alleviating these problems at very young ages in order to prevent secondary disabilities such as the observed problems in psychosocial adjustment, juvenile delinquency, and mental health.

REFERENCES

Aase, J.M.; Jones, K.L.; Clarren, S.K. (1995). Do we need the term "FAE"? *Pediatrics, 95,* 428-430.

Abel, E.L.; Sokol, R.J. (1991). A revised conservative estimate of the incidence of FAS and its economic impact. *Alcoholism: Clinical and Experimental Research, 15,* 514-524.

Ackermann, H.; Graber, S.; Hertrich, I.; Daum, I. (1999). Cerebellar contributions to the perception of temporal cues within the speech and nonspeech domain. *Brain and Language, 67,* 228-241.

Archibald, S.L.; Fennema-Notestine, C.; Gamst, A.; Riley, E.P.; Mattson, S.N.; Jernigan, T.L. (2001). Brain dysmorphology in individuals with severe prenatal alcohol exposure. *Developmental Medicine and Child Neurology, 43,* 148-154.

Bäckman, L.; Robins-Wahlin, T.B.; Lundin, A.; Ginovart, N.; Farde, L. (1997). Cognitive deficits in Huntington's disease are predicted by dopaminergic PET markers and brain volumes. *Brain, 120,* 2207-2217.

Bauman, M.L.; Filipek, P.A.; Kemper, T.L. (1997). Early infantile autism. In J. D. Schmahmann (ed.), *International Review of Neurobiology: Volume 41, The Cerebellum and Cognition* (pp. 367-386). San Diego, CA: Academic Press.

Becker, M.; Warr-Leeper, G.A.; Leeper, H.A. Jr. (1990). Fetal alcohol syndrome: A description of oral motor, articulatory, short-term memory, grammatical, and semantic abilities. *Journal of Communication Disorders, 23,* 97-124.

Berman, R.F.; Hannigan, J.H. (2000). Effects of prenatal alcohol exposure on the hippocampus: Spatial behavior, electrophysiology, and neuroanatomy. *Hippocampus, 10,* 94-110.

Berquin, P.C.; Giedd, J.N.; Jacobsen, L.K.; Hamburger, S.D.; Krain, A.L.; Rapoport, J.L.; Castellanos, F.X. (1998). Cerebellum in attention-deficit hyperactivity disorder: A morphometric MRI study. *Neurology, 50,* 1087-1093.

Bonthius, D.J.; West, J.R. (1990). Alcohol-induced neuronal loss in developing rats: Increased brain damage with binge exposure. *Alcoholism: Clinical and Experimental Research, 14,* 107-118.

Carney, L.J.; Chermak, G.D. (1991). Performance of American Indian children with fetal alcohol syndrome on the test of language development. *Journal of Communication Disorders, 24,* 123-134.

Centers for Disease Control (CDC) (1995). Update: Trends in fetal alcohol syndrome. *Morbidity and Mortality Weekly Report, 44,* 249-251.

Church, M.W.; Eldis, F.; Blakley, B.W.; Bawle, E.V. (1997). Hearing, language, speech, vestibular, and dentofacial disorders in fetal alcohol syndrome. *Alcoholism: Clinical and Experimental Research, 21,* 227-237.

Clark, C.M.; Li, D.; Conry, J.; Conry, R.; Loock, C. (2000). Structural and functional brain integrity of fetal alcohol syndrome in nonretarded cases. *Pediatrics, 105,* 1096-1099.

Clarren, S.K. (1986). Neuropathology in fetal alcohol syndrome. In J.R. West (ed.), *Alcohol and Brain Development* (pp. 158-166). New York: Oxford University Press.

Clarren, S.K.; Alvord, E.C.; Sumi, S.M.; Streissguth, A.P.; Smith, D.W. (1978). Brain malformations related to prenatal exposure to ethanol. *Journal of Pediatrics, 92,* 64-67.

Clarren, S.K.; Astley, S.J. (1992). Pregnancy outcomes after weekly oral administration of ethanol during gestation in the pig-tailed macaque: Comparing early gestational exposure to full gestational exposure. *Teratology, 45,* 1-9.

Clarren, S.K.; Bowden, D.M.; Astley, S.J. (1987). Pregnancy outcomes after weekly oral administration of ethanol during gestation in the pig-tailed macaque *(Macaca nemestrina). Teratology, 35,* 345-354.

Coles, C.D.; Platzman, K.A.; Raskind-Hood, C.L.; Brown, R.T.; Falek, A.; Smith, I.E. (1997). A comparison of children affected by prenatal alcohol exposure and attention deficit, hyperactivity disorder. *Alcoholism: Clinical and Experimental Research, 21,* 150-161.

Connor, P.D.; Streissguth, A.P.; Sampson, P.D.; Bookstein, F.L.; Barr, H.M. (1999). Individual differences in auditory and visual attention among fetal alcohol-affected adults. *Alcoholism: Clinical and Experimental Research, 23,* 1395-1402.

Coulter, C.L.; Leech, R.W.; Schaefer, B.; Scheithauer, B.W.; Brumback, R.A. (1993). Midline cerebral dysgenesis, dysfunction of the hypothalamic-pituitary axis, and fetal alcohol effects. *Archives of Neurology, 50,* 771-775.

Courchesne, E.; Townsend, J.; Saitoh, O. (1994). The brain in infantile autism: Posterior fossa structures are abnormal. *Neurology, 44,* 214-223.

Cragg, B.; Phillips, S. (1985). Natural loss of Purkinje cells during development and increased loss with alcohol. *Brain Research, 325,* 151-160.

Delis, D.C.; Kaplan, E.; Kramer, J.H.; Ober, B.A. (2001). *Delis-Kaplan Executive Function Scale.* San Antonio, TX: The Psychological Corporation.

Diener, H.C.; Hore, J.; Ivry, R.; Dichgans, J. (1993). Cerebellar dysfunction of movement and perception. *The Canadian Journal of Neurological Sciences, 20,* S62-S69.

Gabrielli, O.; Salvolini, U.; Coppa, G.V.; Catassi, C.; Rossi, R.; Manca, A.; Lanza, R.; Giorgi, P.L. (1990). Magnetic resonance imaging in the malformative syndromes with mental retardation. *Pediatric Radiology, 21,* 16-19.

Goel, V.; Grafman, J. (1995). Are the frontal lobes implicated in "planning" functions? Interpreting data from the tower of Hanoi. *Neuropsychologia 33,* 623-642.

Goldstein, G.; Arulanantham, K. (1978). Neural tube defect and renal anomalies in a child with fetal alcohol syndrome. *Journal of Pediatrics, 93,* 636-637.

Goodlett, C.R.; Marcussen, B.L.; West, J.R. (1990). A single day of alcohol exposure during the brain growth spurt induces brain weight restriction and cerebellar Purkinje cell loss. *Alcohol, 7,* 107-114.

Guerri, C. (1998). Neuroanatomical and neurophysiological mechanisms involved in central nervous system dysfunctions induced by prenatal alcohol exposure. *Alcoholism: Clinical and Experimental Research, 22,* 304-312.

Hallett, M.; Grafman, J. (1997). Executive function and motor skill learning. In J.D. Schmahmann (ed.), *International Review of Neurobiology: Volume 41, The Cerebellum and Cognition* (pp. 297-323). San Diego, CA: Academic Press.

Heimer, L. (1995). *The Human Brain and Spinal Cord: Functional Neuroanatomy and Dissection Guide,* Third Edition. New York: Springer-Verlag.

Hynd, G.W.; Semrud-Clikeman, M.; Lorys, A.R.; Novey, E.S.; Eliopulos, D.; Lyytinen, H. (1991). Corpus callosum morphology in attention deficit-hyperactivity disorder: Morphometric analysis of MRI. *Journal of Learning Disabilities, 24,* 141-146.

Institute of Medicine (1996). *Fetal Alcohol Syndrome: Diagnosis, Epidemiology, Prevention, and Treatment.* Washington, DC: National Academy Press.

Iosub, S.; Fuchs, M.; Bingol, N.; Gromisch, D.S. (1981). Fetal alcohol syndrome revisited. *Pediatrics, 68,* 475-479.

Ivry, R.B.; Baldo, J.V. (1992). Is the cerebellum involved in learning and cognition? *Current Opinion in Neurobiology, 2,* 212-216.

Jellinger, K.; Gross, H.; Kaltenback, E.; Grisold, W. (1981). Holoprosencephaly and agenesis of the corpus callosum: Frequency of associated malformations. *Acta Neuropathology, 55,* 1-10.

Jeret, J.S.; Serur, D.; Wisniewski, K.; Fisch, C. (1986). Frequency of agenesis of the corpus callosum in the developmentally disabled population as determined by computerized tomography. *Pediatric Neuroscience, 12,* 101-103.

Johnson, V.P.; Swayze, V.W.; Sato, Y.; Andreasen, N.C. (1996). Fetal alcohol syndrome: Craniofacial and central nervous system manifestations. *American Journal of Medical Genetics, 61,* 329-339.

Jones, K.L.; Smith, D.W. (1973). Recognition of the fetal alcohol syndrome in early infancy. *Lancet, 2,* 999-1001.

Jones, K.L.; Smith, D.W.; Ulleland, C.N.; Streissguth, A.P. (1973). Pattern of malformation in offspring of chronic alcoholic mothers. *Lancet, 1,* 1267-1271.

Kaneko, W.M.; Ehlers, C.L.; Phillips, E.L.; Riley, E.P. (1996). Auditory event-related potentials in fetal alcohol syndrome and Down's syndrome children. *Alcoholism: Clinical and Experimental Research, 20,* 35-42.

Kaneko, W.M.; Phillips, E.L.; Riley, E.P.; Ehlers, C.L. (1996). EEG findings in fetal alcohol syndrome and Down's syndrome children. *Electroencephalography and Clinical Neurophysiology, 98,* 20-28.

Keele, S.W.; Ivry, R. (1990). Does the cerebellum provide a common computation for diverse tasks? In A. Diamond (ed.), *The Development and Neural Bases of Higher Cognitive Functions,* Vol. 608 (pp. 179-211). New York: New York Academy of Sciences.

Kerns, K.A.; Don, A.; Mateer, C.A.; Streissguth, A.P. (1997). Cognitive deficits in nonretarded adults with fetal alcohol syndrome. *Journal of Learning Disabilities, 30,* 685-693.

Kodituwakku, P.W.; Handmaker, N.S.; Cutler, S.K.; Weathersby, E.K.; Handmaker, S.D. (1995). Specific impairments in self-regulation in children exposed to alcohol prenatally. *Alcohol: Clinical and Experimental Research, 19,* 1558-1564.

Kolb, B.; Whishaw, I.Q. (1996). *Fundamentals of Human Neuropsychology,* Fourth Edition. New York: W. H. Freeman and Company.

Konovalav, H.V.; Kovetsky, N.S.; Bobryshev, Y.V.; Ashwell, K.W.S. (1997). Disorders of brain development in the progeny of mothers who used alcohol during pregnancy. *Early Human Development, 48,* 153-166.

Kopera-Frye, K.; Carmichael Olson, H.; Streissguth, A.P. (1997). Teratogenic effects of alcohol on attention. In J.A. Burack and J.T. Enns (eds.), *Attention, Development, and Psychopathology* (pp. 171-204). New York: The Guilford Press.

Lawrence, A.D.; Watkins, L.H.A.; Sahakian, B.J.; Hodges, J.R.; Robbins, T.W. (2000). Visual object and visuospatial cognition in Huntington's disease: Implications for information processing in corticostriatal circuits. *Brain, 123,* 1349-1364.

Lemoine, P.; Harousseau, H.; Borteryu, J.P.; Menuet, J.C. (1968). Les enfants des parents alcooliques: Anomalies observees. A proposos de 127 cas [Children of alcoholic parents: Abnormalities observed in 127 cases]. *Ouest Medical, 21,* 476-482.

Mattson, S.N.; Goodman, A.M.; Caine, C.; Delis, D.C.; Riley, E.P. (1999). Executive functioning in children with heavy prenatal alcohol exposure. *Alcoholism: Clinical and Experimental Research, 23,* 1808-1815.

Mattson, S.N.; Riley, E.P. (1996). Brain anomalies in fetal alcohol syndrome. In E.L. Abel (ed.), *Fetal Alcohol Syndrome: From Mechanism to Prevention* (pp. 51-68). Boca Raton, FL: CRC Press.

Mattson, S.N.; Riley, E.P. (1997). Neurobehavioral and neuroanatomical effects of heavy prenatal exposure to alcohol. In A. Streissguth and J. Kanter (eds.), *The Challenge of Fetal Alcohol Syndrome: Overcoming Secondary Disabilities.* Seattle, WA: University of Washington Press.

Mattson, S.N.; Riley, E.P. (1999). Implicit and explicit memory functioning in children with heavy prenatal alcohol exposure. *Journal of International Neuropsychological Society, 5,* 462-471.

Mattson, S.N.; Riley, E.P. (2000). Parent ratings of behavior in children with heavy prenatal alcohol exposure and IQ-matched controls. *Alcoholism, Clinical and Experimental Research, 24,* 226-231.

Mattson, S.N.; Riley, E.P.; Delis, D.C.; Stern, C.; Jones, K.L. (1996). Verbal learning and memory in children with fetal alcohol syndrome. *Alcoholism: Clinical and Experimental Research, 20,* 810-816.

Mattson, S.N.; Riley, E.P.; Gramling, L.; Delis, D.C.; Jones, K.L. (1997). Heavy prenatal alcohol exposure with or without physical features of fetal alcohol syndrome leads to IQ deficits. *Journal of Pediatrics, 131,* 718-721.

Mattson, S.N.; Riley, E.P.; Gramling, L.; Delis, D.C.; Jones, K.L. (1998). Neuropsychological comparison of children with or without physical features of fetal alcohol syndrome. *Neuropsychology, 12,* 146-153.

Mattson, S.N.; Riley, E.P.; Jernigan, T.L.; Ehlers, C.L.; Delis, D.C.; Jones, K.L.; Stern, C.; Johnson, K.A.; Hesselink, J.R.; Bellugi, U. (1992). Fetal alcohol syndrome: A case report of neuropsychological, MRI, and EEG assessment of two children. *Alcoholism: Clinical and Experimental Research, 16,* 1001-1003.

Mattson, S.N.; Riley, E.P.; Jernigan, T.L.; Garcia, A.; Kaneko, W.M.; Ehlers, C. L.; Jones, K.L. (1994). A decrease in the size of the basal ganglia following prenatal alcohol exposure: A preliminary report. *Neurotoxicology and Teratology, 16,* 283-289.

Mattson, S.N.; Riley, E.P.; Sowell, E.R.; Jernigan, T.L.; Sobel, D.F.; Jones, K.L. (1996). A decrease in the size of the basal ganglia in children with fetal alcohol syndrome. *Alcoholism: Clinical and Experimental Research, 20,* 1088-1093.

Middleton, F.A.; Strick, P.L. (1994). Anatomical evidence for cerebellar and basal ganglia involvement in higher cognitive function. *Science, 266,* 458-461.

Middleton, F.A.; Strick, P.L. (2000). Basal ganglia and cerebellar loops: Motor and cognitive circuits. *Brain Research Reviews, 31,* 236-250.

Miller, M. (1988). Effect of prenatal exposure to ethanol on the development of cerebral cortex: I. Neuronal generation. *Alcoholism: Clinical and Experimental Research, 12,* 440-449.

Mostofsky, S.H.; Reiss, A.L.; Lockhart, P.; Denckla, M.B. (1998). Evaluation of cerebellar size in attention-deficit hyperactivity disorder. *Journal of Child Neurology, 13,* 434-439.

Nanson, J.L.; Hiscock, M. (1990). Attention deficits in children exposed to alcohol prenatally. *Alcoholism: Clinical and Experimental Research, 14,* 656-661.

Olson, H.C.; Feldman, J.J.; Streissguth, A.P.; Sampson, P.D.; Bookstein, F.L. (1998). Neuropsychological deficits in adolescents with fetal alcohol syndrome: Clinical findings. *Alcoholism: Clinical and Experimental Research, 22,* 1998-2012.

Pearson, D.A.; Lachar, D.; Loveland, K.A.; Santos, C.W.; Faria, L.P.; Azzam, P.N.; Hentges, B.A.; Cleveland, L.A. (2000). Patterns of behavior adjustment and maladjustment in mental retardation: Comparison of children with and without ADHD. *American Journal on Mental Retardation, 105,* 236-251.

Peiffer, J.; Majewski, F.; Fischbach, H.; Bierich, J.R.; Volk, B. (1979). Alcohol embryo- and fetopathy. *Journal of the Neurological Sciences, 41,* 125-137.

Pennington, B.F.; Ozonoff, S. (1996). Executive functions and developmental psychopathology. *Journal of Child Psychology and Psychiatry, 37,* 51-87.

Pierce, D.R.; Goodlett, C.R.; West, J.R. (1989). Differential neuronal loss following early postnatal alcohol exposure. *Teratology, 40,* 113-126.

Pulsifer, M.B. (1996). The neuropsychology of mental retardation. *Journal of the International Neuropsychological Society, 2,* 159-176.

Rao, S.M.; Bobholz, J.A.; Hammeke, T.A.; Rose, A.C.; Woodley, S.J.; Cunningham, J.M.; Cox, R.W.; Stein, E.A.; Binder, J.R. (1997). Functional MRI evidence for subcortical participation in conceptual reasoning skills. *Neuroreport, 8,* 1987-1993.

Riikonen, R.; Salonen, I.; Partanen, K.; Verho, S. (1999). Brain perfusion SPECT and MRI in foetal alcohol syndrome. *Developmental Medicine and Child Neurology, 41,* 652-659.

Riley, E.P.; Mattson, S.N.; Sowell, E.R.; Jernigan, T.L.; Sobel, D.F.; Jones, K.L. (1995). Abnormalities of the corpus callosum in children prenatally exposed to alcohol. *Alcoholism: Clinical and Experimental Research, 19,* 1198-1202.

Robin, N.H.; Zachai, E.H. (1994). Unusual craniofacial dysmorphia due to prenatal alcohol and cocaine exposure. *Teratology, 50,* 160-164.

Roebuck, T.M.; Mattson, S.N.; Riley, E.P. (1998). A review of the neuroanatomical findings in children with fetal alcohol syndrome or prenatal exposure to alcohol. *Alcoholism: Clinical and Experimental Research, 22,* 339-344.

Roebuck, T.M.; Mattson, S.N.; Riley, E.P. (1999). Behavioral and psychosocial profiles of alcohol-exposed children. *Alcoholism: Clinical and Experimental Research, 23,* 1070-1076.

Ronen, G.M.; Andrews, W.L. (1991). Holoprosencephaly as a possible embryonic alcohol effect. *American Journal of Medical Genetics, 40,* 151-154.

Sampson, P.D.; Streissguth, A.P.; Bookstein, F.L.; Little, R.E.; Clarren, S.K.; Dehaene, P.; Hanson, J.W.; Graham, J.M. Jr. (1997). Incidence of fetal alcohol syndrome and prevalence of alcohol-related neurodevelopmental disorder. *Teratology, 56,* 317-326.

Samson, H.H. (1986). Microcephaly and fetal alcohol syndrome: Human and animal studies. In J.R. West (ed.), *Alcohol and Brain Development* (pp. 167-183). New York: Oxford University Press.

Schaefer, G.B.; Bodensteiner, J.B.; Thompson, J.N.; Wilson, D.A. (1991). Clinical and morphometric analysis of the hypoplastic corpus callosum. *Archives of Neurology, 48,* 933-936.

Schmahmann, J.D. (1997). *International Review of Neurobiology: Volume 41, The Cerebellum and Cognition.* San Diego, CA: Academic Press.

Schmahmann, J.D.; Pandya, D.N. (1997). The cerebrocerebellar system. In J.D. Schmahmann (ed.), *International Review of Neurobiology: Volume 41, The Cerebellum and Cognition* (pp. 31-60). San Diego, CA: Academic Press.

Shaywitz, S.E.; Caparulo, B.K.; Hodgson, E.S. (1981). Developmental language disability as a consequence of prenatal exposure to ethanol. *Pediatrics, 68,* 850-855.

Siebert, J.R.; Astley, S.J.; Clarren, S.K. (1991). Holoprosencephaly in a fetal macaque *(Macaca nemestrina)* following weekly exposure to ethanol. *Teratology, 44,* 29-36.

Smith, M.L.; Milner, B. (1981). The role of the right hippocampus in the recall of spatial location. *Neuropsychologia, 27,* 781-793.

Sowell, E.R.; Jernigan, T.L.; Mattson, S.N.; Riley, E.P.; Sobel, D.F.; Jones, K.L. (1996). Abnormal development of the cerebellar vermis in children prenatally exposed to alcohol: Size reduction in lobules I-V. *Alcoholism: Clinical and Experimental Research, 20,* 31-34.

Sowell, E.R.; Thompson, P.M.; Mattson, S.N.; Tessner, K.D.; Jernigan, T.L.; Riley, E.P.; Toga, A.W. (2001). Voxel-based morphometric analyses of the brain in children and adolescents prenatally exposed to alcohol. *Neuroreport, 12,* 515-523.

Steinhausen, H.C.; Spohr, H.L. (1998). Long-term outcome of children with fetal alcohol syndrome: Psychopathology, behavior, and intelligence. *Alcoholism: Clinical and Experimental Research, 22,* 334-338.

Steinhausen, H.C.; Willms, J.; Spohr, H.L. (1993). Long-term psychopathological and cognitive outcome of children with fetal alcohol syndrome. *Journal of the American Academy of Child and Adolescent Psychiatry, 32,* 990-994.

Steinhausen, H.C.; Willms, J.; Spohr, H.L. (1994). Correlates of psychopathology and intelligence in children with fetal alcohol syndrome. *Journal of Child Psychology and Psychiatry, 35,* 323-331.

Streissguth, A. (1997). *Fetal Alcohol Syndrome: A Guide for Families and Communities.* Baltimore, MD: Paul H. Brooks Publishing.

Streissguth, A.; Barr, H.; Kogan, J.; Bookstein, F. (1997). Primary and secondary disabilities in fetal alcohol syndrome. In A. Streissguth and J. Kanter (eds.), *The Challenge of Fetal Alcohol Syndrome: Overcoming Secondary Disabilities* (pp. 25-39). Seattle, WA: University of Washington Press.

Streissguth, A.P.; Randels, S.P.; Smith, D.F. (1991). A test-retest study of intelligence in patients with fetal alcohol syndrome: Implications for care. *Journal of the American Academy of Child and Adolescent Psychiatry, 30,* 584-587.

Sulik, K.K.; Johnston, M.C. (1982). Embryonic origin of holoprosencephaly: Interrelationship of the developing brain and face. *Scanning Electron Microscopy, Pt 1,* 309-322.

Swayze, V.W. II.; Johnson, V.P.; Hanson, J.W.; Piven, J.; Sato, Y.; Giedd, J.N.; Mosnik, D.; Andreasen, N.C. (1997). Magnetic resonance imaging of brain anomalies in fetal alcohol syndrome. *Pediatrics, 99,* 232-240.

Thomas, S.E.; Kelly, S.J.; Mattson, S.N.; Riley, E.P. (1998). Comparison of social abilities of children with fetal alcohol syndrome to those of children with similar IQ scores and normal controls. *Alcoholism: Clinical and Experimental Research, 22,* 528-533.

Townsend, J.; Courchesne, E.; Covington, J.; Westerfield, M.; Harris, N.S.; Lyden, P.; Lowry, T.P.; Press, G.A. (1999). Spatial attention deficits in patients with acquired or developmental cerebellar abnormality. *The Journal of Neuroscience, 19,* 5632-5643.

Uecker, A.; Nadel, L. (1996). Spatial locations gone awry: Object and spatial memory deficits in children with fetal alcohol syndrome. *Neuropsychologia, 34,* 209-223.

Uecker, A.; Nadel, L. (1998). Spatial but not object memory impairments in children with fetal alcohol syndrome. *American Journal on Mental Retardation, 103,* 12-18.

Wang, P.P.; Doherty, S.; Hesselink, J.R.; Bellugi, U. (1992). Callosal morphology concurs with neurobehavioral and neuropathological findings in two neurodevelopmental disorders. *Archives of Neurology, 49,* 407-411.

Watkins, L.H.A.; Rogers, R.D.; Lawrence, A.D.; Sahakian, B.J.; Rosser, A.E.; Robbins, T.W. (2000). Impaired planning but intact decision making in early Huntington's disease: Implications for specific fronto-striatal pathology. *Neuropsychologia, 38,* 1112-1125.

Wechsler, D. (1991). *WISC-III Manual: Wechsler Intelligence Scale for Children, Third Edition.* New York: The Psychological Corporation.

Welsh, M.C.; Pennington, B.F. (1988). Assessing frontal lobe functioning in children: Views from developmental psychology. *Developmental Neuropsychology, 4,* 199-230.

Wisniewski, K.; Dambska, M.; Sher, J.H.; Qazi, Q. (1983). A clinical neuropathological study of the fetal alcohol syndrome. *Neuropediatrics, 14,* 197-201.

Woodruff-Pak, D.S. (1997). Classical conditioning. In J.D. Schmahmann (ed.), *International Review of Neurobiology: Volume 41, The Cerebellum and Cognition* (pp. 342-366). San Diego, CA: Academic Press.

Chapter 6

Health Consequences of Marijuana Use

Alan J. Budney
Brent A. Moore
Ryan Vandrey

Marijuana smoking remains the most prevalent form of illicit drug use in the United States, Canada, Australia, New Zealand, and some European countries, and rates of heavy marijuana smoking are high in other countries where accurate epidemiological data are not available (Black and Casswell, 1993; Hall, Johnston, et al., 1999; Substance Abuse and Mental Health Services Administration [SAMHSA], 1999). In the United States, conservative estimates indicate that more than 11 million people smoked marijuana during the last month, and approximately 20 percent of these smoke almost daily (SAMHSA, 2000). The types of problems associated with regular marijuana use have been well documented. Heavy use has been linked to impairment in memory, concentration, motivation, health, interpersonal relationships, and employment, as well as decreased participation in conventional roles of adulthood, history of psychiatric symptoms and hospitalizations, and participation in deviant activities (Haas and Hendin, 1987; Halikas et al., 1983; Jones, 1980; Kandel, 1984; Rainone et al., 1987; Roffman and Barnhart, 1987). Given the large cohort of frequent marijuana users, it is vital that we have available clear, scientific information concerning the risks and consequences of acute and chronic use of marijuana and other forms of cannabis.

Cannabis is the generic name for the psychoactive substance(s) derived from the plant *Cannabis sativa*. Marijuana and hashish are the common forms of cannabis used to obtain psychoactive effects. Cannabis contains numerous chemical substances, but the one usually of primary interest is delta-9-tetrahydrocannabinol (THC). THC has been identified as the predominant substance in marijuana that produces the subjective "high" asso-

Preparation of this chapter was supported, in part, by grants DA12471 and DA12157 from the National Institute on Drug Abuse.

ciated with smoking the plant. Some debate exists regarding whether other compounds in cannabis have direct psychoactive effects or whether they interact with THC to produce other physical or psychological effects. This distinction is important, as "pure" forms of THC that are used orally in medical settings (dronabinol, Marinol) may not have identical effects to smoked or orally ingested cannabis. Moreover, because the most common method of using cannabinoids is smoking (marijuana or hashish), the other substances present in the smoke (e.g., carcinogens, tar) are relevant to a discussion of the health consequences of marijuana use (see sections on the respiratory, immune, and cardiovascular systems in this chapter).

Cannabis was used in the Western Hemisphere both medically and recreationally as early as the eighteenth century. Yet, it was not until the 1930s that scientific investigation began in response to concern over its nonmedical use. Two reports on the health consequences of marijuana use appeared in the mid-1900s (Mayor's Committee on Marijuana [MCM], 1944; Walton, 1938), and the Marijuana Tax Act of 1937 functionally served to prohibit the recreational use of marijuana in the United States. Subsequent to these reports, scientific efforts were limited until the 1960s and 1970s when the prevalence of marijuana use and abuse increased in Western cultures.

Cannabis use in the United States and other countries has long been a topic of controversy. Groups such as NORML (National Organization for the Reform of Marijuana Laws) have led an ongoing effort to decriminalize and legalize marijuana use, and a number of respected medical professionals have argued for legitimizing the medical use of marijuana (Grinspoon and Bakalar, 1997; Hollister, 2000). Marijuana supporters argue that cannabis (1) has many positive effects and benefits, (2) has few and minor adverse consequences, and (3) is less harmful than other legalized drugs such as alcohol. They further argue that government obstructionism and propaganda have misled the public regarding the adverse effects of cannabis.

Such controversy can bias the evaluation and interpretation of scientific findings regarding the health effects of cannabis use, creating general misperceptions and confusion about the current state of knowledge. Conflicting and inconclusive scientific findings have fueled the controversy. As this chapter will indicate, there is much still unknown about the effects of cannabis on human psychological and physical health. Epidemiological and experimental studies have provided clear evidence that many people experience problems related to cannabis use and that ingestion of cannabis is associated with multiple adverse effects. However, demonstrating causal relationships between cannabis use and many of these effects has proven difficult due to methodological challenges. The magnitude of risk and functional significance of such effects also remains elusive.

This chapter summarizes the scientific literature regarding the effects of cannabis on physical health, cognitive and behavioral functioning, and mental/behavioral health. Data relevant to the addictive potential of cannabis use are also presented. We focus on areas with a substantial research base that have provided some indication of definite findings. The space provided to each topic corresponds somewhat to the scope of the literature in that area. We comment on the strength and quality of data supporting the connection between cannabis use and specific effects, but, generally, detailed critical analyses of individual studies or purported causal mechanisms are not provided. Rather, the reader is referred to original sources and previous reviews.

RESPIRATORY SYSTEM

Perhaps the most significant health effects of cannabis are those that impact the respiratory system. Smoking is the primary method for use of cannabis, and almost all chronic users smoke either marijuana cigarettes ("joints") or use pipes to smoke marijuana or hashish. Chronic cannabis smoking has potential for significant respiratory health consequences comparable to tobacco cigarette smoking. The smokes of marijuana and tobacco have similar levels of tar and respiratory toxic chemicals. Marijuana smoke contains up to 50 percent more carcinogens and results in substantially greater tar deposits in the lungs than filtered tobacco cigarettes. Such increased effects likely occur because marijuana users smoke unfiltered material, inhale the smoke more deeply, and hold the smoke longer in their lungs than tobacco smokers (Hoffman et al., 1975; Institute of Medicine, 1982; Roth et al., 1998; Tashkin et al., 1991; Tashkin et al., 1987; Wu et al., 1988). However, marijuana smokers tend to smoke significantly less material per day than tobacco smokers, which serves to counter its impact on the lungs.

Acute Effects

The most significant acute effect of smoking marijuana is its action as a bronchodilator, which increases vulnerability to the smoke by decreasing airway resistance and increasing specific airway conductance (Tashkin et al., 1973; Vachon et al., 1973). Marijuana-induced bronchodilation has been demonstrated with healthy control participants and asthmatics, and under conditions of experimentally induced asthma (Tashkin et al., 1975). Placebo-controlled studies suggest that bronchodilation is due to the THC content in marijuana (Tashkin et al., 1975). Of note, marijuana's effect on brochodilation distinguishes it from tobacco smoking, which produces bronchoconstriction.

Marijuana smoking also increases absorption of carbon monoxide, resulting in elevated levels of blood carboxyhemoglobin (COHb) (Wu et al., 1988; Tilles et al., 1986). Although smoking tobacco also boosts COHb, the increase found with smoking marijuana is as much as four times greater than with tobacco. These elevated levels of COHb lead to reduced oxygen in the blood and impairment in oxygen release from hemoglobin. Reduced blood oxygen levels can stress a number of organs including the heart (see section on cardiovascular effects this chapter). In placebo-controlled studies, examinations of other short-term aspects of respiration such as breathing rate, breath depth, CO_2 production, respiratory exchange ratio, and arterial blood gasses have revealed no significant effects of marijuana smoking (Shapiro et al., 1976).

Chronic Effects

The impact of chronic marijuana smoking on respiratory health has many similarities to that of tobacco smoking (Tashkin, 1999; VanHoozen and Cross, 1997). Compared to nonsmokers, chronic marijuana smokers show increased likelihood of outpatient visits for respiratory illness and exhibit respiratory symptoms of bronchitis at comparable rates to tobacco smokers (Tashkin et al., 1987; Bloom et al., 1987; Polen et al., 1993; Taylor et al., 2000). Chronic bronchitis can be moderately debilitating and increases the risk of additional infections. Because THC appears to suppress immune system function, recurrent bronchitis may further increase the risk of opportunistic respiratory infections such as pneumonia and aspergillosis (see the following section on immune systems effects). This is of concern particularly for those individuals with already compromised immune functions such as cancer and AIDS patients.

Airway obstruction and symptoms of chronic cough, sputum production, and wheezing characterize chronic bronchitis. These symptoms are the result of airway inflammation and tissue damage caused by marijuana smoke that results in increased fluid production, cellular abnormalities, and reduced aveolar permeability (Tashkin et al., 1987; Gil et al., 1995). This damage begins long before overt symptoms such as cough or wheezing are evident (Roth et al., 1998). Cellular abnormalities include reductions in ciliating surface cells of the lungs that function to clear fluid from the lungs to the mouth and throat. As a result, marijuana smokers have substantially higher bronchitis index scores than nonsmokers, and comparable scores to tobacco smokers, even at young ages with only short histories of marijuana use (Taylor et al., 2000).

Investigations of chronic obstructive pulmonary disease (COPD) in chronic marijuana smokers have been inconclusive. A common severe consequence of tobacco smoking, COPD includes chronic *obstructive* bronchitis or emphysema, and is characterized by impairment in small airway function rather than large airways. Marijuana smokers exhibit almost identical degrees of histopathologic and molecular abnormalities associated with progression to COPD in tobacco smokers (Barsky et al., 1998; Fligiel et al., 1991, 1997; Mao and Oh, 1998). However, two large-scale studies of COPD in chronic marijuana users have been inconclusive. Bloom and colleagues (1987) reported some indication of reduced small-airway function suggestive of COPD, while Tashkin and colleagues (1987) found no evidence of small airway obstruction or other indicators of COPD.

Chronic cannabis smoking is likely associated with respiratory cancer, although this link is not definitive (see section on immune system effects). Cannabis smoking is clearly associated with similar processes and patterns of disease that lead to aerodigestive cancers among tobacco smokers (Mao and Oh, 1998; MacPhee, 1999). As noted previously, marijuana smoke contains more carcinogens than cigarette smoke (Hoffman et al., 1975). Marijuana interferes with normal cell function, including synthesis and functions of DNA and RNA (Tahir and Zimmerman, 1991), and appears to activate an enzyme that converts inactive carcinogens found in marijuana smoke into active carcinogens (Marques-Magallanes et al., 1997). Chronic marijuana smokers also show substantial cellular mutation associated with tumor progression (Barsky et al., 1998; Fligiel et al., 1997; Gong et al., 1987; Sherman et al., 1995). Marijuana also reduces the ability of pulmonary alveolar macrophages to kill pathogens, including tumor cells, allowing tumors to grow more rapidly (Baldwin et al., 1997; Zhu et al., 2000).

Clinical reports of aerodigestive cancers in individuals who had a history of marijuana smoking with limited or no tobacco exposure have provided suggestive evidence of a link between marijuana use and cancer (Caplan and Brigham, 1990; Donald, 1991; Fung et al., 1999; Sridhar et al., 1995; Taylor, 1988). In addition, Zhang and colleagues (1999) found increased risk for squamous-cell carcinoma of the head and neck for marijuana smokers compared to nonsmokers when tobacco smoking was statistically controlled. The only epidemiological study that directly examined the risk of aerodigestive cancer in marijuana users reported no significant risk associated with cannabis (Sidney et al., 1997). This study, however, included a relatively young cohort comprised of primarily experimental and light marijuana users rather than chronic heavy users. Individuals who began smoking marijuana in the late 1960s are now approaching ages that are more likely to be associated with aerodigestive cancer, hence, future epidemiological studies should better clarify the risk of cancer associated with chronic cannabis use.

Smoking both cannabis and tobacco warrants mention as this combination most likely produces an additive adverse effect on the respiratory system (Roth et al., 1998; Barsky et al., 1998). Tobacco smoking is common among cannabis users, as almost half of daily marijuana users also smoke tobacco (SAMHSA, 2000; Moore and Budney, 2001). This subgroup of marijuana smokers merits careful study since they may be at particularly high risk for respiratory disease.

IMMUNE SYSTEM

Chronic use of cannabis appears to compromise the immune system, particularly the immune defense systems of the lungs (Baldwin et al., 1997; Klein, 1999; Sherman, Campbell, et al., 1991). This suppressive effect occurs in a variety of immune cells including killer cells, T cells, and macrophages (Kusher et al., 1994; Klein et al., 1998; Newton et al., 1994). Most research has focused on pulmonary alveolar macrophages (PAMs) which are the killer cells that destroy infectious microorganisms in the lungs (Sherman, Campbell, et al., 1991; Huber et al., 1991). Compared to tobacco smokers and nonsmokers, PAMs of chronic cannabis smokers exhibit a reduced ability to kill tumor cells and many microorganisms, including fungi and bacteria (Baldwin et al., 1997; Zhu et al., 2000; Sherman, Campbell, et al., 1991). As with tobacco, cannabis smoking produces an inflammatory response in the lungs which increases growth in the number and concentration of PAMs. However, their efficacy for destroying microorganisms is compromised (Barbers et al., 1991; Wallace et al., 1994). Cannabis smoking also appears to impair phagocytosis and cytokine function of the PAMs (Baldwin et al., 1997). A recent study has identified a specific cannabinoid receptor-mediated pathway that may be involved in the inhibitory responses associated with chronic cannabis smoking (Zhu et al., 2000).

The functional consequences of cannabis's effect on the suppression of the immune system in humans is poorly understood. Nonetheless, clinical findings suggest that such effects warrant some concern. Chronic cannabis smoking is associated with increased bronchitis and other respiratory illnesses. Chronic use may also increase risk of exposure to infectious organisms, since cannabis and tobacco plants are often contaminated with a variety of fungi and molds including aspergillus (Verweij et al., 2000). Lung illnesses in marijuana smokers have been attributed to fungal infection (Verweij et al., 2000; Caiaffa et al., 1994; Marks et al., 1996). Decreased immune system response could increase the vulnerability and risk of developing these respiratory illnesses and lung diseases. More research is needed to determine whether chronic marijuana use is directly responsible for an increased incidence of disease via its effects on immune system function.

Of note, medical use of marijuana has now been legalized in two U.S. states and legislation is pending in others. Many of the patients deemed appropriate candidates for medical marijuana have illnesses that involve already compromised immune systems such as AIDS wasting syndrome and chronic pain from various types of cancer (Grinspoon and Bakalar, 1997; Hollister, 2000; Joy et al., 1999). A better understanding of the functional significance of marijuana's effects on the immune system is imperative as attempts are made to develop safe and effective models for the medical use of marijuana.

CARDIOVASCULAR SYSTEM

Relatively little research has examined long-term cardiovascular effects of chronic cannabis use. Most studies have focused on acute changes and suggest a limited cardiovascular health impact associated with cannabis use. The primary acute effect of smoked marijuana or oral THC is tachycardia (Beaconsfield et al., 1972; Perez-Reyes et al., 1973). The increase in heart rate appears dose dependent, is observed with nonusers and chronic users, and is reduced as tolerance develops (Benowitz and Jones, 1975; Jones and Benowitz, 1976).

Cannabis or oral THC can produce small increases in supine blood pressure and impair vascular reflexes (Jones and Benowitz, 1976; Perez-Reyes et al., 1991; Maddock et al., 1979). Smoking marijuana also results in increased inhalation of carbon monoxide and subsequent COHb, which in combination with tachycardia, increases the work required of the heart. Cannabis use also may reduce exercise tolerance, which is likely due to the combination of tachycardia, reduced thermoregulation caused by decreased vascular reflexes, and the increase in carbon monoxide (Renaud and Cormier, 1986).

Although these findings show clear changes in cardiovascular functioning due to marijuana or THC use, the effects have not been associated with short-term or long-term cardiovascular or cerebrovascular injury or disease. Case reports suggest that regular cannabis smoking may increase risk for some severe disorders such as arteritis and transient ischemic attacks (Mouzak et al., 2000; Goldschmidt et al., 2000), but no controlled studies support these reports. For most healthy young marijuana smokers the stress to the heart produced by marijuana use does not appear clinically detrimental (Institute of Medicine, 1982). However, for individuals with cardiovascular or cerebrovascular disease the additional cardiac stress may increase the risk for chest pain, heart attack, or stroke. Additional research is needed to further elucidate the effects of chronic cannabis use on cardiovascular health, including interactions with other risk factors.

REPRODUCTIVE FUNCTION

Hormones and Fertility

Research examining the effects of cannabis use on reproductive function in women or men has been sparse. In women, marijuana smoking can affect some reproductive hormones (e.g., luteinizing hormone, prolactin), but this effect may occur only when smoking takes place during specific phases of the menstrual cycle (Mendelson et al., 1985, 1986; Block et al., 1991). Chronic cannabis use appears to alter male reproductive hormones, but these effects are not conclusive. Some studies have demonstrated marijuana-related decreased levels of gonadotropin, testosterone, prolactin, and luteinizing hormones in men, while others have reported negative findings (Murphy, 1999). For both men and women the functional significance of these findings remains elusive. Although one might suspect that these purported effects on the reproductive system would adversely influence fertility, this has not been carefully studied in humans.

Perinatal Effects

Pregnant women who use cannabis expose the fetus to its effects, as THC is known to cross the placenta (Howell, Coles, and Kable address the prenatal effects of cannabis use in Chapter 9 of this book). Here we provide an overview of perinatal effects of cannabis use, focused primarily on cognitive functioning. It is estimated that 10 to 20 percent of women use marijuana during pregnancy (Chasnoff, 1990; Fried et al., 1985; Zuckerman et al., 1989). Thus, understanding the effects on fetal development is vital. Studying cannabis use during pregnancy in humans has proven difficult, as pregnant users generally have many additional risk factors for adverse effects such as tobacco smoking, alcohol use, other illicit drug use, poorer nutrition, and lower SES. Moreover, multiple factors deterring self-disclosure in this population raise concern regarding the validity of self-reports of cannabis use.

Studies have attempted to control for these confounds, hence, certain tentative conclusions appear justified. Risk of major congenital anomalies is not increased due to cannabis use in pregnant women (Zuckerman et al., 1989; Tennes et al., 1985). However, some reports suggest that risk of developing minor anomalies, particularly related to the visual system, may be related to heavy cannabis use, but these data are not robust (O'Connell and Fried, 1984; Hingson et al., 1982). Cannabis use during pregnancy may be related to reduced birth weight and length, and possibly shortened length of gestation, although studies have reported conflicting findings (Zuckerman et al., 1989; Day and Richardson, 1991; Gibson et al., 1983; Hatch and Bracken, 1986; Witter and Niebyl, 1990). Overall, these perinatal effects, if valid, are clearly not as severe as those observed with tobacco smokers.

The cognitive and behavioral effects of prenatal exposure to cannabis are perhaps best addressed in one study, the Ottawa Prenatal Prospective Study (OPPS) (Fried, 1980). This study collected birth data on 700 women and has periodically assessed the children of a subsample of 150 to 200. Adverse effects of prenatal cannabis use were observed in testing of the neonate during the first month. Possible indicators of an impact on the nervous system included increased tremors, decreased visual habituation, exaggerated startle, and increased hand-to-mouth behavior. However, at one and two years of age, no cannabis-related effects were observed when children were assessed using the Bayley Scales (Fried and Watkinson, 1988). No cannabis-related effects were observed at three years on tests of language expression, comprehension, and other general cognitive abilities, after controlling for confounding variables (Fried and Watkinson, 1990).

Age four assessments of OPPS children revealed cannabis-related performance decrements on verbal and memory tasks (Fried and Watkinson, 1990). These deficits were similar in type to another study of three-year-olds whose mothers smoked marijuana while pregnant (Day et al., 1994). One hypothesis for why impairment was not observed until age four is the possibility that such deficits may not be detectable until individuals reach a developmental age that allows for testing of more subtle effects on complex processes (Hutchings and Fried, 1999). However, similar testing at five and six years did not reveal any cannabis-related deficits. The authors suggested that environmental exposure to positive influences on cognitive abilities (e.g., school) might have obviated the subtle effects observed a year earlier. Thus, the researchers initiated additional testing of six-year-olds to assess other, more general aspects of cognitive performance such as sustained attention and impulse control. Evidence of a deficit in sustained attention was observed in children whose mothers used marijuana heavily during pregnancy (O'Connell and Fried, 1991).

Testing at nine and twelve years of age showed marijuana-related deficits in measures of higher order or executive functioning that the investigators characterized as involving visual analysis, problem solving, hypothesis testing, and impulse control (Hutchings and Fried, 1999; Fried and Watkinson, 2000). Of note, these types of complex functioning deficits are similar to those observed in some studies of chronic adolescent and adult marijuana users (reviewed later in this chapter). Goldschmidt and colleagues (2000) also reported adverse effects of prenatal marijuana use in ten-year-olds. Increased hyperactivity, impulsivity, inattention, and delinquency were associated with prenatal marijuana use after controlling for extraneous variables. Because of the limitations of their sample and other methodological issues, interpretation of these results warrants caution pending replication in other samples.

The observed effects of prenatal cannabis use on cognitive functioning appear subtle, and determining causality is difficult since genetic predispositions and multiple environmental factors after birth may interact with prenatal effects specific to cannabis use. The functional significance of these subtle deficits is also unclear; however, the types of impairment observed in the OPPS study could potentially affect general behavioral and cognitive performance abilities. Although these data are far from conclusive, they do raise concern regarding prenatal cannabis use and its effects on human offspring. As such, recommendations that pregnant women abstain from marijuana use appear warranted.

PSYCHOLOGICAL CONSEQUENCES

Acute Effects

A number of behavioral and emotional symptoms are associated with the intoxicating effects of cannabis. Generally, cannabis users experience mild euphoria, relaxation, and perceive an overall positive change of sensation and experience (food, music, interpersonal). Mild problems in thought and speech (loss of train of thought, loose associations, distortion in time perception) commonly occur, but these are not deemed aversive by most users, rather they are perceived as a positive aspect of the "high."

Cannabis intoxication appears to influence several aspects of social behavior, although relatively little research has been conducted in this area. The most consistent finding is some degree of introverted behavior (decreased verbal interactions), an effect that is uncommon among most drugs of abuse (Foltin and Fischman, 1988; Higgins and Stitzer, 1986; Kelly et al., 1990, 1994). In laboratory studies, cannabis intoxication generally does not change the amount of time individuals spend engaging in social activities (Kelly et al., 1990, 1994; Heishman et al., 1989). Rather, subjects tend to choose activities that do not require verbal communication (e.g., watching a movie with others). Cannabis intoxication may also increase the distance subjects maintain from each other in social situations (Rachlinski et al., 1989). These social effects of cannabis intoxication might be considered consistent with the increased anxiety and mild paranoia reported by some users. In addition, such effects among frequent users could potentially impact adolescent peer development and the quality of adult social relationships.

The most common adverse psychological reactions to acute intoxication include anxiety attacks, mild paranoia, and increased general anxiety (Schuckit, 1990). Little data on prevalence exist regarding these acute reactions, but they appear to occur in less experienced users, or in experienced users who ingest unusually high doses or use in a novel environment. These symptoms are typically of short duration and subside within hours of their onset. Most times they do not result in help-seeking, although they may be associated with marijuana-related emergency room visits. Such effects are typically managed with education, empathic support, and reassurance. With much less frequency, cannabis ingestion has been associated with more severe psychotic reactions such as hallucinations and delusions (see the following section on psychosis for further information).

Mental Health/Nonpsychotic Disorders

Cross-sectional and longitudinal studies have reported a clear association between chronic cannabis use and impaired psychological functioning (Kandel, 1984; Brooks et al., 1999; Deykin et al., 1986; Fergusson and Horwood, 1997; Kandel et al., 1986; Miller-Johnson et al., 1998; McGee et al., 2000). In particular, cannabis use has been associated with poorer life satisfaction, increased mental health treatment and hospitalization, higher rates of depression, anxiety disorders, suicide attempts, and conduct disorder.

Whether cannabis use contributes to or causes these mental health problems, or the converse, is not clear. Controlling for risk factors common to both problems appears to reduce but not eliminate the positive association (Ferguson and Horwood, 1997; Kandel et al., 1986; McGee et al., 2000). Recent research suggests that the direction of influence may depend on the age of onset of cannabis use (McGee et al., 2000). Early onset of cannabis use is a strong predictor of later mental health problems, but such early onset may itself be predicted from prior mental health problems. Of note, the types of mental health problems that remain associated with cannabis use, once common etiological factors are adequately controlled in longitudinal studies, are typically externalizing problems such as conduct/antisocial disorder or drug dependence disorders.

Cannabis use can be considered a risk factor for mental health problems and, as such, a target for prevention and intervention. Mental health problems and early cannabis use appear to share a common pathway predicted by socioeconomic disadvantage and child behavior problems (McGee et al., 2000). Data on the causal nature of this relationship remain equivocal.

Psychosis

Whether or not marijuana use can induce psychosis (hallucinations, delusions, thought disorder, impaired reality testing) or psychotic disorders (e.g., schizophrenia) remains controversial. Here we discuss data addressing the relationship between acute psychosis and cannabis, followed by a more extensive discussion of the relationship between cannabis and schizophrenia.

Acute Psychosis

Clinical case reports frequent the literature with examples of patients with psychotic symptoms whose onset closely follows ingestion of cannabis and whose symptoms remit within days or, at most, a few weeks of abstinence from cannabis (Schuckit, 1990). Typical symptoms include hallucinations, delusions, confusion, amnesia, paranoia, hypomania, and labile mood, although case reports vary regarding which and how many of these symptoms are observed across patients. Prevalence data on this phenomenon do not appear available.

Suggestive evidence for a causal relationship between cannabis use and acute psychosis is of three types. First, in most case reports, the psychosis appears to involve large doses of cannabis. Large doses of THC have been shown to produce hallucinations in human and nonhuman laboratory studies (Kaymakcalan, 1973; Georgotas and Zeidenberg, 1979). Second, many cases of purported cannabis-induced psychosis involve patients without previous psychiatric histories. Third, the psychotic symptoms usually remit within days. Nonetheless, the literature linking cannabis use and acute psychosis includes only uncontrolled studies, thus other causes for the psychosis cannot be ruled out. One could reasonably conclude that high doses of cannabis can precipitate psychosis in some individuals, but whether or not a predisposition to psychotic illness or some other baseline factor is necessary for psychosis to occur is unknown.

Of note, some researchers have attempted to differentiate acute toxic psychosis (due to direct intoxicating effects) from acute functional psychosis that is precipitated by chronic cannabis but not necessarily due to its intoxicating effects (Thacore and Shukla, 1976). This distinction is difficult to operationalize since acute psychotic effects described across studies typically continue well after (days to weeks) the known duration of the direct effects of cannabis (hours). Hence, discriminating between "functional" or "toxic" effects presents a most difficult methodological challenge. Although studies have attempted to do so by examining differences in cannabis-use patterns, responses to medication, and patterns of psychotic symptoms, results remain inconclusive (Thornicroft, 1990).

Schizophrenia

A number of research studies indicate that cannabis use has some relation to the development and course of schizophrenia, however, the causal nature of this association is difficult to study and remains unfounded. The argument for cannabis use precipitating schizophrenia is primarily supported by research showing that drug-abusing schizophrenics (1) have an earlier onset of the disorder and drug use usually precedes reports of psychotic symptoms, (2) show fewer negative symptoms, and (3) show better response to medications than those schizophrenics who do not abuse drugs (Mueser et al., 1990; Andreasson et al., 1989). The most well-cited study on this topic is a 15-year prospective study conducted in Sweden (Andreasson et al., 1987). Researchers found that cannabis use at age 18 significantly increased risk for development of schizophrenia after controlling for other premorbid characteristics related to risk of schizophrenia, and the more frequent the cannabis use, the greater the risk.

Even this prospective study has methodological weaknesses that preclude drawing conclusions regarding the causal influence of cannabis. This literature has been critically reviewed in detail elsewhere (Channabasavanna et al., 1999), thus, here we offer just a few limitations inherent to this research. First, cannabis use may be initiated due to a prodromal syndrome of schizophrenia, or conversely, as might be the case in the Swedish study, good premorbid adjustment of future schizophrenics might increase the likelihood of contact with peers who use illicit drugs. Second, use of other drugs that can produce acute psychosis, such as amphetamines, has typically not been accounted for in most studies. Third, some studies do a poor job of differentiating schizophrenia from acute psychotic episodes which results in the inclusion of acute, cannabis-associated psychoses when documenting cases of schizophrenia.

Course of illness. How ongoing cannabis use affects the course of schizophrenia has important implications for the treatment and management of schizophrenia, since the rate of cannabis use among schizophrenics exceeds that of the general population and those with other types of psychiatric disorders (Negrete and Gill, 1999). The direct effects of cannabis intoxication, such as distorted time perception, cognitive impairment, and increased paranoia, along with reports of high doses causing hallucinations, delusions, and hypomania, would suggest that regular marijuana use may exacerbate psychiatric problems, particularly in those with major mental illnesses such as schizophrenia. Significant associations between drug use and increased use of treatment resources (hospitalizations and emergency room visits) and poor treatment compliance have been reported in psychiatric patients in general (Bartels et al., 1993; Leon et al., 1998; Richardson et al., 1985). The role of cannabis in most studies, however, has not been isolated from use of other types of drugs. Marijuana use has been associated with increased rates of recurrent psychiatric symptomatology and relapse among schizophrenics (Linszen et al., 1994; Linszen et al., 1997; Jablensky et al., 1991; Martinez-Arevalo et al., 1994; Negrete, 1989; Soni and Brownlee, 1991), but again, effects of other drug use cannot be completely ruled out in these studies. Of note, heavy cannabis use may also result in a misdiagnosis of cannabis-related psychosis resulting in a concomitant delay of a diagnosis and treatment of schizophrenia (Mathers et al., 1991).

Similar to the general population, cannabis use among psychiatric patients is associated with poorer psychosocial adjustment, criminal behavior, homelessness, and suicidality, but the causal direction of this association is unclear. These factors may contribute to the poor psychiatric outcome observed in schizophrenic cannabis users. As with the data on cannabis use and the development of psychotic disorders, a relatively strong association exists between cannabis use and a negative outcome in schizophrenics. Thus, cannabis use can be considered a risk factor for schizophrenia and a predictor of poor outcome in schizophrenic patients, but its role as an etiological factor remains uncertain.

COGNITIVE EFFECTS

Marijuana has long been thought to affect cognitive function. Early reviews, however, concluded that the scientific evidence for long-term deficits was inconclusive (Wert and Raulin, 1986a,b). This conclusion remains appropriate if one is referring to gross deficits with severe impairment of functioning. More recent findings from well-controlled studies indicate that cannabis use can lead to subtle, selective cognitive impairment (Solowij,

1999), although the functional significance of these deficits remains unclear. Specifically, tasks requiring "higher cognitive function" show significant deficits associated with chronic and frequent use of cannabis. The ability to organize and integrate complex information appears compromised, most likely due to an impact of cannabis on memory and attentional processes. A considerable research literature in this area has accumulated. Here, we provide a summary of the types of deficits associated with marijuana use in more recent studies and comment on the possible mechanisms involved.

Psychomotor Performance

Psychomotor performance measures provide a means of evaluating basic cognitive functions such as response slowing. We begin with a summary of this literature because general deficits in this area can affect performance on most other cognitive tasks. The Digit Symbol Substitution Task (DSST) (Lezak, 1995) has been the most commonly used measure of psychomotor performance in cannabis studies. Marijuana- or oral-THC-produced decrements in DSST response speed and accuracy have been observed in some studies, but not in others (Kelly et al., 1990; Azorlosa et al., 1992; Foltin et al., 1993; Heishman et al., 1988, 1997; Kamien et al., 1994; Kelly et al., 1993; Pickworth et al., 1997). Marijuana's effects on other psychomotor tasks have also proved inconclusive. Performance decreases on circular lights, standing steadiness, and pursuit rotor-tracking tasks have been reported in some studies (Cone et al., 1986; Chesher et al., 1990), while others have found no significant effects on circular light, tracking, card sorting, or reaction time tasks (Heishman et al., 1988, 1997; Pickworth et al., 1997).

With some exceptions, dose appears to partially account for between-study differences. Significant adverse effects are typically observed with higher doses, and dose-response effects have been observed in some studies that used multiple-dosing procedures. In summary, there appears to be moderately strong evidence that marijuana or THC used at higher doses can impair performance on some psychomotor tasks. This literature does not indicate a pervasive response slowing, such as decrements on simple reaction time tasks. Rather, tasks that are affected appear to depend more heavily on attention and motivation. As discussed later, cannabis intoxication may reduce the steady state of motivation. Because performance on most cognitive tests is influenced by the degree of attention and motivation directed toward the specific task, determining how cannabis affects these processes is necessary for better understanding its influence on cognitive processing.

Attention and Memory

Acute Effects

Laboratory research on the acute effects of cannabis use on memory has generally shown subtle effects that appear linked to dose and an associated attention or learning deficit. Research on immediate word recall, digit span, and digit recognition tasks has produced equivocal results. Some studies show evidence of impaired performance on short-term memory tasks following marijuana intoxication (Heishman et al., 1989; Chait, Corwin, et al., 1988; Block et al., 1992; Galanter et al., 1973), while others have not (Heishman et al., 1997; Casswell and Marks, 1973; Hooker and Jones, 1987). Dose-related effects can explain some but not all of these conflicting outcomes, as impairment was evident primarily in studies that examined higher doses.

Cannabis intoxication also affects the subjective perception of time. Time estimates are shorter and time productions are longer in subjects after smoking marijuana compared to placebo or no drug use (Jones and Stone, 1970; Chait, 1990; Cappell and Pliner, 1973). Cannabis intoxication does not appear to affect the ability to reproduce a time interval that has been modeled (Heishman et al., 1997; Dornbush et al., 1971). The mechanism for this temporal processing impairment is not clear, but deficits in attention warrant consideration.

The effects of marijuana on longer-term memory tasks (retrieval of information following a significant lapse in time) have proven more reliable across studies. Smoked marijuana has produced deficits in the recall of word lists and of prose material presented to subjects in placebo-controlled studies (Perez-Reyes et al., 1991; Heishman et al., 1997; Block et al., 1992; Hooker and Jones, 1987; Wetzel et al., 1982; Zacny and Chait, 1989). Interestingly, when retrieval cues are used, the impairment of marijuana on these memory tasks may be obviated (Hooker and Jones, 1987; Block and Wittenborn, 1984a,b). Such findings suggest that effects on attentional or learning processes may be primary mechanisms for memory performance deficits associated with cannabis use. Indeed, marijuana has been shown to disrupt the ability to learn novel tasks (Kamien et al., 1994). Moreover, marijuana- or THC-related deficits have generally been observed on divided attention tasks in which subjects must monitor multiple stimuli concurrently and make responses based on their observations (Heishman et al., 1989; Azorlosa et al., 1992; Kamien et al., 1994; Burns and Moskowitz, 1981; Chait, Corwin, et al., 1988; Marks and MacAvoy, 1989; Perez-Reyes et al., 1988).

Methodological differences across studies make it difficult to interpret findings on cannabis and memory. Nonetheless, this literature indicates that the acute effects of cannabis on memory are moderate at most, and are likely dose-dependent. The mechanism for these effects remains unclear, but deficits in attention and learning appear involved. How motivational factors impact these findings is also not clear. Interestingly, one early study reported that subjects performed better on memory tasks when they knew that the effects of marijuana on memory were being tested (Mendelson et al., 1974).

Chronic Effects

Studies of chronic effects of cannabis on cognitive processes have tried to examine the effects of chronic use while controlling for acute intoxication effects. A series of studies by Solowij (1999) examined the long-term effects of cannabis use on attentional processes. Regular cannabis users' performance on an auditory selective-attention task was measured after at least 24 hours of abstinence from cannabis use. Cannabis users' performances were significantly worse than matched controls, suggesting an inability to filter out complex irrelevant information. These findings were replicated in a second study that also demonstrated an association between years of marijuana use and the severity of attentional focus and information integration deficits. Moreover, a reduction in event-related potentials (P300 amplitude), a purported marker of cognitive processing, coincided with the observed cognitive deficits.

Solowij and colleagues (1997) also reported significant deficits in a study of long-term, heavy cannabis users interested in quitting their marijuana use. Increased perseveration on the Wisconsin Card Sorting Test and decreased memory on a verbal learning task were observed, and the severity of impairment increased with the duration of regular marijuana use. Similarly, Leavitt and colleagues (1993) reported that the duration of chronic cannabis use was related to deficits on tasks of verbal learning, complex reaction time, complex reasoning, and short-term memory. Pope and Yurgelun-Todd (1996) reported similar deficits in a study of heavy versus light marijuana-using college students with shorter histories of cannabis use. Again, a 24-hour abstinence period was required prior to testing. Heavy marijuana users made significantly more perseverative errors on the Wisconsin Card Sorting Test, had poorer recall on a verbal learning task, and showed other deficits on specific tasks compared to light users. The authors characterized their findings as deficits of the attentional/executive system involving mental flexibility, learning, and sustained attention.

Two controlled studies of adolescent marijuana abusers reported deficits in specific types of memory and learning tasks, further extending the potential impact of cannabis use to a younger sample (Millsaps et al., 1994; Schwartz et al., 1989). In addition, early onset of chronic cannabis use has recently been associated with impaired reaction time in visual scanning tasks but this relationship was not observed in late-onset users (Ehrenreich et al., 1999). This finding suggests the possibility of a specific vulnerability for development of an attentional impairment during early adolescence, and raises further concern about the impact of regular cannabis use on cognitive development and school performance.

To our knowledge, only one study has examined whether cognitive impairment related to chronic cannabis use recovers following cessation of use (Solowij et al., 1995). Ex-users (last use ranging from three months to six years), current long- and short-term users, and nonusers performed a selective attention task and event-related potentials were recorded. Findings suggested that ex-cannabis smokers continued to show impairment in their ability to filter out irrelevant information, although some evidence of partial recovery was noted.

Historically, interpretation of findings on the chronic effects of cannabis use has been limited by multiple confounding variables such as possible acute marijuana intoxication effects, variable marijuana use histories, unknown cognitive abilities prior to marijuana exposure, concurrent use of other drugs, demographic influences, and comorbidity with other mental or physical illnesses. Recent studies have made strong efforts to control for many of these variables, however, important confounds remain. For example, some studies have required a brief period of abstinence prior to testing to control for the acute intoxicating effects of cannabis. However, this procedure introduces another potential confound, i.e., whether acute withdrawal effects impact performance testing (Budney et al., 1999; Haney et al., 1999; Kouri and Pope, 2000). Moreover, as in studies of the acute effects of cannabis on cognitive performance tests, adverse effects on motivation may contribute to the deficits observed in studies of chronic cannabis use and performance. That is, chronic users may not expend as much effort toward testing as those in control groups.

Notwithstanding the methodological issues inherent to this research, the literature strongly suggests that chronic marijuana use can impair performance on various types of cognitive tests, specifically those thought to involve complex cognitive processes. These deficits may increase in form and severity in relation to the duration of exposure to cannabis. Future research is needed to better elucidate the processes that cause performance deficits and to determine their functional significance.

Academic Performance

Cannabis use has been linked to low grade-point averages, decreased school satisfaction, negative attitudes toward school, poor overall school performance, and absence from school (Lynskey and Hall, 2000). Early cannabis use (prior to age 16) is associated with dropping out of school before graduating high school (Brooks et al., 1999; Fergusson and Horwood, 1997; Fergusson et al., 1996). However, causality between cannabis use and poor academic achievement has not been established. Cannabis use also correlates significantly with delinquency, other drug problems, poor mental health, family dysfunction, and relationships with deviant peers, each of which is a likely contributor to academic problems. Studies that have statistically controlled for these factors have reported mixed results regarding the impact of cannabis use and academic performance (Ellickson et al., 1998; Krohn et al., 1997; Tanner et al., 1999).

Although one might expect that the adverse effects of cannabis use on attentional and complex cognitive processing would have some direct influence on optimal academic performance, the extent of this influence, if any, is unknown. Similarly, if cannabis use adversely affects motivation, one would expect a subsequent negative impact on academic performance through a decreased effort directed toward school work. The aforementioned other psychosocial problems associated with frequent cannabis use and concomitant effects on motivation to achieve in school would likely have a greater impact on a youth's academic performance than the subtle cannabis-related deficits in complex processing observed in laboratory studies. Whether marijuana use is a primary cause of academic problems or the converse, educational and behavioral problems lead to marijuana use, remains at issue.

Driving Performance

The effects of cannabis intoxication on driving have been examined using driving simulators and road tests during which lane position, emergency decisions (braking latency), and risk-taking behavior (speed, passing attempts, headway distance) are assessed. Studies on lane position have produced mixed results (Casswell, 1977; Hansteen et al., 1976; Klonoff, 1974; Peck et al., 1986; Ramaekers et al., 2000; Robbe and O'Hanlon, 1999; Smiley et al., 1981; Stein et al., 1983). Cannabis intoxication has been shown to adversely affect performance in emergency situations (Smiley et al., 1981; Dott, 1972; Liguori et al., 1998). When no warnings are provided, performance in emergency situations declines and brake latency increases. Cannabis has also been shown to adversely affect one's ability to attend to extraneous stimuli while driving, which may contribute to poor performance in emergency situations (Casswell, 1977; Smiley et al., 1981).

Cannabis use appears to decrease risk-taking behavior in driving situations. An association between cannabis intoxication and a reduction in speed has been observed across studies. In addition, subjects appear more hesitant to perform passing maneuvers and maintain a greater distance from other vehicles when under the influence of cannabis (Robbe and Hanlon, 1999; Smiley et al., 1981, 1986; Dott, 1972; Ellingstad et al., 1973).

Adverse effects on driving performance appear most evident when assessed in close temporal proximity to cannabis ingestion and appear to be dose dependent. Performance decrements have not been shown to persist beyond three hours after ingestion. Negative results have typically been observed in studies that use smaller doses of marijuana, less-complicated driving tests, or less-sensitive assessment techniques. Overall, experimental data suggest that cannabis intoxication can decrease control of automobiles as evidenced by variability in lane position and poor performance in emergency situations. However, drivers may partially compensate for these deficits by engaging in low-risk driving behaviors.

Controlled studies have recently examined the effects of the combination of alcohol and cannabis on driving (Ramaekers et al., 2000; Liguori et al., 2001). Such studies are important as the majority of motor vehicle accidents in which the driver is known to have recently used cannabis also find that alcohol was used by the same driver. One study of driving performance in real-world conditions reported clear synergistic effects of low doses of cannabis and alcohol on road tracking, time out of appropriate lane position, and increased variability in headway distance (Ramaekers et al., 2000). Performance in a driving simulator study, however, did not report such clear combination effects, as adverse performance effects observed with either substance alone were not exacerbated by the addition of the other (Liguori et al., 2001). Such conflicting results are difficult to interpret, and indicate the need for additional studies in this area.

Epidemiological studies have been conducted in the United States and Australia in an attempt to define the role of marijuana in major automobile accidents. A recent review of archival studies using police and laboratory reports assessed the relationship among marijuana use, alcohol use, combined use, and motor vehicle accidents in which serious injuries or fatalities occurred (Bates and Blakely, 1999). The authors concluded that use of marijuana alone was associated with reduced risk of a fatal accident relative to drug-free and alcohol-intoxicated related cases. Alcohol alone and in combination with marijuana was found to be a significant risk factor, with the combination showing slightly higher risk than alcohol alone. Studies of nonfatal injuries provided mixed results regarding the relative risk of marijuana use.

These epidemiological studies have several important limitations. First, it is difficult to determine whether the obtained cannabinoid metabolite levels relate to acute intoxication at the time of the accident. Second, cases in which traces of cannabis and another illicit substance are found are typically excluded from these studies. Since the combination of marijuana and other substances, including alcohol, is the most common finding in accident reviews, the relative contribution of marijuana to these accidents cannot be determined. Third, these studies rarely consider the base rates of cannabis use in comparable populations (young adults) and the concomitant accident rates in that population. More sophisticated methods of detecting marijuana intoxication, well-controlled studies, and inclusion of less severe accidents are needed to more fully understand the role of cannabis use in motor vehicle accidents.

Motivation

Marijuana use has long been associated with an "amotivational syndrome" characterized by lethargy, inactivity, loss of motivation, and decreased goal-directed behavior in heavy marijuana smokers (McGlothlin and West, 1968). Evidence for such amotivational effects comes primarily from case studies and clinical reports. Some chronic cannabis users attribute impaired vocational or academic performance and loss of ambition to their marijuana use (Hendin et al., 1987). Moreover, procrastination and impaired motivation are commonly reported as consequences of using marijuana and as reasons for stopping use among heavy users and those seeking treatment (Jones, 1984; Schwartz, 1987; Stephens, 1993).

Controlled field studies have failed to provide clear evidence of an amotivational syndrome. However, these studies have many methodological limitations relating to sample selection and operational definitions of motivation (Carter et al., 1977; Cohen, 1982; Halikas et al., 1982; Rubin and Comitas, 1976; Stefanis et al., 1977). Most recently, an Australian study of chronic users reported findings that typify this literature (Didcott et al., 1997). Many users appeared to be underemployed based on their education and abilities but were well integrated into family and community activities. Participants tended to attribute these circumstances as a lifestyle choice rather than an adverse effect of cannabis use. Family members provided mixed reports, as some noted amotivational effects in users, while others cited only positive effects.

Laboratory studies suggest that the motivational effects of cannabis intoxication on operant behavior are dependent on environmental context and contingencies. Miles and colleagues (1974) showed increased efficiency and no performance decrements when working for monetary reward while under the influence of marijuana. Pihl and Sigal (1978) found that they could reverse performance decrements induced by marijuana intoxication by providing monetary rewards. Other studies have failed to show adverse effects of marijuana on work output. However, the tasks and conditions of these studies may have been insensitive to cannabis effects as participants tended to show maximal performance across conditions (Mendelson et al., 1974; Foltin et al., 1990).

Cherek and colleagues cited in Budney et al. (1997), used a more sensitive operant measure of motivation in a laboratory study of cannabis intoxication. Subjects could choose to spend time working on a high-demand task that earned monetary reinforcement, or switch to a no-demand task that earned a lower level of reinforcement. With this choice available, subjects spent less time working on the high-demand task when under the influence of marijuana than with placebo, suggesting an amotivational effect. This effect appeared dose dependent and was partially reversed by increasing the magnitude of the reinforcement in the high-demand task. This suggests that amotivational effects of cannabis intoxication may occur by impacting the effects of reinforcement on various types of operant behavior (e.g., change sensitivity). The interaction among cannabis's behavioral effects and environmental variables needs further study to better understand the association between cannabis use and motivation.

There remains little scientific evidence that chronic cannabis use leads to an amotivational syndrome that could not be accounted for by chronic intoxication (Hall et al., 1994). Laboratory studies that compare chronic users with nonusers on performance of operant tasks, while controlling for acute intoxication effects, may provide more important information and address the validity of a chronic effect of cannabis on motivation. Of note, the acute motivational effects on operant performance observed in the laboratory indicate that motivation should be considered when interpreting studies that examine the effects of cannabis on any cognitive or behavioral performance task.

Cannabis Dependence

Whether cannabis use can lead to dependence has been controversial in both the lay and scientific communities. Personal experiences may bias many people toward the perception that cannabis is not addictive. More than one-third of the U.S. population has smoked marijuana in their lifetime. Most have not become addicted and have stopped using without difficulty. Moreover, unlike alcohol, cocaine, heroin, or nicotine dependence, most people are not familiar with personal acquaintances who have had problems with marijuana dependence, nor are sensational accounts of problems associated with marijuana common in the popular media.

The scientific community has also been reluctant to acknowledge the dependence potential of cannabis. Unlike most other drugs that humans abuse, animals do not readily self-administer cannabis (THC) in the laboratory. Because drug-dependence research has a productive history of using animal models to explicate drug dependence, this methodological issue raised serious questions about the abuse potential of cannabis. Further quandries arose when early studies of cannabis (THC) withdrawal did not reveal a syndrome that included substantial physical symptoms such as those observed during classic opioid, barbiturate, or alcohol withdrawal. Until recently, the neurobiology of cannabis was poorly understood, casting further uncertainty on this drug's addictive potential.

In contrast, the past ten years of basic and clinical research has produced strong evidence for concluding that cannabis can and does produce dependence. Here we review data addressing two facets of the dependence phenomenon: functional (behavioral) dependence and biological (physiological) dependence. Although this distinction can be considered artificial, it appears a logical way to organize new information in this area.

Functional (Behavioral) Dependence

Both the DSM-IV (American Psychiatric Association, 1994) and the International Statistical Classification of Diseases and Related Health Problems, tenth revision (ICD-10) (WHO, 1992) consider cannabis dependence a reliable and valid diagnostic category of mental disorder suggesting that individuals in the general population experience cannabis dependence in much the same way as they experience other substance dependence disorders. By definition, a diagnosis of dependence indicates that an individual is experiencing a cluster of cognitive, behavioral, or physiological symptoms associated with substance use, yet continues to use the substance regularly. Two epidemiological studies conducted in the United States and another in New Zealand indicate that the lifetime prevalence of marijuana dependence approximates 4 to 5 percent of the population, the highest of any illicit drug (Hall, Johnston, et al., 1999; Anthony and Helzer, 1991; Anthony et al., 1994; Wells et al., 1992).

Such high prevalence of cannabis dependence in comparison to other illicit drugs is clearly due to the greater overall prevalence of cannabis use. The estimated conditional dependence rate for cannabis dependence is lower than most other drugs of abuse, but certainly is not insignificant. That is, the risk of developing marijuana dependence among those who have used marijuana is approximately 9 percent compared to 12 percent for stimulants, 15 percent for alcohol, 17 percent for cocaine, 23 percent for heroin, and 32 percent for tobacco (Anthony et al., 1994). More frequent cannabis use results in greater risk of dependence. For example, rates of dependence are estimated at 20 to 30 percent among those who have used cannabis at least five times, and even higher (35 to 40 percent) estimates are reported among those who report near daily use (Hall et al., 1994; Kandel and Davis, 1992).

Clinical studies indicate that the majority of individuals who seek treatment for marijuana-related problems clearly meet DSM dependence criteria (Budney et al., 1998, 2000; Stephens et al., 2000). These individuals exhibit substantial psychosocial impairment and psychiatric distress, report multiple adverse consequences, report repeated unsuccessful attempts to stop using, and perceive themselves as unable to quit (Roffman and Barnhart, 1987; Stephens et al., 1993; Budney et al., 1998). A recent report comparing marijuana-dependent outpatients with cocaine-dependent outpatients found that the marijuana patients reported substance-use histories and psychosocial impairment comparable to the cocaine group, but showed less-severe dependence symptoms. The marijuana group was also more ambivalent and less confident about stopping their marijuana use than the cocaine group was about their cocaine use. Although marijuana-dependent outpatients typically do not experience the acute crises or severe consequences that many times drive alcohol-, cocaine-, or heroin-dependent individuals into treatment, they clearly show impairment that warrants clinical attention.

The number of individuals who enroll in treatment for marijuana-related problems is not small. Treatment-seeking for marijuana abuse or dependence increased twofold between 1992 and 1996, such that the percentage of illicit-drug-abuse-treatment admissions in U.S. state-approved agencies for marijuana (23 percent) approximated that for cocaine (27 percent) and heroin (23 percent) (SAMHSA, 1998). The response to treatment and relapse rates observed among marijuana-dependent outpatients appeared similar to those observed with other substances of abuse (Budney et al., 2000; Stephens et al., 1994, 2000). In summary, clinical evidence for a cannabis dependence disorder is strong and indicative of a disorder of substantial severity.

Biological (Physiological) Dependence

Physiological dependence has typically been determined by evidence of tolerance or withdrawal. Tolerance to the physiological, cognitive, and social effects of marijuana or cannabinoids has been well documented. Controlled human laboratory studies have clearly shown that tolerance develops to the subjective high, heart rate increases, social interaction deficits, and some of the cognitive and psychomotor performance deficits associated with cannabis or THC ingestion (Compton et al., 1990). In contrast, many regular marijuana users report a lack of tolerance to the subjective effects of marijuana use, with some reporting a sensitization effect (less of the drug is needed to produce the desired effect). Sensitization has not been demonstrated in controlled studies, and some have suggested that this phenomenon may be related to learning how to smoke more efficiently or to better identify the effects of cannabis (Stephens, 1999).

Withdrawal has generally been deemed a more robust indicator of dependence than tolerance. Early nonhuman studies of cessation of THC administration provided evidence of a withdrawal response, but the effects were mild and inconsistent (Kaymakcalan, 1973; Beardsley et al., 1986). Early studies with humans in residential laboratories also found evidence of withdrawal (Jones and Benowitz, 1976; Mendelson et al., 1984; Nowlan and Cohen, 1977; Georgotas and Zeidenberg, 1979). Common symptoms included decreased appetite, irritability, restlessness, sleep difficulties, and uncooperativeness. These effects were characterized as mild, transient, and without serious medical complications, and thus considered clinically insignificant when compared to the dramatic medical and physiological symptoms associated with severe opiate or alcohol withdrawal.

The discovery of a cannabinoid receptor (Devane et al., 1988) and the synthesis of a cannabinoid antagonist renewed scientific interest in cannabis dependence and withdrawal. Antagonist-challenge studies demonstrated a marked, precipitated withdrawal syndrome in rats and dogs (Aceto et al., 1996; Lichtman et al., 1998). Two placebo-controlled inpatient studies with humans, using moderate doses of oral THC and smoked marijuana, demonstrated withdrawal effects that included anxiety, decreased contentment and food intake, depressed mood, irritability, restlessness, sleep difficulty, and stomach pain (Haney, Comer, et al., 1999; Haney, Ward, et al., 1999). Controlled outpatient studies have now begun to demonstrate the reliability and validity of these withdrawal effects and examine their timecourse (Kouri and Pope, 2000; Budney et al., 2001; Budney et al., in press).

Clinical studies indicate that the majority of persons seeking treatment for cannabis dependence, including adolescents, report histories of cannabis withdrawal (Budney et al., 1998, 1999; Stephens et al., 1994; Crowley et al., 1998). For example, in our research clinic the majority (57 percent) of marijuana-dependent outpatients reported experiencing ≥ 6 symptoms of at least moderate severity during previous abstinence attempts. Severity was associated with more frequent marijuana use (Budney et al., 1999).

Cannabis withdrawal is not currently recognized in the DSM-IV, which concludes that the clinical significance of the syndrome has yet to be established. We expect that findings from recent research will result in its inclusion in the next revision of the DSM. Cannabis withdrawal syndrome resembles behaviors observed during nicotine withdrawal (Budney et al., 2001; Budney et al., in press). It appears common among treatment seekers and may warrant attention in clinical settings. Additional research is needed to better determine its prevalence, timecourse, and severity.

Other recent neurobiological findings further support the conclusion that cannabis can produce dependence. The documentation of an endogenous cannabinoid system with identified cannabinoid receptors (CB1 and CB2) and an endogenous cannabinoid-like substance (anandamide) established that the actions of cannabinoids in the brain occur in a manner similar to that of other drugs with well-recognized addictive potential such as opiates or benzodiazepines. The aforementioned precipitated-withdrawal studies demonstrated that withdrawal from cannabinoids likely occurs via a similar process as other abused drugs. Studies that have examined neurochemical responses in animals following exposure to and withdrawal from cannabinoids have observed reductions in mesolimbic dopamine transmission and elevations in extracellular-releasing-factor concentrations in the limbic system that closely resemble the responses seen with other major drugs of abuse (deFonseca et al., 1997; Diana et al., 1998). The behavioral consequences of these neurobiological changes are consistent with the type of negative affective symptoms reported by patients withdrawing from marijuana and other substances, and may be primary contributing factors to the development and maintenance of drug dependence (Koob et al., 1997). In summary, research findings from the 1990s indicate that the biological risk factors for cannabis dependence appear more similar to other well-recognized addictive drugs than was previously believed.

MEDICAL MARIJUANA

In addition to the adverse consequences on health previously discussed, cannabis may also have beneficial effects for a number of medical conditions. Oral THC (dronabinol) has been approved by the U.S. Food and Drug Administration for use as an appetite- and food-intake stimulant in patients with AIDS wasting syndrome and as an antinausea and antivomiting agent in cancer patients receiving chemotherapy. In 1999, the Institute of Medicine and the National Institutes of Health acknowledged the importance of initiating additional scientific study of the risks and benefits of cannabis use and, in particular, smoked marijuana for specific medical conditions. The interest in the benefits of smoked marijuana in contrast to oral THC arises primarily from differences in the pharmacokinetics of these two routes of administration. Through the oral route, THC absorption is slow and variable, and therefore clinical effects have a slower onset and longer duration than smoked marijuana. In addition, smoked marijuana not only delivers delta-9-THC, but other compounds (e.g., delta-8-THC and cannabidiol) are absorbed that may have direct or interactive effects of therapeutic interest.

Illnesses Involving Appetite, Food Intake, and Nausea Problems

Acute cannabis use can increase appetite and food intake. Single- and multiple-dose studies with marijuana and oral THC reliably show increases in food intake and food choice, since cannabis intoxication appears to result in frequent snacking and increased choice of sweet solid foods (Kelly et al., 1990; Haney, Comer, et al., 1999; Haney, Ward, et al., 1999; Abel, 1971; Foltin et al., 1986; Greenburg et al., 1976; Hollister, 1971). Interestingly, recent studies also show that abrupt discontinuation of oral THC or marijuana can result in decreased appetite and food intake, as well as concomitant weight loss during the first few days of withdrawal (Haney, Comer, et al., 1999; Haney,Ward, et al., 1999; Budney et al., 2001).

Cannabis's ability to facilitate appetite and food consumption prompted consideration of use of oral THC and smoked marijuana in clinical populations such as patients with AIDS wasting syndrome. Controlled case studies suggest some benefit of cannabis and THC for increasing appetite and weight gain in patients with AIDS wasting syndrome, but mixed results best characterize this literature (Beal et al., 1995, 1997; Plasse et al., 1991; Timpone et al., 1997).

Cancer patients' reports of the efficacy of smoked marijuana for relief from the nausea and vomiting associated with chemotherapy have stimulated study of such effects using oral THC and smoked marijuana (Grinspoon and Bakalar, 1997; Hollister, 2000). Placebo-controlled studies demonstrated the efficacy of oral THC (dronabinol) for this purpose, although other antiemetic drugs may work at least as well and are accompanied by fewer side effects (Gralla et al., 1984; Grunberg and Hesketh, 1993; Sallan et al., 1975, 1980; Schwartz and Beveridge, 1994). The efficacy of smoked marijuana in this clinical population has received little systematic study. Case reports commonly indicate the benefits of smoked marijuana, but the only controlled study conducted thus far did not demonstrate it to be superior to oral THC (Grinspoon and Bakalar, 1997; Levitt et al., 1984).

As mentioned earlier, the problem with absorption of THC when taken orally in contrast to the efficiency of THC delivery with smoked marijuana has triggered the call for more systematic study of smoked marijuana as an optimal method for achieving antiemetic and appetite effects in these clinical populations. However, the potential adverse effects of smoked marijuana on immune system function (reviewed previously) must be carefully considered as a contraindication for the use of smoked marijuana with immune-compromised clinical populations. Controlled research comparing the efficacy of oral THC and smoked marijuana is needed to determine whether cannabis should be considered a treatment of choice for severe problems with nausea and appetite in chronically ill populations.

Analgesia

The discovery of the endogenous cannabinoid system has rekindled interest in the use of cannabis for the treatment of pain. Elevated levels of cannabinoid receptors are located in areas of the brain that modulate nociception and can also be found in peripheral tissue. Recent research in nonhumans using animal models of pain indicate that cannabinoid agonists clearly exert analgesic effects in both the CNS and the periphery. The mechanisms for these analgesic effects differ from that of the opioids; hence, the potential use of cannabinoids as an adjunct or alternative treatment for acute or chronic pain has received increased attention.

The evidence for analgesic effects of cannabis in humans is less clear. Historically, the few studies of the effects of cannabis, THC, or other cannabinoid analogues on acute pain (i.e., laboratory induced or surgical) have not produced impressive results (Clark et al., 1981; Hill et al., 1974; Jain et al., 1981; Libman and Stern, 1985; Raft et al., 1977). Greenwald and Stitzer (2000) reported significant dose-dependent antinociceptive effects of smoked marijuana using a radiant-heat pain stimulus. However, the effects on pain reduction were not clinically robust and lasted less than one hour. Unfortunately, most of the research in this area has not been methodologically strong, making interpretation of findings difficult.

Early research on chronic pain demonstrated that oral THC and a nitrogen analogue produced analgesia similar to codeine, but side effects (sedation and depersonalization) were significant (Staquet et al., 1978; Noyes, Brunk, Avery, et al., 1975; Noyes, Brunk, Baram, et al., 1975). To date the most evidence for the efficacy of smoked marijuana for pain reduction in clinical populations experiencing chronic pain comes from case reports and survey studies. Patients have reported relief from cancer-related chronic pain, pain related to neurological disease, muscle spasticity, and headaches as well as phantom limb pain (Grinspoon and Bakalar, 1997; Dunn and Davis, 1974; Consroe et al., 1997). Many of these patients cite the superiority of smoked marijuana when compared to other treatments they have tried. Marijuana's positive effects on nausea and appetite make it particularly attractive for chronic-pain patients who also experience problems in these areas (e.g., cancer chemotherapy or AIDS patients). Moreover, the "positive" effect of cannabis on mood may further add to its desirability among patients with these types of chronic debilitating illnesses.

Again, the potential differences in the effects of delivering THC and the other compounds found in cannabis through smoking compared with oral administration are reason enough to pursue additional study of smoked marijuana as an analgesic agent. Controlled studies are needed to (1) compare smoked cannabis with oral THC, (2) compare cannabis with other analgesics, and (3) examine the effects of combinations of cannabis and other analgesics (e.g., opioids). Of note, there is reason to hope that additional basic research on the analgesic effects of cannabinoids might result in the development of efficacious agents that do not produce the other problematic effects of THC such as sedation, memory problems, and intoxication.

Other Medical Indications

Spasticity Associated with Movement Disorders

Case studies have suggested that cannabis might help alleviate tremors, spasms, or loss of coordination associated with multiple sclerosis or other neurological disorders such as spinal cord injury (Grinspoon and Bakalar, 1997; Consroe et al., 1986, 1997; Clifford, 1983; Malec et al., 1982; Ungerleider et al., 1987; Meinck et al., 1989). Controlled studies have not been conducted. Uncontrolled trials of oral THC have produced some evidence for a reduction in spasticity in patients with multiple sclerosis and spinal cord injury, but the effect has not been uniform and multiple side effects including loss of impaired posture and balance have been reported (Clifford, 1983; Malec et al., 1982; Ungerleider et al., 1987; Greenberg et al., 1994; Petro and Ellenberger, 1981). Conclusions regarding the efficacy of cannabis and other cannabinoids for the treatment of muscle spasticity await data from controlled studies.

Glaucoma

Both smoked marijuana and oral THC can reduce intraocular pressure that contributes to glaucoma and its progression (Joy et al., 1999). Nonetheless, cannabis use is no longer a good choice for treatment of this disease. THC clearly reduces intraocular pressure, but this effect is transient and thus requires chronic, high doses multiple times per day to achieve the desired therapeutic response. Although not the case 10 to 20 years ago, alternative local treatments are now available which require less frequent dosing and have fewer adverse side effects than cannabis. Hence, cannabis should no longer be considered a treatment of choice for glaucoma.

The current literature on medical indications for cannabis includes primarily uncontrolled case studies or open clinical trials with only a handful of controlled studies of oral THC conducted, mostly in the 1970s. Nonetheless, a number of medical indications appear to have enough support to warrant additional investigation. Much more data on the efficacy of smoked marijuana and oral THC for various medical conditions will soon become available, as the NIH and other funding sources (e.g., Center for Medicinal Cannabis Research, UCSD, San Diego, CA) have initiated focused efforts to stimulate research in this area.

CONCLUSIONS

Cannabis use engenders health risks across many areas of functioning. The magnitude of such effects and their clinical significance remains difficult to discern in most domains. The probability of experiencing many of the adverse health effects mentioned in this chapter is also not clear. We know that dose, frequency, and duration of cannabis use increase risk, but this relationship has not been well quantified. We also remain uncertain regarding the etiologic role of cannabis use in the occurrence of many of the negative effects reported in the literature. Heavy cannabis users typically have numerous other characteristics that are known risk factors for health and behavior problems. Continued investigation directed toward a better understanding of the interaction between these factors and cannabis use is necessary to more fully understand the impact of cannabis use on human functioning and health.

Despite these caveats, the scientific evidence for substantial cannabis-related adverse effects appears strong enough that individuals who use or who are considering using cannabis should be made aware of these potential negative outcomes. Overall, such outcomes appear less severe than those associated with alcohol, tobacco, heroin, or cocaine abuse (Hall, Room, et al., 1999). However, that does not mean they should be ignored. As with other substances of abuse, many individuals use cannabis without significant consequence, but others misuse, abuse, or become dependent and experience adverse outcomes. Moreover, cannabis use may have positive effects and even legitimate medical benefits for persons with specific types of illnesses, yet this could also be said of the many other substances that are abused.

The ongoing controversy and legalization debate over marijuana has spawned distrust in the scientific data. If we stop treating cannabis as a special case, and consider it as we would other psychoactive substances, a reasonable assumption is that some level of use (i.e., misuse) will result in harmful effects (Hall, 1999). We still have much to learn about the parameters of cannabis use that result in adverse consequences, but a wealth of new knowledge has accumulated during the past decade of research. Our understanding of its potential for harm has increased and these new findings warrant our attention and additional study.

REFERENCES

Abel, E.L. (1971). Effects of marijuana on the solution of anagrams, memory, and appetite. *Nature,* 231:260-261.

Aceto, M.; Scates, S.; Lowe, J.; Martin, B. (1996). Dependence on delta-9 tetrahydrocannabinol: Studies on precipitated and abrupt withdrawal. *J Pharmacol Exp Ther* 278:1290-1295.

American Psychiatric Association (1994). *Diagnostic and Statistical Manual of Mental Disorders,* Fourth Edition. Washington, DC: American Psychiatric Association.

Andreasson, S.; Allebeck, P.; Engstrom, A.; Rydberg, U. (1987). Cannabis and schizophrenia: A longitudinal study of Swedish conscripts. *Lancet,* 2:1483-1486.

Andreasson, S.; Allebeck, P.; Rydberg, U. (1989). Schizophrenia in users and nonusers of cannabis. A longitudinal study in Stockholm County. *Acta Psychiatr Scand,* 79:505-510.

Anthony, J.C.; Helzer, J.E. (1991). Syndromes of drug abuse and dependence. In: Robins, L.N.; Regier, D.A. (eds.), *Psychiatric Disorders in America.* New York: Free Press, 116-154.

Anthony, J.; Warner, L.; Kessler, R. (1994). Comparative epidemiology of dependence on tobacco, alcohol, controlled substances, and inhalants: Basic findings from the National Comorbidity Survey. *Exp Clin Psychopharmacol,* 2:244-268.

Azorlosa, J.L.; Heishman, S.J.; Stitzer, M.L.; Mahaffey, J.M. (1992). Marijuana smoking: Effect of varying delta-9-tetrahydrocannabinol content and number of puffs. *J Pharmacol Exp Ther,* 261:114-122.

Baldwin, G.C.; Tashkin, D.P.; Buckley, D.M.; Park, A.N.; Dubinett, S.M.; Roth, M.D. (1997). Marijuana and cocaine impair alveolar macrophage function and cytokine production. *Am J Respir Crit Care Med,* 156:1606-1613.

Barbers, R.G.; Evans, M.J.; Gong, H.; Tashkin, D.P. (1991). Enhanced alveolar monocytic phagocyte (macrophage) proliferation in tobacco and marijuana smokers. *Am Rev Respir Dis,* 143:1092-1095.

Barsky, S.F.; Roth, M.D.; Kleerup, E.C.; Simmons, M.; Tashkin, D.P. (1998). Histopathologic and molecular alterations in bronchial epithelium in habitual smokers of marijuana, cocaine, and/or tobacco. *J Natl Cancer Inst,* 90:1198-1205.

Bartels, S.J.; Teague, G.B.; Drake, R.E.; Clark, R.E.; Bush, P.W.; Noordsy, D.L. (1993). Substance abuse in schizophrenia: Service utilization and costs. *J Nerv Ment Dis,* 181:227-232.

Bates, M.N.; Blakely, T.A. (1999). Role of cannabis in motor vehicle crashes. *Epidemiol Rev,* 21:222-232.

Beaconsfield, P.; Ginsburg, J.; Rainsbury, R. (1972). Marijuana smoking: Cardiovascular effects in man and possible mechanisms. *N Engl J Med,* 287:209-212.

Beal, J.F.; Olson, R.; Laubenstein, L.; Morales, J.O.; Bellman, P.; Yango, B.; Lefkowitz, L.; Plasse, T.F.; and Shepard, K.V. (1995). Dronabinol as a treatment for anorexia associated with weight loss in patients with AIDS. *J Pain Symptom Manage,* 10:89-97.

Beal, J.F.; Olson, R.; Lefkowitz, L.; Laubenstein, L.; Bellman, P.; Yango, B.; Morales, J.O.; Murphy, R.; Powderly, W.; Plasse; et al. (1997). Long-term efficacy and safety of dronabinol for anorexia. *J Pain Symptom Manage,* 14:7-14.

Beardsley, P.M.; Balster, R.L.; Harris, L.S. (1986). Dependence on tetrahydrocannabinol in rhesus monkeys. *J Pharmacol Exp Ther,* 239:311-319.

Benowitz, N.L.; Jones, R.T. (1975). Cardiovascular effects of prolonged delta-9-tetrahydrocannabinol ingestion. *Clin Pharmacol Ther,* 18:287-297.

Black, S.; Casswell, S. (1993). *Drugs in New Zealand: A survey in 1990.* Auckland, New Zealand: University of Auckland, Alcohol and Public Health Research Unit.

Block, R.I.; Wittenborn, J.R. (1984a). Marijuana effects on semantic memory: Verification of common and uncommon category members. *Psychol Rep,* 55:503-512.

Block, R.I.; Wittenborn, J.R. (1984b). Marijuana effects on visual imagery in a paired-associate task. *Percept Mot Skills,* 58:759-766.

Block, R.; Farinpour, R.; Braverman, K. (1992). Acute effects of marijuana on cognition: Relationships to chronic effects and smoking techniques. *Pharmacol Biochem Behav,* 43:907-917.

Block, R.I.; Farinpour, R.; Schelchtem, J.A. (1991). Effects of chronic marijuana use on testosterone, luteinizing hormone, follicle stimulating hormone, prolactin and cortisol in men and women. *Drug Alcohol Depend,* 28:121-128.

Bloom, J.W.; Kaltenborn, W.T.; Paoletti, P.; Camilli, A.; Lebowitz, M.D. (1987). Respiratory effects of non-tobacco cigarettes. *Br Med J,* 295:1516-1518.

Brooks, J.S.; Balka, E.B., Whiteman, M. (1999). The risks for late adolescence of early adolescent marijuana use. *Am J Public Health,* 89(10):1549-1554.

Budney, A.J.; Higgins, S.T.; Radonovich, K.J.; Novy, P.L. (2000). Adding voucher-based incentives to coping-skills and motivational enhancement improves outcomes during treatment for marijuana dependence. *J Consult Clin Psychol,* 68:1051-1061.

Budney, A.J.; Hughes, J.R.; Moore, B.A.; Novy, P.L. (2001). Marijuana abstinence effects in marijuana smokers maintained in their home environment. *Arch Gen Psychiatry,* 58:917-924.

Budney, A.J.; Kandel, D.; Cherek, D.R.; Martin, B.R.; Stephens, R.S.; Roffman, R. (1997). Marijuana use and dependence: College on problems of drug dependence annual meeting, Puerto Rico (June, 1996). *Drug Alcohol Depend,* 45:1-11.

Budney, A.J.; Moore, B.A.; Vandrey, R.; Hughes, J.R. (in press). Timecourse and significance of cannabis withdrawal. *Journal of Abnormal Psychology.*

Budney, A.J.; Novy, P.; Hughes, J.R. (1999). Marijuana withdrawal among adults seeking treatment for marijuana dependence. *Addiction,* 94(9):1311-1322.

Budney, A.J.; Radonovich, K.J.; Higgins, S.T.; Wong, C.J. (1998). Adults seeking treatment for marijuana dependence: A comparison to cocaine-dependent treatment seekers. *Exp Clin Psychopharmacol,* 6:419-426.

Burns, M.; Moskowitz, H. (1981). Alcohol, marijuana, and skills performance. In: Goldburg, L. (ed.), *Alcohol, Drugs and Traffic Safety* (pp. 954-968). Stockholm: Almqvist and Wiksell International.

Caiaffa, W.T.; Vlahov, D.; Graham, N.M.; Astemborski, J.; Solomon, L.; Nelson, K.E.; Munoz, A. (1994). Drug smoking, pneumocystis carinii pneumonia and immunosuppression increase risk of bacterial pneumonia in human immunodeficiency virus-seropositive injection drug users. *Am J Respir Crit Care Med,* 150:1493-1498.

Caplan, G.A.; Brigham, B.A. (1990). Marijuana smoking and carcinoma of the tongue: Is there an association? *Cancer,* 66:1005-1006.

Cappell, H.D.; Pliner, P.L. (1973). Volitional control of marijuana intoxication: A study of the ability to come down on command. *J Abnorm Psychol,* 1:428-434.

Carter, W.E.; Coggins, W.; Doughty, P.L. (1977). *Cannabis in Costa Rica: A Study of Chronic Marijuana Use.* Philadelphia: Institute for the Study of Human Issues.

Casswell, S. (1977). Cannabis and alcohol: Effects on closed course driving behaviour. In: Johnson, I. (ed.) *Seventh International Conference on Alcohol, Drugs, and Traffic Safety* (pp. 238-246). Melbourne, Australia.

Casswell, S.; Marks, D.F. (1973). Cannabis and temporal disintegration in experienced and naive subjects. *Science,* 179:803-805.

Chait, L.D. (1990). Subjective and behavioral effects of marijuana the morning after smoking. *Psychopharmacology (Berl),* 100:328-333.

Chait, L.D.; Corwin, R.L.; Johanson, C.E. (1988). A cumulative dosing procedure for administering marijuana smoke to humans. *Pharmacol Biochem Beh,* 29: 553-557.

Chait, L.D.; Evans, S.M.; Grant, K.A.; Kamien, J.B.; Johanson, C.E.; Schuster, C.R. (1988). Discriminative stimulus and subjective effects of smoked marijuana in humans. *Psychopharmacology (Berl),* 94:206-212.

Channabasavanna, S.M.; Paes, M.; Hall, W. (1999). Mental and behavioral disorders due to cannabis. In: Kalant, H.; Corrigall, W.A.; Hall, W.; Smart, R.G. (eds.), *The Health Effects of Cannabis.* Toronto: Centre for Addictions and Mental Health, 267-290.

Chasnoff, I.J. (1990). *Cocaine use in pregnancy: Effect on infant neurobehavioural functioning.* Paper presented at the American Society for Pharmacology and Experimental Therapeutics. Washington, DC.

Chesher, G.B.; Bird, K.D.; Jackson, D.M.; Perrignon, A.; Starmer, G.A. (1990). The effects of orally administered delta-9-tetrahydrocannabinol in man on mood and performance measures: A dose-response study. *Pharmacol Biochem Behav,* 35:861-864.

Clark, W.C.; Janal, M.N.; Zeidenberg, P.; Nahas, G.G. (1981). Effects of moderate and high doses of marijuana on thermal pain: A sensory decision theory analysis. *J Clin Pharmacol,* 21.

Clifford, D.B. (1983). Tetrahydrocannabinol for tremor in multiple sclerosis. *Ann Neurol,* 13:669-671.

Cohen, S. (1982). Cannabis effects upon adolescent motivation. *Marijuana and Youth: Clinical Observations on Motivation and Learning* (pp. 2-10). Rockville, MD: National Institute on Drug Abuse.

Compton, D.R.; Dewey, W.L.; Martin, B.R. (1990). Cannabis dependence and tolerance production. *Adv Alcohol Subst Abuse,* 9:129-147.

Cone, E.J.; Johnson, R.E.; Moore, J.D.; Roache, J.D. (1986). Acute effects of smoking marijuana on hormones subjective effects and performance in male human subjects. *Pharmacol Biochem Behav,* 24:1749-1754.

Consroe, P.; Musty, R.; Rein, J.; Tillery, W.; Pertwee, R. (1997). The perceived effects of smoked cannabis on patients with multiple sclerosis. *Eur Neurol,* 38: 44-48.

Consroe, P.; Sandyk, R.; Snider, S.R. (1986). Open label evaluation of cannabidiol in dystonic movement disorders. *Int J Neurosci,* 30:277-282.

Crowley, T.J.; MacDonald, M.J.; Whitmore, E.A.; Mikulich, S.K. (1998). Cannabis dependence, withdrawal, and reinforcing effects among adolescents with conduct disorder symptoms and substance use disorders. *Drug Alcohol Depend,* 50:27-37.

Day, N.; Richardson, G.A. (1991). Prenatal marijuana use: Epidemiology, methodological issues and infant outcome. In: Chasnoff, I. (ed.), *Clinics in Perinatology.* Philadelphia: W.B. Saunders, 77-92.

Day, N.; Richardson, G.A.; Goldschmidt, L.; Robles, N.; Taylor, P.M.; Stoffer, D.S.; Cornelius, M.D.; Geva, D. (1994). The effect of prenatal exposure on the cognitive development of offspring at age three. *Neurotoxicol Teratol,* 16:169-176.

DeFonseca, F.R.; Carrera, M.R.A.; Navarro, M.; Koob, G.F.; Weiss, F. (1997). Activation of corticotropin-releasing factor in the limbic system during cannabinoid withdrawal. *Science,* 276:2050-2054.

Devane, W.A.; Dysarz, F.A.; Johnson, M.R.; Melvin, L.S.; Howlett, A.C. (1988). Determination and characterization of a cannabinoid receptor in rat brain. *Mol Pharmacol,* 34:605-613.

Deykin, E.Y.; Levy, J.C.; Wells, V. (1986). Adolescent depression, alcohol, and drug abuse. *Am J Public Health,* 76:178-182.

Diana, M.; Melis, M.; Muntoni, A.L.; Gessa, G.L. (1998). Mesolimbic dopaminergic decline after cannabinoid withdrawal. *Proc Natl Acad Sci USA,* 95: 10269-10273.

Didcott, P.; Reilly, D.; Swift, W.; Hall, W. (1997). *Long Term Cannabis Users on the New South Wales North Coast.* Sydney: National Drug and Alcohol Research Centre.

Donald, P.J. (1991). Advanced malignancy in the young marijuana smoker. *Adv Exp Med Biol,* 288:33-46.

Dornbush, R.L.; Fink, M.; Freedman, A.M. (1971). Marijuana memory and perception. *Am J Psychiatry,* 128:194-197.

Dott, A.B. (1972). *Effect of Marijuana on Risk Acceptance in a Simulated Passing Task.* Washington, DC: U.S. Government Printing Office.

Dunn, M.; Davis, R. (1974). The perceived effects of marijuana on spinal cord injured males. *Paraplegia,* 12:175.

Ehrenreich, H.; Rinn, T.; Kunert, H.J.; Moeller, M.R.; Poser, W.; Schilling, L.; Gigerenzer, G.; Hoehe, M.R. (1999). Specific attentional dysfunction in adults following early start of cannabis use. *Psychopharmacology (Berl),* 142:295-301.

Ellickson, P.; Bui, K.; Bell, R.; McGuigan, K.A. (1998). Does early drug use increase the risk of dropping out of high school? *Journal of Drug Issues,* 28:357-380.

Ellingstad, V.S.; McFarling, L.H.; Struckman, D.L. (1973). Alcohol, marijuana, and risk taking. Vermillion, SD: South Dakota University, Vermillion Human Factors Laboratory.

Fergusson, D.M.; Horwood, L.J. (1997). Early onset cannabis use and psychosocial adjustment in young adults. *Addiction,* 92(3):279-296.

Fergusson, D.M.; Lynskey, M.T.; Horwood, L.J. (1996). The short-term consequences of early cannabis use. *J Abnorm Child Psychol,* 24(4):499-512.

Fligiel, S.E.G.; Beals, T.F.; Tashkin, D.P.; Paule, M.G.; Scallet, A.L.; Ali, S.F.; Bailey, J.R.; and Slikker, W. Jr. (1991). Marijuana exposure and pulmonary alterations in primates. *Pharmaco Biochem Behav,* 40:637-642.

Fligiel, S.E.G.; Roth, M.D.; Kleerup, E.C.; Barsky, S.H.; Simmons, M.S.; Tashkin, D.P. (1997). Tracheobronchial histopathology in habitual smokers of cocaine, marijuana, and/or tobacco. *Chest,* 112:319-326.

Foltin, R.W.; Brady, J.V.; Fischman, M.W. (1986). Behavioral analysis of marijuana effects on food intake in humans. *Pharmacol Biochem Behav,* 25:577-582.

Foltin, R.W.; Fischman, M.W. (1988). Effects of smoked marijuana on human social behavior in small groups. *Pharmacol Biochem Behav,* 30:539-541.

Foltin, R.W.; Fischman, M.W.; Brady, J.V.; Bernstein, D.J.; Capriotti, R.M.; Nellis, M.J.; Kelly, T.H. (1990). Motivational effects of smoked marijuana: Behavioral contingencies and low-probability activities. *J Exp Anal Behav,* 53(1):5-19.

Foltin, R.W.; Fischman, M.W.; Pippen, P.A.; Kelly, T.H. (1993). Behavioral effects of cocaine alone and in combination with ethanol or marijuana in humans. *Drug Alcohol Depend,* 32:93-106.

Fried, P.A. (1980). Marijuana use by pregnant women: Neurobehavioral effects in neonates. *Drug Alcohol Depend,* 6:415-424.

Fried, P.A.; Barnes, M.V.; Drake, E.R. (1985). Soft drug use after pregnancy compared to use before and during pregnancy. *Am J Obstet Gynecol,* 151:787-792.

Fried, P.A.; Watkinson, B. (1988). 12- and 24-month neurobehavioral follow-up of children prenatally exposed to marijuana, cigarettes, and alcohol. *Neurotoxicol Teratol,* 10:305-313.

Fried, P.A.; Watkinson, B. (1990). 36- and 48-month neurobehavioural follow-up of children prenatally exposed to marijuana, cigarettes, and alcohol. *J Dev Behav Pediatr,* 11:49-58.

Fried, P.A.; Watkinson, B. (2000). Visuoperceptual functioning differs in 9- to 12-year olds prenatally exposed to cigarettes and marihuana. *Neurotoxicol Teratol,* 22:11-20.

Fung, M.; Gallagher, C.; Machtay, M. (1999). Lung and aero-digestive cancers in young marijuana smokers. *Tumori,* 85:140-142.

Galanter, M.; Weingartner, H.; Vaughn, T.B.; Roth, W.T.; Wyatt, R.J. (1973). Delta-9-transtetrahydrocannabinol and natural marijuana. *Arch Gen Psychiatry,* 28:278-281.

Georgotas, A.; Zeidenberg, P. (1979). Observations on the effects of four weeks of heavy marijuana smoking on group interaction and individual behavior. *Compr Psychiatry,* 20:427-432.

Gibson, G.T.; Baghurst, P.A.; Colley, D.P. (1983). Maternal alcohol, tobacco and cannabis consumption and the outcome of pregnancy. *Aust NZ J Obstet Gynaecol,* 23:15-19.

Gil, E.; Chen, B.; Kleerup, E.; Webber, M.; Tashkin, D.P. (1995). Acute and chronic effects of marijuana smoking on pulmonary alveolar permeability. *Life Sci,* 56:2193-2199.

Goldschmidt, L.; Day, N.L.; Richardson, G.A. (2000). Effects of prenatal marijuana exposure on child behavior problems at age 10. *Neurotoxicol Teratol,* 22:325-336.

Gong, H.; Fligiel, S.; Tashkin, D.P.; Barbers, R.G. (1987). Tracheobronchial changes in habitual, heavy smokers of marijuana with and without tobacco. *Am Rev Respir Dis,* 136:142-149.

Gralla, R.J.; Tyson, L.B.; Bordin, L.A.; Clark, R.A.; Kelsen, D.P.; Kris, M.G.; Kalman, L.B.; Groshen, S. (1984). Antiemetic therapy: A review of recent studies and a report of a random assignment trial comparing metoclopramide with delta-9-tetrahydrocannabinol. *Cancer Treat Rep,* 68:163-172.

Greenberg, H.S.; Werness, S.A.; Pugh, J.E.; Andrus, R.O.; Anderson, D.J.; Domino, E.F. (1994). Short-term effects of smoking marijuana on balance in patients with multiple sclerosis and normal volunteers. *Clin Pharmacol Ther,* 55:324-328.

Greenburg, I.; Kuehnle, J.; Mendelson, J.H.; Bernstein, J.G. (1976). Effects of marijuana use on body weight and caloric intake in humans. *Psychopharmacology (Berl),* 49:79-84.

Greenwald, M.K.; Stitzer, M.L. (2000). Antinociceptive, subjective and behavioral effects of smoked marijuana in humans. *Drug Alcohol Depend,* 59:261-275.

Grinspoon, L.; Bakalar, J.B. (1997). *Marihuana, the Forbidden Medicine.* New Haven, CT: Yale University Press, 296.

Grunberg, S.M.; Hesketh, P.J. (1993). Control of chemotherapy-induced emesis. *N Engl J Med,* 329:1790-1796.

Haas, A.P.; Hendin, H. (1987). The meaning of chronic marijuana use among adults: A psychosocial perspective. *J Drug Issues,* 17:333-348.

Halikas, J.A.; Weller, R.A.; Morse, C.L.; Hoffman, R.G. (1983). Regular marijuana use and its effects on psychosocial variables: Longitudinal study. *Compr Psychiatry,* 24:229-235.

Halikas, J.A.; Weller, R.A.; Morse, C.; Shapiro, T. (1982). Incidence and characteristics of amotivational syndrome, including associated findings, among chronic marijuana users. *Marijuana and Youth: Clinical Observations on Motivation and Learning* (pp. 11-26). Rockville, MD: National Institute on Drug Abuse.

Hall, W. (1999). Assessing the health and psychological effects of cannabis use. In: Kalant, H.; Corrigall, W.A.; Hall, W.; Smart, R. G. (eds.), *The Health Effects of Cannabis* (pp. 1-18). Toronto: Centre for Addiction and Mental Health.

Hall, W.; Johnston, L.; Donnelly, N. (1999). Epidemiology of cannabis use and its consequences. In: Kalant, H.; Corrigall, W.A.; Hall, W.; Smart, R.G. (eds.), *The Health Effects of Cannabis* (pp. 69-126). Toronto: Centre for Addiction and Mental Health.

Hall, W.; Room, R.; Bondy, S. (1999). Comparing the health and psychological risks of alcohol, cannabis, nicotine, and opiate use. In: Kalant, H.; Corrigall, W.A.; Hall, W.; Smart, R.G. (eds.), *The Health Effects of Cannabis* (pp. 475-495). Toronto: Centre for Addiction and Mental Health.

Hall, W.; Solowij, N.; Lemon, J. (1994). *The Health and Psychological Consequences of Cannabis Use.* Canberra, Australia: Australian Government Publication Services.

Haney, M.; Comer, S.D.; Ward, A.S.; Foltin, R.W.; Fischman, M.W. (1999). Abstinence symptoms following oral THC administration to humans. *Psychopharmacology (Berl),* 14:385-394.

Haney, M.; Ward, A.S.; Comer, S.D.; Foltin, R.W.; Fischman, M.W. (1999). Abstinence symptoms following smoked marijuana in humans. *Psychopharmacology (Berl),* 14:395-404.

Hansteen, R.W.; Miller, R.D.; Lonero, L. (1976). Effects of cannabis and alcohol on automobile driving and psychomotor tracking. *Ann NY Acad Sci,* 282:240-256.

Hatch, E.E.; Bracken, M.B. (1986). Effect of marijuana use in pregnancy on fetal growth. *Am J Epidemiol,* 124:986-993.

Heishman, S.J.; Arasteh, K.; Stitzer, M.L. (1997). Comparative effects of alcohol and marijuana on mood, memory and performance. *Pharmacol Biochem Behav,* 58:93-101.

Heishman, S.J.; Stitzer, M.L.; Bigelow, G.E. (1988). Alcohol and marijuana: Comparative dose effect profiles in humans. *Pharmacol Biochem Behav,* 31:649-655.

Heishman, S.J.; Stitzer, M.L.; Yingling, J.E. (1989). Effects of tetrahydrocannabinol content on marijuana smoking behavior: Subjective reports and performance. *Pharmacol Biochem Behav,* 34:173-179.

Hendin, H.; Haas, A.P.; Singer, P.; Eller, M.; Ulman, R. (1987). *Living High: Daily Marijuana Use Among Adults.* New York: Human Sciences Press.

Higgins, S.T.; Stitzer, M.L. (1986). Acute marijuana effects on social conversation. *Psychopharmacology (Berl),* 89:234-238.

Hill, S.Y.; Schwin, R.; Goodwin, D.W.; Powell, B.J. (1974). Marijuana and pain. *J Pharmacol Exp Ther,* 188:415-418.

Hingson, R.; Alpert, J.; Day, N.; Dooling, E.; Kayne, H.; Morelock, S.; Oppenheimer, E.; and Zuckerman, B. (1982). Effects of maternal drinking and marijuana use on fetal growth and development. *Pediatrics,* 70:539-546.

Hoffmann, D.; Brunnemann, K.D.; Gori, G.B.; Wynder, E.L. (1975). On the carcinogenicity of marijuana smoke. In: Runeckles, V.C. (ed.), *Recent Advances in Phytochemistry* (pp. 63-81). New York: Plenum Press.

Hollister, L.E. (1971). Hunger and appetite after single doses of marijuana, alcohol, and dextroamphetamine. *Clin Pharmacol Ther,* 12:44-49.

Hollister, L.E. (2000). An approach to the medical marijuana controversy. *Drug Alcohol Depend,* 58:3-7.

Hooker, W.D.; Jones, R.T. (1987). Increased susceptibility to memory intrusions and the Stroop interference effect during acute marijuana intoxication. *Psychophamacologia,* 91:20-24.

Huber, G.L.; First, M.W.; Grubner, O. (1991). Marijuana and tobacco smoke gas-phase cytotoxins. *Pharmacol Biochem Behav,* 40:629-636.

Hutchings, D.E.; Fried, P.A. (1999). Cannabis during pregnancy: Neurobehavioral effects in animals and humans. In: Kalant, H.; Corrigall, W.A.; Hall, W.; Smart, R.G. (eds.), *The Health Effects of Cannabis* (pp. 401-434). Toronto: Centre for Addiction and Mental Health.

Institute of Medicine (1982). *Marijuana and Health.* Washington, DC: National Academy Press, Institute of Medicine.

Jablensky, A.; Sartorius, N.; Ernberg, G.; Anker, M.; Korten, A.; Cooper, J.E.; Day, R.; and Bertelsen, A. (1991). *Schizophrenia: Manifestations, Incidence, and Course in Different Cultures. A World Health Organization ten-country study.* Geneva: World Health Organization.

Jain, A.K.; Ryan, J.R.; McMahon, F.G.; Smith, G. (1981). Evaluation of intramuscular levonantradol and placebo in acute postoperative pain. *J Clin Pharmacol,* 21:320S-326S.

Jones, R.T. (1980). Human effects: An overview. In: Peterson, R.C. (ed.), *Marijuana Research Findings: 1980. NIDA Research Monograph 31.* Washington, DC: U.S. Government Printing Office, 54-80.

Jones, R.T. (1984). Marijuana: Health and treatment issues. *Psychiatr Clin North Am,* 7:703-712.

Jones, R.T.; Benowitz, N. (1976). The 30-day trip—Clinical studies of cannabis tolerance and dependence. In: Braude, M.C.; Szara, S. (eds.), *Pharmacology of marihuana.* New York: Raven Press, 627-642.

Jones, R.T.; Stone, G.C. (1970). Psychological studies of marijuana and alcohol in man. *Psychopharmacologia,* 18:108-117.

Joy, J.E.; Watson, S.J.; Benson, J.A. (1999). *Marijuana as Medicine: Assessing the Scientific Base.* Washington, DC: National Academy Press.

Kamien, J.B.; Bickel, W.K.; Higgins, S.T.; Hughes, J.R. (1994). The effects of delta-9-tetrahydrocannabinol on repeated acquisition and performance of response sequences and on self-reports in humans. *Behav Pharmacol,* 5:71-78.

Kandel, D.B. (1984). Marijuana users in young adulthood. *Arch Gen Psychiatry,* 41:200-209.

Kandel, D.B.; Davis, M. (1992). Progression to regular marijuana involvement: Phenomenology and risk factors of near daily use. In: Glantz, M.; Pickens, R. (eds.), *Vulnerability to Drug Abuse.* Washington, DC: American Psychological Association, 221-253.

Kandel, D.B.; Davies, M.; Karus, D.; Yamaguchi, K. (1986). The consequences in young adulthood of adolescent drug involvement. *Arch Gen Psychiatry,* 43:746-754.

Kaymakcalan, S. (1973). Tolerance to and dependence on cannabis. *Bull Narc,* 25: 39-47.

Kelly, T.H.; Foltin, R.W.; Emurian, C.S.; Fischman, M.W. (1990). Multidimensional behavioral effects of marijuana. *Prog Neuropsychopharmacol Biol Psychiatry,* 14:885-902.

Kelly, T.H.; Foltin, R.W.; Fischman, M.W. (1993). Effects of smoked marijuana on heart rate, drug ratings, and task performance by humans. *Behav Pharmacol,* 4:167-178.

Kelly, T.H.; Foltin, R.W.; Mayr, M.T.; Fischman, M.W. (1994). Effects of delta 9-tetrahydrocannabinol and social context on marijuana self-administration by humans. *Pharmacol Biochem Behav,* 49:763-768.

Klein, T.W. (1999). Cannabis and immunity. In: Kalant, H.; Corrigall, W.A.; Hall, W.; Smart, R.G. (eds.), *The Health Effects of Cannabis* (pp. 347-374). Toronto: Centre for Addiction and Mental Health.

Klein, T.W.; Friedman, H.; Specter, S. (1998). Marijuana, immunity, and infection. *J Neuroimmunol,* 83:102-115.

Klonoff, H. (1974). Marijuana and driving in real-life situations. *Science,* 186:317-324.

Koob, G.F.; Caine, S.B.; Parsons, L.; Markou, A.; Weiss, F. (1997). Opponent process model and psychostimulant addiction. *Pharmacol Biochem Behav,* 57: 513-521.

Kouri, E.M.; Pope, H.G. (2000). Abstinence symptoms during withdrawal from chronic marijuana use. *Exp Clin Psychopharmacol,* 8:483-492.

Krohn, M.D.; Lizotte, A.J.; Perez, C.M. (1997). The interrelationship between substance use and precocious transitions to adult statuses. *J Health Soc Behav,* 38(1):87-103.

Kusher, D.I.; Dawson, L.O.; Taylor, A.C.; Djeu, J.Y. (1994). Effect of the psychoactive metabolite of marijuana, delta 9-tetrahydrocannabinol (THC), on the synthesis of tumor necrosis factor by human large granular lymphocytes. *Cell Immunology,* 154:99-108.

Leavitt, J.; Webb, P.; Norris, G.; Struve, F.; Straumanis, J.; Fitz-Gerald, M.; Nixon, F.; Patrick, G.; and Manno, J. (1993). Performance of chronic daily marijuana users on neuropsychological tests. In: Harris, L. (ed.), *Problems of Drug Dependence 1992.* Washington, DC: Government Printing Office, 179.

Leon, S.C.; Lyons, J.S.; Christopher, N.J.; Miller, S.I. (1998). Psychiatric hospital outcomes of dual diagnosis patients under managed care. *Am J Addict,* 7:81-86.

Levitt, M.; Faiman, C.; Hawks, R.; Wilson, A. (1984). Randomized double blind comparison of delta-9-tetrahydrocannabinol (THC) and marijuana as chemotherapy antiemetics. *Proceedings of the Meeting of the American Society of Clinical Oncology,* 3:91.

Lezak, M.D. (1995). *Neurophysical Assessment,* Third Edition. New York: Oxford University Press.

Libman, E.; Stern, M.H. (1985). The effects of delta-9-tetrahydrocannabinol on cutaneous sensitivity and its relation to personality. *Pers Indiv Differ,* 6:169-174.

Lichtman, A.H.; Wiley, J.L.; LaVecchia, K.L.; Niviaser, S.T.; Arthur, D.B.; Wilson, D.M.; Martin, B.R. (1998). Effects of SR 141716A after acute or chronic cannabinoid administration in dogs. *J Pharmacol Exp Ther,* 278:1290-1295.

Liguori, A.; Gatto, C.P.; Jarrett, D.B. (2001). *Effects of Marijuana-Alcohol Combinations on Mood, Equilibrium and Simulated Driving.* Scottsdale, AZ: College on Problems of Drug Dependence.

Liguori, A.; Gatto, C.P.; Robinson, J.H. (1998). Effects of marijuana on equilibrium, psychomotor performance, and simulated driving. *Behavioral Pharmacol,* 9:599-609.

Linszen, D.H.; Dingemans, P.M.; Lenior, M.E. (1994). Cannabis abuse and the course of recent-onset schizophrenic disorders. *Arch Gen Psychiatry,* 51:273-279.

Linszen, D.H.; Dingemans, P.M.; Nugter, M.A.; Does, A.; Scholte, W.F.; Lenior, M.A. (1997). Patient attributes and expressed emotion as risk factors for psychotic relapse. *Schizophr Bull,* 23:119-130.

Lynskey, M.; Hall, W. (2000). The effects of adolescent cannabis use on educational attainment: A review. *Addiction,* 95:1621-1630.

MacPhee, D. (1999). Effects of marijuana on cell nuclei: A review of the literature relating to the genotoxicity of cannabis. In: Kalant, H.; Corrigall, W.A.; Hall, W.; Smart, R.G. (eds.), *The Health Effects of Cannabis* (pp. 291-310). Toronto: Centre for Addiction and Mental Health.

Maddock, R.; Farrell, T.R.; Herning, R.; Jones, R.T. (1979). Marijuana and thermoregulation in a hot environment. In: Cox, B.; Lomax, P.; Milton, A.S.; Schonbaum, E. (eds.), *Thermoregulatory Mechanisms and Their Therapeutic Implications* (pp. 62-64). Basel, NY: Karger.

Malec, J.; Harvey, R.F.; Cayner, J. (1982). Cannabis effect on spasticity in spinal cord injury. *Arch Phys Med Rehabil,* 63:116-118.

Mao, L.; Oh, Y. (1998). Does marijuana or crack cocaine cause cancer? [Comment] *J Natl Cancer Inst,* 90:1182-1183.

Marks, D.F.; MacAvoy, M.F. (1989). Divided attention performance in cannabis users and non-users following alcohol and cannabis separately and in combination. *Psychopharmacology (Berl),* 99:397-401.

Marks, W.H.; Florence, L.; Lieberman, J.; Chapman, P.; Howard, D.; Roberts, P.; Perkinson, D. (1996). Successfully treated invasive pulmonary aspergillosis associated with smoking marijuana in a renal transplant recipient. *Transplantation,* 61:1771-1774.

Marques-Magallanes, J.A.; Tashkin, D.P.; Serafian, T.; Stegeman, J.; Roth, M.D. (1997). In vivo and in vitro activation of cytochrome P4501A1 by marijuana smoke. *1997 Symposium on the Cannabinoids of the International Cannabinoid Research Society*. Stone Mountain, GA.

Martinez-Arevalo, M.J.; Calcedo-Ordonez, A.; Varo-Prieto, J.R. (1994). Cannabis consumption as a prognostic factor in schizophrenia. *Br J Psychiatry,* 164:679-681.

Mathers, D.C.; Ghodse, A.H.; Caan, A.W.; Scott, S.A. (1991). Cannabis use in a large sample of acute psychiatric admissions. *Br J Addict,* 86:779-784.

Mayor's Committee on Marijuana (1944). *The Marijuana Problem in the City of New York*. Lancaster, PA: Jacques Cattell Press.

McGee, R.; Williams, S.; Poulton, R.; Moffitt, T. (2000). A longitudinal study of cannabis use and mental health from adolescence to early adulthood. *Addiction,* 95:491-503.

McGlothlin, W.H.; West, L.J. (1968). The marijuana problem: An overview. *Am J Psychiatry,* 125:370-378.

Meinck, H.M.; Schonle, P.W.; Conrad, B. (1989). Effect of cannabinoids on spasticity and ataxia in multiple sclerosis. *J Neurol,* 236:120-122.

Mendelson, J.H.; Mello, N.K.; Cristofaro, P.; Ellingboe, J.; Benedikt, R. (1985). Acute effects of marijuana on pituitary and gonadal hormones during the periovulatory phase of the menstrual cycle. In: Harris, L.S. (ed.), *Problems of Drug Dependence*. Washington, DC: U.S. Government Printing Office, 24-31.

Mendelson, J.H.; Mello, N.K.; Ellingboe, J.; Skupny, A.T.; Lex, B.W.; Griffin, M. (1986). Marijuana smoking suppresses luteinizing hormone in women. *J Pharmacol Exp Ther,* 237:862-866.

Mendelson, J.H.; Mello, N.K.; Lex, B.W.; Bavli, S. (1984). Marijuana withdrawal syndrome in a woman. *Am J Psychiatry,* 141:1289-1290.

Mendelson, J.H.; Rossi, A.M.; Meyer, R.E. (1974). *The Use of Marijuana: A Psychological and Physiological Inquiry*. New York: Plenum Press.

Miles, C.G.; Congreve, G.R.S.; Gibbins, R.J.; Marshman, J.; Devenyi, P.; Hicks, R.C. (1974). An experimental study of the effects of daily cannabis smoking on behaviour patterns. *Acta Pharmacol Toxicol,* 34(1) 1-43.

Miller-Johnson, S.; Lochman, J.E.; Cone, J.D.; Terry, R.; Hyman, C. (1998). Comorbidity of conduct and depressive problems at sixth grade: Substance use outcomes across adolescence. *J Abnorm Child Psychol,* 26:221-232.

Millsaps, C.L.; Azrin, R.L.; Mittenberg, W. (1994). Neuropsychological effects of chronic cannabis use on the memory and intelligence of adolescents. *J Child Adolesc Sub Abuse,* 3:47-55.

Moore, B.A.; Budney, A.J. (2001). Tobacco smoking in marijuana dependent outpatients. *Journal of Substance Abuse,* 13:585-598.

Mouzak, A.; Agathos, P.; Kerezoudi, E.; Mantas, A.; Vourdeli-Yiannakoura, E. (2000). Transient ischemic attack in heavy cannabis smokers—How "safe" is it? *Eur Neurol,* 44:42-44.

Mueser, K.T.; Yarnold, P.R.; Levinson, D.F.; Singh, H.; Bellack, A.S.; Kec, K.; Morrison, R.L.; Yadalam, K. G. (1990). Prevalence of substance abuse in schizophrenia: Demographic and clinical correlates. *Schizophr Bull,* 16:31-56.

Murphy, L. (1999). Cannabis effects on endocrine and reproductive function. In: Kalant, H.; Corrigall, W.A.; Hall, W.; Smart, R.G. (eds.), *Health Effects of Cannabis* (pp. 375-400). Toronto: Centre for Addiction and Mental Health.

Negrete, J.C. (1989). Cannabis and schizophrenia. *Br J Addict,* 84:349-351.

Negrete, J.C.; Gill, K. (1999). Cannabis and schizophrenia: An overview of the evidence to date. In Nahas, G.G. (ed.), *Marijuana and Medicine.* Totowa, NJ: Humana Press, 671-681.

Newton, C.A.; Klein, T.W.; Friedman, H. (1994). Secondary immunity to *Legionella pneumophila* and Th1 activity are suppressed by Δ^9-tetrahydrocannabinol injection. *Infect Immun,* 62:4015-4020.

Nowlan, R.; Cohen, S. (1977). Tolerance to marijuana: Heart rate and subjective "high." *Clin Pharmacol Ther,* 22:550-556.

Noyes, R. Jr.; Brunk, S.F.; Avery, D.H.; Canter, A. (1975). The analgesic properties of delta-9-tetrahydrocannabinol and codeine. *Clin Pharmacol Ther,* 18:84-89.

Noyes, R. Jr.; Brunk, S.F.; Baram, D.; Canter, A. (1975). Analgesic effect of delta-9-tetrahydrocannabinol. *J Clin Pharmacol,* 15:139-143.

O'Connell, C.M.; Fried, P.A. (1984). An investigation of prenatal cannabis exposure and minor physical anomalies in a low risk population. *Neurotoxicol Teratol,* 6:345-350.

O'Connell, C.M.; Fried, P.A. (1991). Prenatal exposure to cannabis: A preliminary report of postnatal consequences in school-age children. *Neurotoxicol Teratol,* 13:631-639.

Peck, R.C.; Biasotti, A.; Boland, P.N.; Mallory, C.; Reeve, V. (1986). The effects of marijuana and alcohol on actual driving performance. *Alcohol, Drugs and Driving,* 2:135-154.

Perez-Reyes, M.; Hicks, R.E.; Bumberry, J.; Jeffcoat, A.R.; Cook, C.E. (1988). Interaction between marijuana and ethanol: Effects on psychomotor performance. *Alcohol Clin Exp Res,* 12:268-276.

Perez-Reyes, M.; Lipton, M.A.; Timmons, M.C.; Walls, M.E.; Brine, D.R.; Davis, K.H. (1973). Pharmacology of administered delta-9-tetrahydrocannabinol. *Clin Pharmacol Ther,* 14:48-55.

Perez-Reyes, M.; White, W.R.; McDonald, S.A.; Hicks, R.E.; Jeffcoat, A.R.; Cook, C.E. (1991). The pharmocologic effects of daily marijuana smoking in humans. *Pharmacol Biochem Behav,* 40:691-694.

Petro, D.C.; Ellenberger, J. (1981). Treatment of human spasticity with delta 9-tetrahydrocannabinol. *J Clin Pharmacol,* 21:413S-416S.

Pickworth, W.B.; Rohrer, M.S.; Fant, R.V. (1997). Effects of abused drugs on psychomotor performance. *Exp Clin Psychopharmachol,* 5:235-241.

Pihl, R.O.; Sigal, H. (1978). Motivational levels and the marijuana high. *J Abnorm Psychol,* 87(2):280-285.

Plasse, T.F.; Gorter, R.W.; Krasnow, S.H.; Lane, M.; Shepard, K.V.; Wadleigh, R.G. (1991). Recent clinical experience with dronabinol. *Pharmacol Biochem Behav,* 40:695-700.

Polen, M.R.; Sidney, S.; Tekawa, I.S.; Sadler, M.; Friedman, G.D. (1993). Health care use by frequent marijuana smokers who do not smoke tobacco. *West J Med,* 158:596-601.

Pope, H.G.; Yurgelun-Todd, D. (1996). The residual cognitive effects of heavy marijuana use in college students. *JAMA,* 275:521-527.

Rachlinski, J.J.; Foltin, R.W.; Fischman, M.W. (1989). The effects of smoked marijuana on interpersonal distances in small groups. *Drug Alcohol Depend,* 24:183-186.

Raft, D.; Gregg, J.; Ghia, J.; Harris, L. (1977). Effects of intravenous tetrahydrocannabinol on experimental and surgical pain: Psychological correlates of the analgesic response. *Clin Pharmacol Ther,* 21:26-33.

Rainone, G.A.; Deren, S.; Kleinman, P.H.; Wish, E.D. (1987). Heavy marijuana users not in treatment: The continuing search for the "pure" marijuana user. *J Psychoactive Drugs,* 19:353-359.

Ramaekers, J.G.; Robbe, H.W.J.; O'Hanlon, J.F. (2000). Marijuana, alcohol, and actual driving performance. *Human Psychopharmacol,* 15:551-558.

Renaud, A.M.; Cormier, Y. (1986). Acute effects of marijuana smoking on maximal exercise performance. *Med Sci Sports Exerc,* 18:685-689.

Richardson, M.S.; Craig, T.J.; Haugland, G. (1985). Treatment patterns of young chronic schizophrenic patients in the era of deinstitutionalization. *Psychiatr Q,* 57:104-110.

Robbe, H.J.; O'Hanlon, J.F. (1999). Marijuana and actual driving performance. Washington, DC: National Highway Transportation Administration.

Roffman, R.K.; Barnhart, R. (1987). Assessing need for marijuana dependence treatment through an anonymous telephone interview. *Int J Addict,* 22:639-651.

Roth, M.D.; Arora, A.; Barsky, S.H.; Kleerup, E.C.; Simmons, M.; Tashkin, D.P. (1998). Airway inflammation in young marijuana and tobacco smokers. *Am J Respir Crit Care Med,* 157:928-937.

Rubin, F.; Comitas, L. (1976). *Ganja in Jamaica.* Garden City, NY: Doubleday.

Sallan, S.E.; Cronin, C.; Zelen, M.; Zinberg, N.E. (1980). Antiemetics in patients receiving chemotherapy for cancer: A randomized comparison of delta-9-tetrahydrocannabinol and prochlorperazine. *N Engl J Med,* 302:135-138.

Sallan, S.E.; Zinberg, N.E.; Freii, E. (1975). Antiemetic effect of delta-9-tetrahydrocannabinol in patients receiving cancer chemotherapy. *N Engl J Med,* 293:795-797.

Schuckit, M.A. (1990). *Drug Abuse and Alcohol Abuse: A Clinical Guide to Diagnosis and Treatment.* New York: Plenum Medical Book Company.

Schwartz, R.H. (1987). Marijuana: An overview. *Pediatr Clin North Am,* 34(2): 305-317.

Schwartz, R.H.; Beveridge, R.A. (1994). Marijuana as an antiemetic drug: How useful is it today? Opinions from clinical oncologists. *J Addict Dis,* 13:53-65.

Schwartz, R.H.; Gruenewald, P.J.; Klitzner, M.; Fedio, P. (1989). Short-term memory impairment in cannabis-dependent adolescents. *Am J Dis Child,* 143: 1214-1219.

Shapiro, B.J.; Reiss, S.; Sullivan, S.F.; Tashkin, D.P.; Simmons, M.S.; Smith, R.T. (1976). Cardiopulmonary effects of marijuana smoking during exercise. *Chest,* 70:1351-1356.

Sherman, M.P.; Aeberhard, E.E.; Wong, V.Z.; Simmons, M.S.; Roth, M.D.; Tashkin, D.P. (1995). Effects of smoking marijuana, tobacco, or cocaine alone or in combination on DNA damage in human alveolar macrophages. *Life Sci,* 56:2201-2207.

Sherman, M.P.; Campbell, L.A.; Gong, H.J.; Roth, M.D.; Tashkin, D.P. (1991). Antimicrobial and respiratory burst characteristics of pulmonary alveolar macrophages recovered from smokers of marijuana alone, smokers of tobacco alone, smokers of marijuana and tobacco, and nonsmokers. *Am Rev Respir Dis,* 144: 1351-1356.

Sidney, S.; Quesenberry, C.P.; Friedman, G.D.; Tekawa, I.S. (1997). Marijuana use and cancer incidence (California, United States). *Cancer Causes Control,* 8:722-728.

Smiley, A.M.; Moskowitz, H.; Zeidman, K. (1981). Driving simulator studies of marijuana alone and in combination with alcohol. *Proceedings of the 25th Conference of the American Association for Automotive Medicine,* 107-116.

Smiley, A.M.; Noy, Y.I.; Tostowaryk, W. (1986). The effects of marijuana, alone and in combination with alcohol, on driving an instrumented car. *Proceedings of the 10th International Conference on Alcohol, Drugs, and Traffic Safety.* Amsterdam, 203-206.

Solowij, N. (1999). Long-term effects of cannabis on the central nervous system. In: Kalant, H.; Corrigall, W.A.; Hall, W.; Smart, R.G. (eds.), *The Health Effects of Cannabis* (pp. 195-266). Toronto: Centre for Addictions and Mental Health.

Solowij, N.; Grenyer, B.F.S.; Chesher, G.; Lewis, J. (1995). Biopsychosocial changes associated with cessation of cannabis use: A single case study of acute and chronic cognitive effects, withdrawal, and treatment. *Life Sci,* 56:2127-2134.

Solowij, N.; Grenyer, B.F.S.; Peters, R.; Chesher, G. (1997). Long term cannabis use impairs memory processes and frontal lobe function. *1997 Symposium on the Cannabinoids.* Burlington, VT: International Cannabinoid Research Society, 84.

Soni, S.D.; Brownlee, M. (1991). Alcohol abuse in chronic schizophrenics: Implications for management in the community. *Acta Psychiatr Scand,* 84:272-276.

Sridhar, K.S.; Raub, W.A.; Weatherby, N.L.; Metsch, L.R. (1995). Possible role of marijuana smoking as a carcinogen in the development of lung cancer at a young age. *J Psychoactive Drugs,* 26:285-288.

Staquet, M.; Gantt, C.; Machin, D. (1978). Effect of nitrogen analog of tetrahydrocannabinol of cancer pain. *Clin Pharmacol Ther,* 23:397-401.

Stefanis, C.; Dornbush, R.; Fink, M. (1977). *Hashish: Studies of long-term use.* New York: Raven Press.

Stein, A.C.; Allen, R.W.; Cook, M.L.; Karl, R.L. (1983). *A Simulator Study of the Combined Effects of Alcohol and Marijuana on Driving Behaviour.* Hawthorne, CA: National Highway Traffic Safety Administration.

Stephens, R.S. (1999). Cannabis and hallucinogens. In: McCrady, B.S.; Epstein, E.E. (eds.), *Addictions.* New York: Oxford University Press, 121-140.

Stephens, R.S.; Roffman, R.A.; Curtin, L. (2000). Comparison of extended versus brief treatments for marijuana use. *J Consult Clin Psychol,* 68:898-908.

Stephens, R.S.; Roffman, R.A.; Simpson, E.E. (1993). Adult marijuana users seeking treatment. *J Consult Clin Psychol,* 61:1100-1104.

Stephens, R.S.; Roffman, R.A.; Simpson, E.E. (1994). Treating adult marijuana dependence: A test of the relapse prevention model. *J Consult Clin Psychol,* 62:92-99.

Substance Abuse and Mental Health Services Administration (SAMHSA) (1998). *National Admissions to Substance Abuse Treatment Services - The Treatment Episode Data Set (TEDS) 1992-1996.* Rockville, MD: U.S. Department of Health and Human Services.

Substance Abuse and Mental Health Services Administration (SAMHSA) (1999). *Summary of Findings from the 1998 National Household Survey on Drug Abuse.* Rockville, MD: U.S. Department of Health and Human Services.

Substance Abuse and Mental Health Services Administration (SAMHSA) (2000). *National Household Survey on Drug Abuse, 1998* [Computer file], Second ICPSR version. Research Triangle Park, NC: Research Triangle Institute, Inter-university Consortium for Political and Social Research.

Tahir, S.K.; Zimmerman, A.M. (1991). Influence of marijuana on cellular structures and biochemical activities. *Pharmacol Biochem Behav,* 40:617-623.

Tanner, J.; Davies, S.; O'Grady, B. (1999). Whatever happened to yesterday's rebels? Longitudinal effects of youth delinquency on education and employment. *Soc Probl,* 46:250-274.

Tashkin, D.P. (1999). Cannabis effects on the respiratory system. In: Kalant, H.; Corrigall, W.A.; Hall, W.; Smart, R.G. (eds.), *The Health Effects of Cannabis* (pp. 311-346). Toronto: Centre for Addiction and Mental Health.

Tashkin, D.P.; Coulson, A.H.; Clark, V.A.; Simmons, M.; Borque, L.B.; Duann, S.; Spivey, G.H.; Gong, H. (1987). Respiratory symptoms and lung function in habitual heavy smokers of marijuana alone, smokers of marijuana and tobacco, smokers of tobacco alone, and nonsmokers. *Am Rev Respir Dis,* 135:209-216.

Tashkin, D.P.; Gliederer, F.; Rose, J.; Change, P.; Hui, K.K.; Yu, J.L.; Wu, T.C. (1991). Effects of varying marijuana smoking profile on disposition of tar and absorption of CO and delta-9-THC. *Pharmacol Biochem Behav,* 40:651-656.

Tashkin, D.P.; Shapiro, B.J.; Frank, I.M. (1973). Acute pulmonary physiologic effects of smoked marijuana and oral Δ^9-tetrahydrocannabinol in healthy young men. *N Engl J Med,* 289:336-341.

Tashkin, D.P.; Shapiro, B.J.; Lee, Y.E.; Harper, C.E. (1975). Effects of smoked marijuana in experimentally induced asthma. *Am Rev Respir Dis,* 112:377-386.

Taylor, D.R.; Poulton, R.; Moffitt, T.E.; Ramankutty, P.; Sears, M.R. (2000). The respiratory effects of cannabis dependence in young adults. *Addiction,* 95:1669-1677.

Taylor, F.M. (1988). Marijuana as a potential respiratory tract carcinogen: A retrospective analysis of a community hospital population. *South Med J,* 81:1213-1216.

Tennes, K.; Avitable, N.; Blackard, C.; Boyles, C.; Hassoun, B.; Holmes, L.; Kreye, M. (1985). Marijuana: Prenatal and postnatal exposure in the human. In: Pinkert, T.M. (ed.), *Current Research on the Consequences of Maternal Drug Abuse* (pp. 48-60). Washington, DC: U.S. Government Printing Office.

Thacore, V.R.; Shukla, S.P. (1976). Cannabis psychosis and paranoid schizophrenia. *Arch Gen Psychiatry,* 33:383-386.

Thornicroft, G. (1990). Cannabis and psychosis: Is there epidemiological evidence for association? *Br J Psychiatry,* 157:25-33.

Tilles, D.S.; Goldenheim, P.D.; Johnson, D.C.; Mendelson, J.A.; Mellow, N.K.; Hales, C.A. (1986). Marijuana smoking as cause of reduction in single-breath carbon monoxide diffusing capacity. *Am J Med,* 80:601-606.

Timpone, J.G.; Wright, D.J.; Egorin, M.J.; Enama, M.E.; Mayers, J.; Galetto, G. (1997). The safety and pharmacokinetics of single-agent and combination therapy with megestrol acetate and dronabinol for the treatment of HIV wasting syndrome. *AIDS Res Hum Retroviruses,* 13:305-315.

Ungerleider, J.T.; Andrysiak, Y.; Fairbanks, L.; Ellison, G.W.; Myers, L.W. (1987). Delta-9-THC in the treatment for spasticity associated with multiple sclerosis. *Adv Alcohol Subst Abuse,* 7:39-50.

Vachon, L.; Fitzgerald, M.X.; Solliday, N.F.; Gould, I.A.; Gaensler, E.A. (1973). Single-dose effect of marijuana smoke: Bronchial dynamics and respiratory center sensitivity in normal subjects. *N Engl J Med,* 288:985-989.

VanHoozen, B.E.; Cross, C.E. (1997). Marijuana: Respiratory tract effects. *Clin Rev Allergy Immunol,* 15:243-269.

Verweij, P.E.; Kerremans, J.J.; Voss, A.; Meis, J.F. (2000). Fungal contamination of tobacco and marijuana. *JAMA,* 384:2875.

Wallace, J.M.; Oishi, J.S.; Barbers, R.G.; Simmons, M.S.; Tashkin, D.P. (1994). Lymphocytic subpopulation profiles in bronchoalveolar lavage fluid and peripheral blood from tobacco and marijuana smokers. *Chest,* 105:847-852.

Walton, R.P. (1938). *Marijuana—America's New Drug Problem.* Philadelphia: J.P. Lippincott.

Wells, J.E.; Bushnell, J.A.; Joyce, P.R.; Oakley-Browne, M.A.; Hornblow, A.R. (1992). Problems with alcohol, drugs and gambling in Christchurch, New Zealand. In: Abbot, M.; Evans, K. (eds.), *Alcohol and Drug Dependence and Disorders of Impulse Control* (pp. 3-13). Auckland, New Zealand: Alcohol Liquor Advisory Council.

Wert, R.C.; Raulin, M.L. (1986a). The chronic cerebral effects of cannabis use: I. Methodological issues and neurological findings. *Int J Addict,* 21:605-628.

Wert, R.C.; Raulin, M.L. (1986b). The chronic cerebral effects of cannabis use: II. Psychological findings and conclusions. *Int J Addict,* 21:629-642.

Wetzel, C.D.; Janowsky, D.S.; Clopton, P.L. (1982). Remote memory during marijuana intoxication. *Psychopharmacology (Berl),* 76:278-281.

Witter, F.R.; Niebyl, J.R. (1990). Marijuana use in pregnancy and pregnancy outcome. *Am J Perinatol,* 7:36-38.

World Health Organization (WHO) (1992). Classification of mental and behavioural disorders: Clinical description and diagnostic guidelines. In *International Statistical Classification of Diseases and Related Health Programs,* Tenth Revision. Geneva: WHO.

Wu, T.C.; Tashkin, D.P.; Djahed, B.; Rose, J.E. (1988). Pulmonary hazards of smoking marijuana as compared with tobacco. *N Engl J Med,* 318:347-351.

Zacny, J.P.; Chait, L.D. (1989). Breathhold duration and response to marijuana smoke. *Pharmacol Biochem Behav,* 33:481-484.

Zhang, Z.F.; Morgenstern, H.; Spitz, M.R.; Tashkin, D.P.; Yu, G.P.; Marshall, J.R.; Hsu, T.C. (1999). Marijuana use and increased risk of squamous cell carcinoma of the head and neck. *Cancer Epidemiol Biomarkers Prev,* 8:1071-1078.

Zhu, L.X.; Sharma, S.; Stolina, M.; Gardner, B.; Roth, M.D.; Tashkin, D.P.; Dubinett, S.M. (2000). Delta-9-tetrahydrocannabinol inhibits antitumor immunity by a CB2 receptor-mediated, cytokine-dependent pathway. *J Immunol,* 165:373-380.

Zuckerman, B.; Frank, D.; Hingson, R.; Amaro, H.; Levenson, S.; Kayne, H.; Parker, S.; Vinci, R.; Aboagye, K.; Fried, L.; Cabral, H.; Timperi, R.; Bauchner, S. (1989). Effects of maternal marijuana and cocaine use on fetal growth. *N Engl J Med,* 320:762-768.

Chapter 7

The Medical Consequences
of Opiate Abuse and Addiction
and Methadone Pharmacotherapy

Pauline F. McHugh
Mary Jeanne Kreek

OVERVIEW

The incomparable ability of opium and its derivatives to kill pain, both physical and mental, has led to their use throughout recorded history as much for medicinal as for "recreational" purposes. For as long as opiates have been used, they have also been abused, and the dangers inherent in opiate abuse and addiction have long been recognized. The introduction in 1898 of the highly lipid-soluble, injectable opiate diacetylmorphine, or heroin, has led to problems of opiate abuse and addiction on a grand scale. The rapid onset of heroin and its powerful reinforcing properties have made it the most commonly abused opiate in the United States (Kreek, 1996). In recent reports from the National Institute of Drug Abuse and the Substance Abuse and Mental Health Services Administration, about 2.7 million people in the United States were reported to have used heroin at some time in their lives, and an estimated 800,000 to 1 million were currently hard-core addicts, only a fraction of whom were in methadone treatment programs (Kreek, 1996; Karch and Stephens, 2000). Although 1998 is the last year for which such statistics are available, reports indicate that these numbers are rising (Perrone et al., 1999). The costs to society have been enormous. In 1996 alone, 70,500 emergency room visits in the United States were directly attributable to heroin use, while in 1993, heroin was held to be directly responsible for approximately 4,000 deaths by overdose (Sporer, 1999). The number of deaths for which heroin has been indirectly responsi-

Supported in part by NIH grants NIDA P50-DA-05130, K05 DA00049, NCRR M01-RR00102, and OASAS-NYS. Thanks to Dr. James Schluger for reviewing the manuscript.

ble, due to the transmission of HIV-1 or the development of other medical complications, as well as from high-risk psychosocial behavior associated with drug abuse and addiction, is much harder to calculate. The estimated cost to society in the United States of the medical and legal consequences of drug addiction was $246 billion in 1992, for which a significant percentage was due to heroin (Kreek, 1996). The cost in terms of human suffering is incalculable.

Apart from the vast psychosocial risks associated with drug abuse and addiction, the medical consequences of addiction to any drug can be attributed to several factors: the pharmacological properties of the drug itself, the problems inherent in the routes of self-administration, and the various diluents and adulterants which are used to extend the resale value of the drug on the streets or sometimes used to enhance the quality of the drug's intended effects (Kreek et al., 1972; Kreek, 1973b; Furst, 2000). Drugs can exacerbate underlying medical problems, or, alternatively, can cause medical problems to be neglected. In already dire social situations such as homelessness, the additional presence of a drug addiction significantly increases an individual's likelihood of premature death (Hwang et al., 1998; Gunne and Gronbladh, 1981).

Opiates are set apart from other drugs of abuse by the diverse sites of opiate receptors throughout human tissues and organ systems, including vital centers in the brain. Thus medical problems due to direct pharmacological effects of opiates involve multiple organ systems and have a higher lethality in the case of overdose than other drugs of abuse. Findings about the effects of opiates on specific biochemical functions, such as neuroendocrine functioning or immune response, suggest other ways in which opiates differ from other drugs of abuse. There appears to be an even greater risk for complications and infections in addicted individuals because of the suppressive effect opiates have on the immune response and endocrine functioning (Kreek, 1990a,b; Kreek et al., 1990).

The opiates most commonly abused tend to be those with rapid onset and short half-lives, as is the case with heroin. The half-life of heroin in humans is about three minutes. The major metabolite of heroin, morphine, has a half-life of four to six hours (Inturrisi et al., 1984). The rapidity of onset of a drug is related to its rewarding or reinforcing effects, but also to its intoxicating effects. As such, rapidity of onset may also be involved in the neurobiological changes that occur in addiction. The short half-lives of heroin, morphine, and related short-acting opiates also result in a need for multiple doses to be self-administered throughout any given day, in order to maintain the rewarding effect or, as addiction progresses, to avoid the sickness of withdrawal. Multiple daily self-administrations of a drug in unhygienic conditions increase the risk of infection and other complications to the drug user. In addition, this short-acting pharmacokinetic profile results in peaks and troughs of serum opiate levels that are cycling several times a day, and the corresponding waxing and waning of functionality in an opiate-addicted individual (see Figure 7.1).

This cycling of serum opiate level in cases of abuse and addiction appears to cause some of the deleterious pharmacological effects of opiates. The "on-off" cycles of opiates lead to a dysregulation of those physiological systems which are at least partly modulated by opiate receptors. This is most striking in the immune system and the neuroendocrine system, both of which appear to be suppressed in opiate abuse and addiction (Kreek et al., 1972; Kreek, 1973a,b,c; Cushman and Kreek, 1974a). These systems may slowly recover when drug use is stopped, but in the hard-core addict for whom stopping opiate use is unlikely or impossible, pharmacotherapy with a long-acting opioid such as methadone or l-α-acetylmethadone (LAAM) may ameliorate physiological changes by eliminating the "on-off" cycle

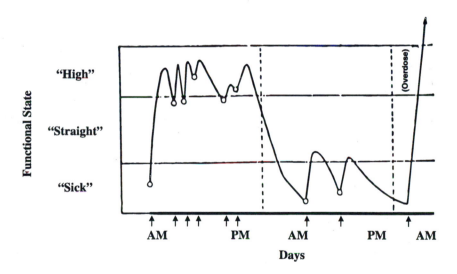

FIGURE 7.1. Diagrammatic summary of the functional state of a typical intravenous heroin user. Dashed lines indicate new days. Arrows show the repetitive injection of uncertain doses of heroin, usually 10 to 30 mg but sometimes much more. The addict is hardly ever in a state of normal function. (*Source:* Adapted from Dole et al., 1966.)

(Kreek, 1990a, 1996; Novick et al., 1993).* The half-lives of these medications are significantly longer than those of the commonly abused opiates. Racemic methadone has a half-life of 24 hours and the active l-enantiomer of methadone has a half-life of 36 to 48 hours, while LAAM has a half-life of two days or longer (Kreek, 1973c, 2000). The slow onset times and long half-lives of these medications allow for a physiological steady-state of opioid stimulation in the hard-core addict. Thus multiple daily cycles of euphoria and withdrawal are eliminated and normal functioning is restored (see Figure 7.2).

This chapter is intended to describe the medical consequences attributable to abuse of and addiction to short-acting opiates such as heroin. The medical consequences of the pharmacotherapy of opiate addiction with long-acting opiates such as methadone and LAAM will also be discussed. Because death is the worst direct medical consequence of heroin abuse and addiction, it is covered first, followed by the direct pathophysiological effects of opiates on tissues and organ systems that result in significant morbidity for this patient population. Indirect causes of medical illness resulting from heroin use, such as infection and contamination with adulterants used to cut the drug, are covered last. Psychosocial problems resulting in medical consequences with this population, including prostitution and violence, are not specifically covered here, since those problems are common to all varieties of addictions and resolve with treatment of the addiction, including the methadone pharmacotherapy that is the current treatment of choice for people addicted to heroin. Finally, the medical consequences of methadone pharmacotherapy are included with each section, to provide a comparison with the medical problems so often seen in people addicted to short-acting opiates.

PHARMACOLOGICAL EFFECTS OF OPIATES: DEATH

The mortality rate for opiate abusers and addicts has been estimated at 6 to 20 times that of the non-drug-using population. While much of the morbidity and mortality associated with opiate abuse and addiction is from secondary causes such as infection or other complications, a significant percentage is due to direct effects of the drug itself. In people who regularly inject heroin, for example, the annual mortality rate is estimated to be 2 percent, half of which is attributable to overdose (Sporer, 1999; Gunne and

---

*Buprenorphine, a mixed opioid agonist/antagonist with long-acting activity at opiate receptors, is also currently being investigated as another medication for the treatment of opiate addiction.

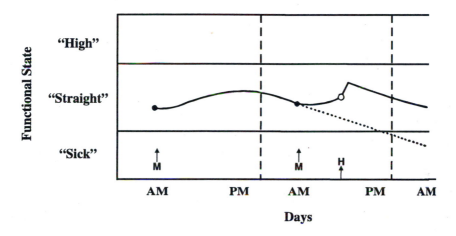

FIGURE 7.2. Methadone maintenance: Functional state of a former heroin addict treated with a single daily oral dose of methadone pharmacotherapy (M). The effect of an intravenous injection of heroin (H) in the methadone-treated patient is shown in the second day. The dotted line indicates the course if methadone is omitted. (*Source:* Adapted from Dole et al., 1966.)

Gronbladh, 1981). While overdose is the most common acute cause of death in the opiate-abusing population, other physiological mechanisms have also been reported, although the rates of these causes of death are unclear. When opioid pharmacotherapy such as methadone is made available, the death rates from opiate abuse and addiction drop precipitously (Karch and Stephens, 2000).

Overdose Deaths

Overdose Deaths Due to Heroin and Other Short-Acting Opiates

Overdose by short-acting opiates results in central respiratory depression and coma due to the direct effects of opiate agonists on central nervous system opiate receptors. Overdose is most commonly reported in intravenous opiate abusers, although cases of fatal overdose by intranasal, subcutaneous, intramuscular, and oral self-administration have also been reported (Sporer, 1999; Karch and Stephens, 2000). The majority of opiate overdose deaths occur in experienced users and are due to unexpectedly high purity of the drug contained in the usual "dose" (or purchased packet), interactions between opiates and very large amounts of other drugs, especially alcohol and benzodiazepines (which can exacerbate the respiratory depression effects of the opiates) or, alternatively, the deliberate self-administration of an over-dose in a suicide attempt (Karch and Stephens, 2000). Accidental overdoses have also been reported in naïve users and "body packers," people who transport quantities of drugs in packages by swallowing them or inserting them rectally. Body packers are susceptible to overdose if a package breaks en route (Utecht et al., 1993; Wetli et al., 1997).

The mechanism of overdose death is respiratory depression. Most intra-venous opiate deaths occur within one to three hours of intravenous admin-istration, although some occur with the needle used to intravenously inject heroin still in the vein. Central respiratory depression is reversible with opi-ate antagonists such as naloxone or nalmefene, which are administered by bolus followed by continuous intravenous drip until the opiate agonist has been adequately cleared. Because of the different half-lives of the various opiates, or the interactions of other drugs with the opiates, clearance rates may vary. In addition, the duration of antagonistic effects of opiate antago-nists varies. The duration of effectiveness of naloxone is one to four hours, while the duration of effectiveness of nalmefene is four to ten hours. Clear-ance times of opiates as well as duration of action of opiate antagonists must be taken into account in the treatment of overdose, and overdose victims must be monitored for several hours before the opiate antagonist treatment can be discontinued (Hartman and Kreek, 1983; Finfer, 1996). Withdrawal symptoms following opiate antagonist administration can be severe and sei-zures (though rare) have been reported in connection with acute and severe opiate withdrawal (Delanty et al., 1998; Kaplan et al., 1999).

Because of the widespread use of opiates in both addictive diseases and the treatment of pain, administration of opiate antagonists should be admin-istered to anyone presenting with unconsciousness of unknown origin. Monitoring of the patient should continue following discontinuation of opi-ate antagonist therapy, since complications such as aspiration or recurrent respiratory depression with resultant hypoxia or anoxia can lead to further morbidity and mortality. About 3 to 7 percent of opiate overdose patients treated emergently will develop complications requiring hospitalization (Karch and Stephens, 2000; Kumar et al., 1999).

Overdose Deaths Due to Methadone

Deaths that have been reported from methadone or LAAM overdose fre-quently have been iatrogenic, secondary to a too-rapid increase in dose by methadone treatment providers in persons who have only a modest opioid tolerance. Other methadone-related overdose deaths are attributable to accidental causes, such as the combination of illicit methadone with very large amounts of alcohol or benzodiazepines or accidental ingestion, as well as deliberate causes such as overdose suicide attempts (Perret et al., 2000; Karch and Stephens, 2000). Death is again attributable to respiratory depression, with both pulmonary and cerebral edema found postmortem (Perret et al., 2000). Because of the long half-life of these medications, opiate antagonist therapy must be instituted for up to twenty-four hours in the event of an overdose, and the patient must be monitored closely for at least one day, rather than a few hours (Hartman and Kreek, 1983; Finfer, 1996).

Positional Asphyxia and Muscular Necrosis

Positional Asphyxia Due to Heroin and Other Short-Acting Opiates

Because of the rapid onset of short-acting opiates, the sedating effects of these drugs are profound and occur very quickly following self-administration of the drug. Numerous case reports describe unusual or awkward positions in which acutely intoxicated people have remained for long periods of time following self-administration. A mechanism for death in these individuals has been attributed to some form of respiratory compromise that can result from a compressed position, particularly in combination with the central respiratory depression characteristic of opiates. This cause of death has been presumed in many cases where serum levels of opiates measured postmortem were too low to be lethal in and of themselves and no other mechanism of death was apparent. However, in many other cases the sedated position in which the victim was found was more clearly involved in the mechanism of death. A syndrome consisting of hypoxia, vascular thromboses, and necrosis of skeletal muscle has been seen in case reports of deaths following acute intoxication while sitting in the lotus or other constricted positions (Howard and Reay, 1998; Klockgether et al., 1997; Rabl and Markwalder, 1996). A certain number of deaths of opiate addicts in police custody have been attributed to police procedures of restraining acutely intoxicated heroin addicts in "hogtie" positions, although this finding has been the subject of much debate (Karch and Stephens, 1999; Howard and Reay, 1998; Rabl and Markwalder, 1996).

Positional Asphyxia and Methadone

There are apparently no reports of positional asphyxia occurring in the presence of methadone pharmacotherapy alone. The sedating effects of methadone are less profound and of much slower onset than those of the short-acting opiates, and therefore the chances of an individual suddenly collapsing into an awkward position are very low.

"Anaphylactoid" Shock Due to Direct or Indirect Effects of Opiates

"Anaphylactoid" Shock Due to Heroin and Other Short-Acting Opiates

Some immediate deaths following opiate self-administration appear to have an acute hypersensitivity-like response as their cause. In one study of heroin addicts who died suddenly following injection of heroin, Edston and van Hage-Hamsten (1997) found increased levels of mast-cell tryptase in the serum and pulmonary tissue. This is sometimes described as an "anaphylactoid reaction" to the drug, due to the well-known effects of opioids in causing mast-cell degranulation and related histamine release. Alternatively, an adulterant in the drug may be present that causes an actual allergic response (Edston and van Hage-Hamsten, 1997).

It has been shown that in all individuals, morphine administered subcutaneously will cause a wheal-and-flare response secondary to mast-cell degranulation and histamine release (Novick et al., 1989). Likewise, acute opiate administration can also cause acute release of histamine in lung tissue, thus triggering an allergic-like response that can have rapid effects on pulmonary and systemic capillaries. This can lead to a drop in blood pressure and further respiratory compromise in a patient who already has central respiratory depression as a result of the direct effects of the opiate (Karch, 1998; Remskar et al., 1998). In these cases, death from respiratory failure appears to occur more rapidly than in uncomplicated overdose. While it has been speculated that this mechanism may account for many opiate deaths that have been ascribed to overdose, the rate of "anaphylactoid" death for opiate abuses is unknown. Pulmonary edema due to this mechanism is implicated in many or most overdose deaths. True "allergic" response to heroin, morphine, and related drugs is probably rare.

"Anaphylactoid" Shock Due to Methadone

The oral route of administration of methadone and slow onset time markedly decrease the chance of an individual having a fulminant mast cell degranulation and reaction to acute histamine release. Methadone induces histamine release to a modest extent, but again the slow onset time decreases the chances of acute bronchospasm, capillary insufficiency, and related sequelae.

DIRECT MEDICAL CONSEQUENCES OF OPIATES

It has been documented that opiates have no known direct toxic effect on tissues and organ systems in humans apart from the risk of overdose. Adulterants in the drugs and the unhygienic methods used in the course of their self-administration, as well as the relative hypoxia or anoxia resulting from central respiratory depression in overdose, are the principle causes of tissue damage in opiate addicts. However, the direct effects of short-acting opiates on opiate receptor systems when self-administered chronically can lead to physiological disruption of metabolic pathways and organ system functioning. Some of these opiate-induced tissue alterations in normal physiological function, while not potentially fatal or debilitating in and of themselves, may predispose an individual to be at greater risk for the indirect effects of drug addiction. One of the most clinically relevant functional alterations is the effect of opiates on the immune response. Studies have suggested that this effect may functionally decrease an individual's resistance to infection when exposed to an infectious agent (Thomas et al., 1995; Cherubin and Sapira, 1993). Other physiological changes resulting from opiate addiction may also have great clinical relevance, both in their effects on normal systemic and metabolic function, and perhaps also in the acquisition and perpetuation of the addiction itself (Kreek, 1996).

The Effects of Opiates on the Immune Response

The Effects of Heroin and Other Short-Acting Opiates on the Immune Response

Among the earliest indications that chronic opiate abuse had effects on the human immune response were the lymphadenopathy, lymphocytosis, hyperimmunoglobulinemia, and altered T-cell function noted in untreated heroin addicts in early studies prior to the advent of HIV-1 but after hepatitis B had been recognized (Kreek et al., 1972; Kreek, 1973a,b, 1990a). While the actions of the opiates themselves were suspected, it was initially held that chronic bouts of bacteremia, repeated exposure to inert adulterants, and infection with hepatitis B virus, all results of intravenous drug use, could be the causes of the immune system changes seen in heroin addicts. More recently, extensive studies performed in a variety of in vitro, animal, and a few human models suggest that opiates can directly modulate the immune response through opiate receptors located on immune cell surfaces. In laboratory models these effects appear to be dose dependent and are reversible by opiate antagonists such as naloxone (Singhal et al., 2000; Singhal et al., 1995). A number of different mechanisms for these effects have been proposed, but the evidence from these models is often conflicting, and their relevance to human disease is unclear at this time.

In humans, short-acting opiates may additionally affect the immune system through modulation of the hypothalamic-pituitary-adrenal axis via changes in the levels of serum cortisol that are released through that endocrine cascade (Novick et al., 1989; Culpepper-Morgan and Kreek, 1997). Both of these actions result in changes in immune function that are generally suppressive in nature. However, specific immune cell activation induced by morphine and morphine withdrawal has also been reported (Singhal et al., 1999). Dose and chronicity of administration may play a role in the specific immune functions that are induced or suppressed. The immune alterations that have been found in humans to date include: attenuation of lymphocyte proliferation (Govitrapong et al., 1998); increased levels of serum immunoglobulins (Novick et al., 1989); suppression of bone marrow macrophage colony formation (Govitrapong et al., 1998); suppression of natural killer-cell activity (Yeager et al., 1995); suppression of phagocytosis of *Candida albicans* (Carr et al., 1996); the presence in the circulation of heroin addicts of elevated levels of immune complexes (Lazzarin et al., 1984); destruction of thymocytes (Glavina-Durdov and Definis-Gojanovic, 1999); and a change in total number of B cells (Fletcher et al., 1993; Novick et al., 1989). Such immune impairments have been seen in chronic, untreated heroin addicts, in the absence of any evidence of hepatitis B markers, HIV-1, HTLV-I, or HTLV-II infection (Fletcher et al., 1993).

Natural killer-cell activity seems particularly vulnerable to the acute effects of opiates. Suppression occurs within hours of the initial dose, and will persist for some time following cessation of opiate administration in the opiate naïve subject. Natural killer-cell activity appears to be suppressed in opiate addicts in the absence of HIV-1 or other viral infections. This may, in fact, predispose opiate addicts to acquire a retroviral infection (Novick et al., 1989; Yeager et al., 1995).

The Effects of Methadone on the Immune Response

Some, although not all, of the functions altered in short-acting opiate addiction appear to return to normal when patients are treated with a long-acting opioid pharmacotherapy such as methadone. Natural killer-cell activity in particular appears to normalize with methadone treatment (Novick et al., 1989). Methadone does not appear to have the same immunosuppressive potential as heroin or other commonly abused short-acting opiates. This may be due to methadone's efficacy in preventing opiate withdrawal, a result of normalization of the HPA axis, or possibly due to pharmacokinetic differences at the level of immune cell surface opiate receptors (Thomas et al., 1995; Kreek, 1996; Novick et al., 1989).

The Effects of Opiates on Neuroendocrine Functioning

The Effects of Heroin and Other Short-Acting Opiates
on Neuroendocrine Functioning

The stress hormone cortisol is regulated by the hormone cascade produced by the hypothalamic-pituitary-adrenal (HPA) axis. The release of corticotrophin releasing factor (CRF) from the hypothalamus induces the synthesis and release of adrenocorticotrophin (ACTH) and β-endorphin, major peptides derived from pro-opiomelanocortin (POMC) in the pituitary gland. ACTH then induces the release of cortisol from the adrenal glands. The major modulator of the HPA axis is cortisol, which acts at the levels of the pituitary and the hypothalamus in a negative feedback mode to reduce CRF release from the hypothalamus. Furthermore, endogenous opioids have been found to modulate this hormone axis by their inhibitory action on opiate receptors present in the pituitary and the hypothalamus (Kreek, 1987; Kreek, 2000). Therefore, endogenous opioids are intimately involved with the regulation of the stress response.

Addiction to short-acting opiates results in a chronically fluctuating dysregulation of the HPA axis and abnormal release of cortisol throughout the course of the day. Irregular release of cortisol is a factor that may contribute to the immune response abnormalities seen in opiate addicts. The physiological dysregulation of stress hormones also leads to disruptions in the sleep-wake cycle as well as regulations of mood states, thus contributing to the decrease in daily functioning experienced by opiate addicts (Novick et al., 1997; Novick and Kreek, 1992; Kreek, 1987; Kreek, 2000).

The feedback mechanism for the hypothalamic-pituitary-gonadal (HPG) axis is similarly impaired. Acute administration of opiates can suppress pulsatile leutinizing hormone (LH) release from the hypothalamus, resulting in irregularities of sex hormone levels (Mendelson and Mello, 1978). Therefore, ovarian function in women may be impaired, with resultant anovulation and amenorrhea, and in men decreased libido and erectile dysfunction are frequently reported (Santen et al., 1975; Mendelson and Mello, 1978; Thomas et al., 1977; Melman and Gingell, 1999). Some evidence indicates that other hormone systems involving hypothalamic releasing factors, such as the thyroid and parathyroid hormone systems, are also subject to dysregulation in the presence of opiates. The mechanisms, while presumably similar to those for the HPA and HPG axes, have not been well established (Surks and Sievert, 1995; Tagliaro et al., 1984).

The Effects of Methadone on Neuroendocrine Functioning

Most of the dysregulations of the neuroendocrine axis occurring in heroin addiction appear to be normalized following successful treatment of heroin addiction with methadone. The HPA axis in particular appears to normalize, in part due to the steady-state pharmacokinetics of the long-acting opioids, but also to the elimination of the stress-inducing lifestyle that accompanies heroin addiction (Kreek, 1973a,b, 1996; Novick and Kreek, 1992). Some reduction in pulsatile secretion of LH persists with methadone treatment, although absolute values are no different from those of normal controls. Nevertheless, some ovulatory or erectile dysfunction may persist with methadone treatment, although not to the degree that is seen in active heroin addiction (Cushman and Kreek, 1974a). Thyroid-stimulating-hormone levels appear to be reduced with methadone treatment, as well as in active addiction. In neither case does this appear to have much clinical significance (Cushman and Kreek, 1974b; Surks and Sievert, 1995).

Effects of Opiates on Organ Systems

The Effects of Heroin and Other Short-Acting Opiates on Organ Systems

The majority of toxic effects from opiate abuse and addiction come from adulterants and inert diluents used to cut the drug on the street or from the relative hypoxia or anoxia resulting from opiate overdose. However, some questions remain as to whether there are any toxic effects of opiates themselves. In vitro and animal studies have suggested that there may be a specific toxicity of short-acting opiates such as pure morphine or pure heroin on various tissue types. However, direct toxic effects of opiates on organ systems are generally not seen in opiate-addicted humans. The organ system changes seen in opiate-addicted humans are instead due to an expected regulatory effect of endogenous opioids that is dysregulated in the presence of illicit opiates.

Neuropathies. The rate of peripheral neuropathies and plexopathies in HIV-negative intravenous heroin users is nearly 25 times higher than the general population (Berger et al., 1999). Mechanisms that have been proposed for opiate-related neuropathies have included chronic inflammation, neurotoxic adulterants, nutritional deficiencies, and comorbid alcoholism, all of which doubtlessly contribute to neurological damage in opiate addicts (Berger et al., 1999; Evans and Millington, 1993; Hillstrom et al., 1990). However, similar neuropathic symptoms may also be seen in non-drug-abusing cancer patients who are being treated for chronic pain with large doses of morphine. It has been hypothesized from a small series of patients that the morphine metabolite morphine-3-glucuronide (M-3-G), which constitutes a small percentage of the metabolites of morphine but is highly neuroexcitatory and possibly neurotoxic, is responsible for neuronal damage in patients who are regularly receiving large doses of morphine. In these patients, the neuropathies were reversible when the morphine doses were stopped (Sjogren et al., 1998; Inturrisi et al., 1984). Morphine is the primary metabolite of heroin. Diacetylmorphine breaks down to morphine in the liver, which is further broken down into M-3-G. Therefore, heroin users may also be subject to direct neurotoxic effects from heroin's metabolites, compounded by or perhaps even predisposed to them by the nutritional deficiencies and other problems that commonly occur in addictions. However, this hypothesis has not been confirmed.

Pulmonary effects. The acute, rapid administration of opiates directly triggers the release of histamines in lung tissue, causing acute broncho-constriction, inflammation, and increased capillary permeability (Cruz et al., 1998; Benson and Bentley, 1995). By this mechanism, short-acting opiate use by asthmatic opiate users can result in sudden asphyxic asthma, although as with the "anaphylactoid" syndrome described earlier, asthma-like symptoms may similarly be triggered in opiate users who have no prior asthma history (Cygan et al., 2000; Levenson et al., 1996).

Even in the absence of acute bronchoconstriction, the increased permeability of the pulmonary capillary bed caused by opiate-induced histamine release can result in a noncardiogenic pulmonary edema. Pulmonary edema as a result of opiate abuse is most often described as a complication of overdose, independent of the route by which the overdose was administered. However, with the increasing popularity of inhaled heroin, cases of acute pulmonary edema following heroin inhalation or insufflation in the absence of overdose have been reported (Karne et al., 1999; Benson and Bentley, 1995; Cruz et al., 1998).

In some individuals, the inflammation accompanying the pulmonary edema can present as an acute pneumonia. The inflammation is often found by bronchial lavage to consist of eosinophils, thus attesting to the origin of the pneumonia as a hypersensitivity-like response rather than an infection (Pope-Harman et al., 1996). Circulating immune complexes have also been found deposited in alveolar capillary membranes in association with this edema (Smith et al., 1978). The infiltrates caused by eosinophilic pneumonia may persist as long as drug use persists. When chronic, this can eventually result in an interstitial pneumonitis that is responsive to steroids (Benson and Bentley, 1995; Brander and Tukiainen, 1993). The central respiratory depression characteristic of opiate abuse and addiction doubtlessly contributes to the development of such pulmonary problems (O'Donnell et al., 1995).

Skeletal-muscle toxicity. Rhabdomyolysis, a disease in which massive skeletal-muscle-cell breakdown causes the release of intracellular myoglobin into the bloodstream, is one cause of severe medical complications in drug addicts. Severe myoglobinemia resulting from acute rhabdomyolysis can cause renal damage, which can progress to end-stage renal failure (Deighan et al., 2000; Kumar et al., 1999). This has been reported in intravenous drug users, irrespective of the drug that is being injected. For this reason, rhabdomyolysis is often attributed to the use of contaminated needles, drug adulterants, or skeletomuscular injuries sustained while intoxicated.

In opiate-addicted individuals, rhabdomyolysis is again most commonly reported in intravenous heroin users. However, there have been reports of rhabdomyolysis also occurring in heroin addicts who inhale rather than inject heroin (Otero et al., 1992; Annane et al., 1990; Rabl and Markwalder, 1996). It is likely that the pharmacological properties of opiates contribute further risks for the development of rhabdomyolysis. The anoxia or hypoxia caused by opiate overdose and the muscular breakdown that can accompany long periods of immobility while intoxicated with opiates are predisposing factors for rhabdomyolysis (Novick et al., 1997; Richards, 2000). Furthermore, recent animal model studies have suggested that short-acting opiates may have a direct toxic effect on skeletal-muscle cell membranes (Pena et al., 1993; Pena et al., 1990). Although the relevance of these findings is not clear in regard to human illness, they raise the possibility that short-acting opiates may play a more directly causal role in the development of rhabdomyolysis.

Renal effects. Apart from the risk of renal failure secondary to rhabdomyolysis, renal illness is increased in heroin addicts, particularly among intravenous drug users. Heroin-associated nephropathy occurs as focal segmental glomerulosclerosis (predominantly in young African-American men who have been using heroin for several years, and as such may be related to a genetic predisposition), but may also present as a membranous glomerulopathy or a chronic interstitial nephritis irrespective of ethnicity or gender (Haskell et al., 1988; Dettmeyer et al., 1998). While the etiologies of heroin-associated nephropathies remain largely idiopathic, both in vitro and postmortem human studies have suggested that elevated amounts of circulating immune complexes formed in response to opiates may play a role in their genesis (Singhal et al., 1995; Sanders and Marshall, 1989). The mechanisms remain unclear, but may have to do with mesangial deposition of circulating immune complexes or the formation of antiglomerulomembrane antibodies (Savige et al., 1989).

Teratogenicity and fetal development. Babies born to heroin-addicted mothers have been found to be significantly smaller in terms of head circumference and lower birth weight than babies born to non-drug-using mothers (Vance et al., 1997). However, it is not clear whether the low birth weight is an effect of heroin itself, or a consequence of nicotine dependence. The rate of cigarette smoking, which has been linked with low birth weight in numerous studies, is nearly 100 percent in the heroin-addicted population (Kenner and D'Apolito, 1997; Miller et al., 1991). Poor nutrition, also commonly seen in this population, may be another contributing factor to low birth weight.

Opiates, and heroin in particular, readily cross the placenta, and heroin will appear in fetal tissue within one hour of maternal use (Kenner and D'Apolito, 1997). For pregnant women who are addicted to short-acting opiates such as heroin, the fetus experiences multiple daily cycles of intoxication and withdrawal. The increased catecholamine release accompanying opiate withdrawal, which is generally well-tolerated by the mother, can be fatal to the developing fetus. In addition, short-acting opiate abuse and dependence during pregnancy has been associated with a number of complications, including spontaneous abortion, placental insufficiency, pre-term labor, premature rupture of membranes, breech presentation, chorioamnionitis, meconium passage, fetal distress during labor, pre-eclampsia, and eclampsia (Archie, 1998). The likelihood of a fetus surviving to term appears largely dependent on the pharmacokinetics of the opiate. Longer-acting opiates do not have the continuous cycle of intoxication and withdrawal of the short-acting opiates and are not associated with increased risk to fetal survival. For these reasons, a long-acting opiate pharmacotherapy such as methadone maintenance continues to be the treatment of choice for opiate-addicted mothers (Archie, 1998; American Academy of Pediatrics, 1998).

Neonates may undergo opiate withdrawal, usually beginning several hours after delivery. Infants have much greater difficulty than adults in tolerating withdrawal. The increased catecholamine release that accompanies opiate withdrawal causes a central nervous system irritability, with seizures and respiratory difficulties that in rare instances can be fatal to the neonate. Subacute withdrawal symptoms may resemble colic: gastrointestinal distress, sleeplessness, continuous crying, fever, and weight loss may persist in infants for weeks or months after birth (Vance et al., 1997; American Academy of Pediatrics, 1998).

Development after birth proceeds at a normal pace, and generally by six months to a year, the infant's growth has "caught up" with its peers. Developmental abnormalities not attributable to social factors such as poverty, neglect, or comorbid alcohol or cocaine abuse have not been seen in children born to opiate-addicted mothers (Vance et al., 1997).

Gastrointestinal effects. Opiate receptors found along the musculature of the gastrointestinal tract appear to play a regulatory role in gastrointestinal motility. Stimulation of these receptors leads to marked functional slowing of the gastrointestinal tract, resulting in decreased gastric emptying, prolonged transit time, and increased absorption of water by the large bowel. This frequently results in constipation that can be severe and debilitating. Tolerance to these effects does not appear to fully develop over time (Yuan et al., 2000; Quigley, 1999).

Drug-drug interactions. Many short-acting opiates are substrates of the 2D6 enzyme of the P450 enzyme system, an enzyme for which many common antidepressants and other medications are also substrates. Thus, opiates can act as competitive inhibitors of this enzyme system in the presence of other drugs. Conversely, other drugs may act as competitive inhibitors at this enzyme system with respect to the opiates. Other drugs may interact with short-acting opiates by activating or inhibiting the P450 enzyme system's biotransformational properties (Goldberg, 1996). This can lead to drug-drug interactions in the medically or psychiatrically ill addict who is taking prescribed medications, and may increase the chances of accidental overdose. This effect is sometimes exploited by "street doctors," who use empirical knowledge of these drug-drug interactions to prolong the effects of heroin by cutting it with antidepressants or other competitive inhibitors, a practice which may also have lethal consequences (Furst, 2000). Presently, researchers have little knowledge of these interactions, and few drug-drug interactions with heroin and other short-acting opiates are well understood.

Street drugs and alcohol may also interact with short-acting opiates. Large amounts of alcohol used in combination with heroin may increase morbidity and mortality by inhibiting the P450 enzyme system (Goldberg, 1996). Cocaine's known attenuating effect on heroin intoxication and withdrawal is also exploited by "street doctors," and many heroin addicts will begin using cocaine as a means of "titrating" the effects of the opiate. The increasing appearance of heroin in nightclubs has encouraged the admixture of heroin and "club drugs" including amphetamines and hallucinogens, and at least one death associated with the concurrent use of heroin and the club drug γ-hydroxybutyrate (GHB) has been reported (Ferrara et al., 1995).

Antinociception, tolerance, and withdrawal. Some medical consequences of opiate abuse and addiction are inadvertent results of expected opiate effects. The most commonly expected, and indeed anticipated, effect of opiates is antinociception stemming from the activity of the abused opiate on central opioid receptors that mediate the perception of pain. Although lack of awareness of pain is one of the prime motivators in the induction of opiate abuse and addiction, it may also lead to neglect of injury and illness, particularly those sustained early in the course of an addiction. Tolerance developing over periods of chronic opiate use can diminish the antinociceptive effect of the opiates as well as interfere with induction of anesthesia, potential problems for an ill or injured opiate addict who may require surgery for an injury that has been neglected. The development of tolerance also predisposes opiate-addicted people to overdose, as greater amounts of drug are needed to induce the same desired effect.

Physical dependence is the inevitable result of chronic self-administration of opiates. Thus, withdrawal ensues when the opiates are stopped or when opiate antagonists are given. Withdrawal from opiates is not lethal in and of itself and rarely causes seizures or other significant morbidity. However, it is remarkably uncomfortable and frequently associated with feelings of desperation and a fear of dying, which is extraordinarily aversive to the patient experiencing it and is the other prime motivator for ongoing opiate use once addiction has been established. This may be due in part to the increased release of catecholamines that accompanies opiate withdrawal, although the dysregulation of the stress hormone axis and other physiological mechanisms may also play a role (Kreek, 1996).

The Effects of Methadone on Organ Systems

Some, although not all, of the physiological functions that are dysregulated by short-acting opiates appear to return to normal when patients are treated with a long-acting opiate pharmacotherapy such as methadone.

Neuropathies

Methadone is not broken down into any known neurotoxic metabolites, nor are there reports of neuropathies attributable to methadone seen in the literature. Neurological injury or impairment does not appear to be a result of methadone treatment.

Pulmonary Effects

Although methadone induces some modest histamine release from mast cells, its effects on histamine release in lung tissue are negligible, and rapid bronchospasm or clinically significant changes in capillary permeability are not seen in successful methadone treatment. Pulmonary morbidity does not appear in methadone pharmacotherapy (Novick et al., 1997).

Skeletal-Muscle Toxicity

There are no reports of skeletal-muscle toxicity or rhabdomyolysis in successful methadone pharmacotherapy. Myoglobinuria and myoglobulinemia are not seen as a consequence of methadone treatment.

Renal Effects

Since methadone and other long-acting opiates do not appear to precipitate the immune complexes seen in heroin addiction, there is no risk for immune-complex deposition in renal tissues once heroin use has stopped. Renal illness has not been identified as a consequence of chronic methadone pharmacotherapy (Novick et al., 1997).

Teratogenicity and Fetal Development

Reports of low birth weight in some babies born to methadone-maintained mothers are confounded by the high prevalence of nicotine dependence and other drug comorbidities seen in methadone-treated populations. Although cigarette smoking is a known risk factor for decreased birth weight, methadone is not known to cause reduction of birth weight in and of itself. As mentioned above, treatment of heroin-addicted pregnant women with methadone reduces the multiple daily cycles of intoxication and withdrawal experienced by the fetus, and thus increases the chances of the fetus surviving to term. The reduction of intravenous drug use by the mother occasioned by adequate treatment with methadone further decreases the risk to the fetus of viral and bacterial infections, as well as exposure to toxic adulterants that may cross the placental barrier or obstruct blood vessels.

Babies born to methadone-treated mothers may experience methadone withdrawal within the first few days of life. Methadone withdrawal is usually modest in severity, but more protracted in neonates because of the longer half-life of the drug. Methadone lacks the potential fatality that heroin withdrawal has, since catecholamine release is much less severe in methadone withdrawal. Because of the increase in health benefits to the mother, as well as the increase in viability and health of the fetus and neonate, methadone remains the treatment of choice for heroin-addicted pregnant women (Vance et al., 1997; American Academy of Pediatrics, 1998).

Gastrointestinal Effects

As with other opiates, methadone does not appear to be hepatotoxic (Kreek et al., 1972; Novick et al., 1993). Gastrointestinal slowing persists in methadone pharmacotherapy, and chronic constipation is a significant problem for many patients treated with methadone. Tolerance to the gastrointestinal effects of methadone develops very slowly, however, with less than 20 percent of persons experiencing relief from gastrointestinal slowing and constipation after three years of moderate-to-high dose treatment (Kreek, 1973a,b). Methadone-induced constipation can be treated effectively by oral doses of naloxone or by methylated naltrexone, which are not readily absorbed into the bloodstream from the gut, and therefore reverse the gastrointestinal effects of methadone without placing an individual at risk for withdrawal (Culpepper-Morgan et al., 1992; Yuan et al., 2000).

Drug-Drug Interactions

Methadone is metabolized by different P450 enzymes than the short-acting opiates, and therefore, competitive-inhibition drug-drug-interaction profiles are somewhat different from those of the short-acting opiates (Goldberg, 1996; Kreek, 1990b). For example, while heroin may be more likely to interfere with the metabolism of tricyclic antidepressants, methadone has been found to interfere with the metabolism of selective serotonin reuptake inhibitors such as fluoxetine and fluvoxamine (Borg and Kreek, 1995). Significant drug-drug interactions between methadone and other medications include the antitubercular drug rifampin and the anticonvulsant phenytoin, both of which accelerate the biotransformation of methadone and result in lower plasma levels and mild-to-moderate withdrawal symptoms if the methadone dose is not adjusted (Kreek et al., 1976; Tong et al., 1981). Methadone may also interfere with the biotransformation of antiretroviral drugs such as retronavir or zidovudine (Borg and Kreek, 1995; Tooley et al., 1999; McCance-Katz et al., 1998), a significant issue for HIV-seropositive former heroin addicts whose addictions are being treated with methadone.

Street drugs and alcohol may also interact with methadone. Alcohol in particular may have a bimodal effect, that is, it may inhibit the metabolism of methadone when very high blood levels of alcohol are present. When people who were regular, heavy users of alcohol stop drinking, the metabolism of methadone may be accelerated due to the resultant enhancement of P450 enzymes (Kreek, 2000).

Antinociception, Tolerance, and Withdrawal

The antinociceptive effects of methadone are well documented. Through its long-acting properties, methadone can be used effectively for the management of chronic pain. Because of its slow onset time and paucity of intoxicating effects, as well as the regular monitoring of former heroin addicts in methadone treatment programs, injuries and other pain-producing ailments are not neglected in methadone-maintained former addicts, and increased morbidity from untreated physical illness does not appear to be an issue in successfully treated addicted populations (Novick et al., 1993).

Tolerance does not appear to develop in former addicts being treated with methadone, in that larger doses of methadone are not continually required to produce the same opiate blockade effect, even in patients treated with methadone for 20 or 30 years. When adequate doses of methadone are administered to former heroin addicts, drug craving and symptoms of opiate withdrawal are eliminated. Barring changes in methadone serum level due to physical illness or drug-drug interactions, no further increase of methadone dose is necessary (Kreek, 2000).

Withdrawal from long-acting opiates may be protracted, because of their long half-lives, but also involves less acute catecholamine release, and may be somewhat less uncomfortable than withdrawal from short-acting opiates for that reason. However, withdrawal from methadone requires very slow dose reduction to avoid signs and symptoms of opiate withdrawal (Kreek, 1996).

INDIRECT MEDICAL CONSEQUENCES
OF OPIATE ABUSE AND ADDICTION

As described previously, the direct effects of opiate abuse and addiction on the immune system can predispose an individual to be at higher risk for indirect medical problems associated with drug addiction. Many of these problems stem from the means of self-administration of the drug. Intravenous drug use in particular has been associated with increases in morbidity and mortality in this population. The vast majority of medical problems associated with opiate addiction stem from exposure to microorganisms or foreign matter via the use of shared or contaminated needles in nonsterile environments. The suppressed immune response associated with short-acting opiate addiction may contribute to the development of disease following exposure. Exposure to infectious agents and contaminants is of equal likelihood in improperly used opioid pharmacotherapy, i.e., if injectable methadone preparations (generally stolen from hospitals) are used illicitly or the oral methadone preparations used in clinics are solubilized and injected. It is unknown at this time whether persons injecting only long-acting opioids are at lesser risk for the development of disease than persons injecting short-acting opiates.

However, other routes of self-administration also have risks associated with them, as will be described; attempts to stave off medical consequences in the era of AIDS by avoiding needle use has unmasked other medical conditions that accompany intranasal use or inhalation of opiate smoke. In addition, methods of diluting and enhancing the effects of drugs with adulterants have become more complicated in the past decade, resulting in mini-epidemics of medical syndromes in places where noxious adulterants are used. Because these kinds of problems are seen so commonly with heroin use in particular, this section will focus specifically on the indirect medical consequences of heroin, in comparison with methadone pharmacotherapy.

It should be understood that "successful" methadone pharmacotherapy in these cases refers to the complete elimination of all illicit substances in the context of methadone treatment. In cases in which illicit drug use or other high-risk behavior persists despite methadone treatment (a possibility that is not rare: 20-30 percent of methadone-treated individuals in well-run programs using adequate doses of methadone report comorbid alcohol, cocaine, or other illicit drug use, which includes occasional heroin use), the risks of indirect medical consequences probably remain the same (Kreek et al., 1986). Patients successfully treated with methadone outlive their untreated counterparts. One study of long-term medical follow-ups of patients treated for eight or more years with methadone had difficulty finding an age-matched cohort of ongoing heroin addicts (Novick et al., 1993). The long-term methadone patients in this study showed medical problems consistent with a normal aging population with a sedentary lifestyle. Non-insulin-dependent diabetes mellitus, obesity, and hypertension were problems for these patients while debilitating infections, abscesses, renal failure, pulmonary compromise, and neurological complaints were not.

Viral Infections

Heroin and Viral Infections

Intravenous drug use in particular is associated with an increased risk of transmission of blood-borne viruses, particularly HIV, HTLV-I and HTLV-II, hepatitis B virus (HBV), and hepatitis C virus (HCV). The considerable morbidity and mortality of illnesses caused by these viral infections have been well documented and are beyond the scope of this chapter. It has been demonstrated, however, that the complications of these viral infections tend to be more severe and more lethal in affected individuals whose abuse and addiction remain untreated (Borg et al., 1999; Des Jarlais et al., 1984; Friedman et al., 1996; Modahl et al., 1997; Muga et al., 2000; Novick et al., 1986). This may be a result of nutritional deficiencies and poor self-care seen in people with active addictions, although the additional immune function impairments seen in opiate addiction may also play a role.

The prevalence of these viral infections in IV drug users is high. At their peak periods, before the effects of AIDS awareness education and needle-exchange programs took hold in 1985-1986, 55 percent of IV drug users were HIV positive, 65 percent were hepatitis B and C (HBC) positive, and as many as 98 percent were positive for HCV when blood samples were tested retrospectively (Borg et al., 1999; Kreek, 1996; Novick et al., 1988). The high-risk sexual behaviors often associated with addictions may also predispose individuals to these infections in the presence of opiate-induced T-cell immunosuppression.

Methadone and Viral Infections

The number of blood-borne viral infections in opiate addiction currently appear to be decreasing, especially in the context of methadone pharmacotherapy (Novick et al., 1993; Piccolo et al., 2000). By eliminating the use of needles and decreasing the likelihood of high-risk sexual behaviors associated with active heroin addiction, methadone pharmacotherapy is associated with much lower risks for infection with HIV-1, HBC, and HCV in seronegative individuals (Des Jarlais et al., 1984; Piccolo et al., 2000). Whether the improved immune functioning seen in methadone-treated former heroin addicts is also a protective factor against viral infection is still unknown.

Bacterial and Fungal Infections

Heroin and Bacterial and Fungal Infections

Seeding of microorganisms into the bloodstream is produced by intravenous or subcutaneous drug use, or through injuries sustained in the course of an addiction. The sources of infective microorganisms may be skin or saliva, or they may be harbored in the drug itself. Repeated bouts of bacteriemia or fungemia due to multiple daily intravenous self-administrations of the drug may lead to systemic infections and debilitating complications. The classic example of this is infective endocarditis caused most often by seeding of skin and oral flora directly into blood vessels by unsterilized needles, which can have a rate of serious cardiovascular complications as high as 70 percent (Mathew et al., 1995). Poor dentition, reduced brachiotracheal clearance, and high-risk sexual behavior may also account for sources of infection (Scheidegger and Zimmerli, 1989).

More unusual varieties of infection, of the kind seen in immunocompromised patients and held to be opportunistic in nature, are also seen in HIV-seronegative opiate addicts. Systemic fungal infections, for example, can be seen in intravenous heroin abusers. Systemic candidiasis due to infection with *Candida albicans* in the absence of HIV seropositivity has been linked specifically with intravenous heroin abuse, as opposed to intravenous drug use in general (LaFont et al., 1994). More recently, outbreaks of systemic infections with a newly emerging fungal pathogen, *Scedosporium prolificans,* have been reported in heroin addicts in California, the United Kingdom, Australia, and Spain (Berenguer et al., 1997). Tuberculosis is endemic among opiate addicts in some areas, particularly among untreated homeless heroin addicts. Opiates may also interfere with the metabolism of antitubercular medications (Borg and Kreek, 1995; Friedman et al., 1996).

Relatively unusual presentations of bacterial infections also may be seen in opiate addicts. Group B streptococcal infections, generally quite rare in adult populations, are more common among intravenous opiate abusers (Garcia-Lechuz et al., 1999). Group B streptococcal infections and more common staphylococcal infections may present as osteomyelitis in the absence of any history of injury, or as septic arthritis, most notably in the knee and hip (Goldenberg, 1998; Lossos et al., 1998). Abscesses caused by any number of organisms have been reported in every organ in the bodies of intravenous heroin users, including the brain, liver, skin, and lungs (Novick et al., 1997; Cherubin and Sapira, 1993).

Subcutaneous opiate use provides an anaerobic environment for other bacteria, notably *Clostridium tetani* and *Clostridium botulinum,* to propagate. The prevalence of tetanus and botulism occurring in heroin addicts currently appears to be increasing (Shapiro et al., 1998; Talan and Moran, 1998). Street preparations of heroin can harbor *Clostridium* spores, which are not killed by the boiling process used to prepare the drug for injection. Injection of contaminated heroin into subcutaneous spaces provides an environment for spores to hatch and reproduce, resulting in systemic illness or death due to the toxins secreted. The fatality rate of tetanus in this population in one study was 25 percent (Sun et al., 1994). Preventative vaccination, at least to tetanus, may not be protective in this population. Cases of fatal tetanus in opiate-addicted patients with therapeutic antitetanus titer levels have been documented (Abrahamian et al., 2000).

Methadone and Bacterial and Fungal Infections

Again, the elimination of needle use in successful methadone pharmacotherapy markedly reduces the risk of exposure to bacterial and fungal pathogens. It is unknown whether the improved immune status of methadone-treated former heroin addicts provides additional protection against pathogens introduced by routes other than needle use. However, the unusual and opportunistic infections seen in heroin addiction are not reported in methadone-maintained populations (Novick et al., 1986; Kreek, 2000).

Systemic Toxic/Metabolic Syndromes

Heroin and Systemic Toxic/Metabolic Syndromes

The presence of adulterants and contaminants in the needles used for intravenous administration or in the drug itself, may lead to contaminant-specific toxic or metabolic syndromes. Many of these are poisonings due to deliberate adulteration of the street preparation with other drugs such as scopolamine. Street drugs are often cut with others to produce a specific drug-drug interaction and effect (Furst, 2000). Accidental poisonings due to contamination of needles with heavy metals such as lead or mercury have also been reported (Antonini et al., 1989; Haffner et al., 1991).

Talcosis is a systemic syndrome frequently reported in individuals who have injected opiates containing talc, particularly when oral preparations of opiates are ground and injected intravenously. The talc or other inert material used to bind opiate pills is disseminated widely by intravenous injection and lodges in capillary beds where granulomas form around talc deposits. Pulmonary capillary beds are particularly vulnerable to talc deposition and granuloma formation, and respiratory compromise or failure may result (Pare et al., 1989; Ben-Haim et al., 1988).

Repeated injection of inert materials as well as multiple bouts of bacteremia has been associated with the deposition of amyloid in tissues, leading to a systemic amyloidosis that is symptomatic depending on the size and locations of the amyloid deposits. Although the mechanism for this is unknown, a predisposing genetic factor appears to be required (Neugarten et al., 1986).

Methadone and Toxic/Metabolic Syndromes

The elimination of needle use and use of street drugs containing adulterants eliminates the risk for toxic and metabolic syndromes in persons successfully treated with methadone pharmacotherapy. Toxic/metabolic syndromes are not reported as a consequence of successful methadone treatment (Novick et al., 1993).

Neurological Sequelae

Neurological Sequelae of Heroin

Apart from the peripheral neuropathies and plexopathies seen in heroin addiction that may be due to a combination of alcohol or other drug comorbidities and/or nutritional deficiencies, indirect neurological complications of opiate addiction seem relatively rare. Seizures are rarely reported in the context of heroin use and, when present, have most often been attributed to other underlying causes. Cerebrovascular accidents are more commonly reported in heroin addicts and have been attributed to intracerebral vasculitis induced by opiate use or infarcts caused by infective emboli in patients with endocarditis stemming from intravenous drug use (Sloan et al., 1998; Brust, 1998; Niehaus and Meyer, 1998; Calabrese et al., 1997; Adams et al., 1995).

More recently, reports of a progressive leukoencephalopathy have been seen in individuals who inhale the heated vapor of heroin, a practice known as "huffing" or "chasing the dragon," and which appears to be on the rise in an attempt by opiate abusers to avoid the risks of needle use. The leukoencephalopathy consists of a vacuolization of white matter, which can be generalized throughout the central nervous system, although some reports suggest lesions are more likely to be seen in regions of poor blood perfusion, particularly the basal ganglia and cerebellum. The mechanism of the leukoencephalopathy is not known. The fact that it is most often seen in mini-epidemics suggests that a particular unidentified contaminant may be to blame, although reports that only a certain few individuals using a particular supply of heroin have been affected suggest that an underlying genetic predisposition may also be necessary to developing the syndrome. Speculation that a toxic metabolite of heroin produced by heat vaporization may be a causative factor seems to have been invalidated by a report of an identical progressive leukoencephalopathy in an addict who was using heroin intranasally. Initially seen as pockets of miniepidemics in Europe over the past decade, cases have recently been reported in the United States (Hill et al., 2000; Rizzuto et al., 1997; Kreigstien et al., 1998; Celius and Andersson, 1996).

Neurological Sequelae of Methadone

The elimination of intravenous or inhalation routes of administration of street drugs, as well as the elimination of exposure to toxic adulterants by successful treatment with orally administered methadone, appears to eliminate the risks of neurological complications. Neurological sequelae are not associated with successful methadone treatment (Novick et al., 1993; Brust, 1998).

Cardiovascular Sequelae

Cardiovascular Sequelae of Heroin

Postmortem studies of heroin addicts have revealed very little gross cardiac pathology (Kringsholm and Christoffersen, 1987). However, one study of asymptomatic intravenous heroin users showed changes in mitral and tricuspid heart valve function that were detectable by echocardiograph. It was speculated that contaminants found in heroin caused microscopic damage to heart valves that is cumulative over time, and may form toeholds for the bacteria that result in endocarditis (Pons-Llado et al., 1992). A combination of microscopic cardiovascular damage from adulterants, fungemia, and immune suppression may also contribute to the mycotic aneurysms that are sometimes seen in intravenous heroin addicts (Tsao et al., 1999; Spirito et al., 1999).

Cardiovascular Sequelae of Methadone

Cardiovascular tone may actually be improved with methadone pharmacotherapy, both because the catecholamine release accompanying multiple daily withdrawals is avoided, and because opiates when at steady-state appear to have a protective or preconditioning effect on cardiac function (Barron, 2000; Liang and Gross, 1999).

Renal Sequelae

Renal Sequelae of Heroin

Along with the direct opiate-induced interstitial injuries seen in renal tissue, and the potential for renal failure as a consequence of opiate-induced rhabdomyolysis, some of the adulterants contained in street opiates have been implicated in mechanisms of renal damage, particularly when injected intravenously. Much of this appears in the form of insoluble diluents that are deposited in the capillary beds of glomeruli, resulting in progressive glomerulonephropathy and consequent nephrotic syndrome. Tissue pathology has varied and tends to occur in miniepidemics seen in specific localizations, suggesting again that locally introduced adulterants are the culprits (Crowe et al., 2000; Peces et al., 1998; Lynn et al., 1998). Other immune-related kidney damage, including reports of mixed cryoglobulinemia and hemolytic uremic syndrome, necrotizing angiitis, and chronic interstitial nephritis have been speculated to be caused by adulterants found in injectable opiates, although the action of opiates themselves on immune cells cannot be ruled out as a causative factor (Ramos et al., 1994; Peces et al., 1998; Crowe et al., 2000).

Renal Sequelae of Methadone

The elimination of needle use and use of street drugs containing adulterants eliminates the risk for renal damage in persons successfully treated with methadone pharmacotherapy. Renal syndromes are not reported as a consequence of successful methadone treatment (Novick et al., 1993).

Dermatological Sequelae

Dermatological Sequelae of Heroin

The dermatological manifestations of heroin addiction are related to intravenous and subcutaneous heroin use. Bacterial infections and abscesses in the skin are a common finding in opiate addicts using needles in unhygienic conditions. Stigmata of chronic opiate use include multiple round scars resulting from abscesses caused by subcutaneous injection, as well as "track marks," scars resulting from repeated IV needle injury along the paths of veins. These marks are often darkened by a tattooing effect produced by the introduction of carbonized contaminants into the skin during injection (Novick et al., 1997).

Dermatological Sequelae of Methadone

Methadone pharmacotherapy is administered orally, and thus no dermatological symptoms have been associated with methadone in the therapeutic setting.

SUMMARY

Since many of the medical problems seen as a result of opiate abuse and addiction are common with other drugs of abuse, and are clearly related to the mechanisms of administration of the drugs and psychosocial complications, it has been largely assumed that the opiates themselves were reasonably medically benign. More recent studies, however, have continued to support our findings that short-acting opiates such as heroin may directly alter normal physiological function (and also, as seen in animal models, molecular, neurobiological, and cellular functions) that not only lead to problems in and of themselves, but also may predispose an individual to some of the secondary effects of drug addiction. The most striking findings have been studies suggesting that short-acting opiates actively alter the immune response and neuroendocrine functioning, rendering opiate addicts more susceptible to infection, hypersensitivity-like responses, and organ damage from the deposition of immune complexes. In addition, microscopic damage to tissues caused by adulterants or inert substances in the drugs are less likely to be repaired with an altered immune response, especially when multiple daily self-administrations of the drug cause repeated injuries to the tissues.

Recent attempts by opiate addicts to avoid the medical problems associated with needle use, likely as a result of HIV-awareness education, have led to a recent increase in reports of medical complications associated with other routes of opiate self-administration, particularly smoking. Reports of heroin-associated pulmonary edema, interstitial pneumonitis, and progressive leukoencephalopathy appear to be on the rise as a result of the increasing popularity of smoking and intranasal use of heroin as substitutes for intravenous and subcutaneous needle use.

Whatever the route of administration, the harmful effects of short-acting opiates continue to be associated with their pharmacokinetics. The "on-off" pattern of multiple daily intoxications and withdrawals seem to place opiate addicts at greater risk for medical complications. The ameliorating effects of steady-state pharmacokinetics of the long-term opiate pharmacotherapies such as methadone are associated with the prolongation of life and the diminution of morbidity. Methadone thus continues to be the treatment of choice for chronic opiate addiction.

REFERENCES

Abrahamian, F.M.; Pollack, C.V.; LoVecchio, F.; Nanda, R.; Carlson, R.W. (2000). Fatal tetanus in a drug abuser with "protective" antitetanus antibodies. *The Journal of Emergency Medicine,* 18(2):189-193.

Adams, H.P.; Kappelle, L.J.; Biller, J.; Gordon, D.L.; Love, B.B.; Gomez, F.; Heffner, M. (1995). Ischemic stroke in young adults. *Archives of Neurology,* 52:491-495.

American Academy of Pediatrics Committee on Drugs (1998). Neonatal drug withdrawal. *Pediatrics,* 101(6):1079-1088.

Annane, D.; Teboul, J.L.; Richard, C.; Auzepy, P. (1990). Severe rhabdomyolysis related to heroin sniffing [letter]. *Intensive Care Medicine,* 16(6):410.

Antonini, G.; Palmieri, G.; Spagnoli, L.G.; Millefiorini, M. (1989). Lead brachial neuropathy in heroin addiction. A case report. *Clinical Neurology and Neurosurgery,* 91(2):167-170.

Archie, C. (1998). Methadone in the management of narcotic addiction in pregnancy. *Current Opinion in Obstetrics and Gynecology,* 10:435-440.

Barron, B.A. (2000). Cardiac opioids. *Proceedings of the Society for Experimental Biology and Medicine,* 224:1-7.

Ben-Haim, S.A.; Ben-Ami, H.; Edoute, Y.; Goldstien, N.; Barzilai, D. (1988). Talcosis presenting as pulmonary infiltrates in an HIV-positive heroin addict. *Chest,* 94(3):656-658.

Benson, M.K.; Bentley, A.M. (1995). Lung disease induced by drug addiction. *Thorax,* 50:1125-1127.

Berenguer, J.; Rodriguez-Tudela, J.L.; Richard, C.; Alvarez, M.; Sanz, M.A.; Gaztelurrutia, L.; Ayats, J.; Martinez-Suarez, J.V.; the *Scedosporium prolificans* Spanish Study Group (1997). Deep infections caused by *Scedosporium prolificans. Medicine,* 76:256-265.

Berger, A.R.; Schaumburg, H.H.; Gourevitch, M.N.; Freeman, K.; Herskovitz, S.; Arezzo, J.C. (1999). Prevalence of peripheral neuropathy in injection drug users. *Neurology,* 53:592-597.

Borg, L.; Khuri, E.; Wells, A.; Melia, D.; Bergasa, N.; Ho, A.; Kreek, M.J. (1999). Methadone-maintained former heroin addicts, including those who are anti-HIV-1 seropositive, comply with and respond to hepatitis B vaccination. *Addiction,* 94(4):489-493.

Borg, L.; Kreek, M.J. (1995). Clinical problems associated with interactions between methadone pharmacotherapy and medications used in the treatment of HIV-1-positive and AIDS patients. *Current Opinion in Psychiatry,* 8:199-202.

Brander, P.E.; Tukiainen, P. (1993). Acute eosinophilic pneumonia in a heroin smoker. *European Respiratory Journal,* 6:750-752.

Brust, J.C.M. (1998). Acute neurologic complications of drug and alcohol abuse. *Neurologic Clinics of North America,* 16(2):503-519.

Calabrese, L.H.; Duna, G.F.; Lie, J.T. (1997). Vasculitis in the central nervous system. *Arthritis and Rheumatism,* 40(7):1189-1201.

Carr, D.J.J.; Rogers, T.J.; Weber, R.J. (1996). The relevance of opioids and opioid receptors on immunocompetence and immune homeostasis. *Proceedings of the Society for Experimental Biology and Medicine,* 213:248-257.

Celius, E.G.; Andersson, S. (1996). Leucoencephalopathy after inhalation of heroin: a case report. *Journal of Neurology, Neurosurgery, and Psychiatry,* 60(6): 694-695.

Cherubin, C.E.; Sapira, J.D. (1993). The medical complications of drug addiction and the medical assessment of the intravenous drug user: 25 years later. *Annals of Internal Medicine,* 119(10):1017-1028.

Coffey, R.M.; Mark, T.; King, E.; Harwood, H.; McKusiack, D.; Genuardi, J.; Dilonardo, J.; Chalk, M. (2001). *National Estimates of Expenditures for Substance Abuse Treatment,* 1997. Rockville, MD: U.S. Department of Health and Human Services, Substance Abuse and Mental Health Services Administration (SAMHSA).

Crowe, A.V.; Howse, M.; Bell, G.M.; Henry, J.A. (2000). Substance abuse and the kidney. *Quarterly Journal of Medicine,* 93:147-152.

Cruz, R.; Davis, M.; O'Neil, H.; Tamarin, F.; Brandstetter, R.D.; Karetzky, M. (1998). Pulmonary manifestations of inhaled street drugs. *Heart and Lung,* 27(5):297-305.

Culpepper-Morgan, J.A.; Inturrisi, C.E.; Portenoy, R.K.; Foley, K.; Houde, R.W.; Marsh, F.; Kreek, M.J. (1992). Treatment of opioid-induced constipation with oral naloxone: A pilot study. *Clinical Pharmacology and Therapeutics,* 52(1):90-95.

Culpepper-Morgan, J.A.; Kreek, M.J. (1997). Hypothalamic-pituitary-adrenal axis hypersensitivity to naloxone in opioid dependence: A case of naloxone-induced withdrawal. *Metabolism,* 46(2):130-134.

Cushman, P.; Kreek, M.J. (1974a). Methadone-maintained patients: Effect of methadone on plasma testosterone, FSH, LH, and prolactin. *New York State Journal of Medicine,* 74(11):1970-1973.

Cushman, P.; Kreek, M.J. (1974b). Some endocrinologic observations in narcotic addicts. In: Zimmerman, E.; George, R. (eds.), *Narcotics and the Hypothalamus,* New York: Raven Press, pp. 161-173.

Cygan, J.; Trunsky, M.; Corbridge, T. (2000). Inhaled heroin-induced status asthmaticus: Five cases and a review of the literature. *Chest,* 117(1):272-275.

Deighan, C.J.; Wong, K.M.; McLaughlin, K.J.; Harden, P. (2000). Rhabdomyolysis and acute renal failure resulting from alcohol and drug abuse. *Quarterly Journal of Medicine,* 93:29-33.

Delanty, N.; Vaughan, C.J.; French, J.A. (1998). Medical causes of seizures. *The Lancet,* 352:383-390.

Des Jarlais, D.C.; Marmor, M.; Cohen, H.; Yancovitz, S.; Garber, J; Friedman, S.; Kreek, M.J.; Miescher, A.; Khuri, E.; Friedman, S.M.; et al. (1984). Antibodies to a retrovirus etiologically associated with acquired immunodeficiency syndrome (AIDS) in populations with increased incidences of the syndrome. *Morbidity and Mortality Weekly Report,* 33:377-379.

Dettmeyer, R.; Wessling, B.; Madea, B. (1998). Heroin associated nephropathy—A post-mortem study. *Forensic Science International,* 95(2):109-116.

Dole, V.P.; Nyswander, M.E.; Kreek, M.J. (1966). Narcotic blockade. *Archives of Internal Medicine,* 118(4):304-309.

Edston, E.; van Hage-Hamsten, M. (1997). Anaphylactoid shock—A common cause of death in heroin addicts? *Allergy,* 52(9):950-954.

Evans, P.A.; Millington, H.T. (1993). Atraumatic brachial plexopathy following intravenous heroin use. *Archives of Emergency Medicine,* 10(3):209-211.

Ferrara, S.D.; Tedeschi, L.; Frison, G.; Rossi, A (1995). Fatality due to gamma-hydroxybutyric acid (GHB) and heroin intoxication. *Journal of Forensic Sciences,* 40(3):501-504.

Finfer, S. (1996). Fatal methadone overdose. Close observation in intensive care unit is required when naloxone infusion ends. *BMJ,* 313(7070):1480.

Fletcher, M.A.; Klimas, N.G.; Morgan, R.O. (1993). Immune function and drug treatment in anti-retrovirus negative intravenous drug users. *Advances in Experimental Medicine and Biology,* 335:241-246.

Friedman, L.N.; Williams, M.T.; Singh, T.P.; Frieden, T.R. (1996). Tuberculosis, AIDS, and death among substance abusers on welfare in New York City. *The New England Journal of Medicine,* 334:828-833.

Furst, R.T. (2000). The re-engineering of heroin: An emerging heroin "cutting" trend in New York City. *Addiction Research,* 8(4):357-379.

Garcia-Lechuz, J.M.; Bachiller, P.; Vasallo, F.J.; Munoz, P.; Padilla, B.; Bouza, E. (1999). Group B streptococcal osteomyelitis in adults. *Medicine,* 78:191-199.

Glavina-Durdov, M.; Definis-Gojanovic, M. (1999). Thymus alterations related to intravenous drug abuse. *The American Journal of Forensic Medicine and Pathology,* 20(2):150-153.

Goldberg, R.J. (1996). The P-450 system. *Archives of Family Medicine,* 5:406-412.

Goldenberg, D.L. (1998). Septic arthritis. *The Lancet,* 351:197-202.

Govitrapong, R.; Suttitum, T.; Kotchabhakdi, N.; Uneklabh, T. (1998). Alterations of immune functions in heroin addicts and heroin withdrawal subjects. *The Journal of Pharmacology and Experimental Therapeutics,* 286(2):883-889.

Gunne, L.M.; Gronbladh, L. (1981). The Swedish methadone program: A controlled study. *Drug and Alcohol Dependence,* 7(3):249-256.

Haffner, H.T.; Erdelkamp, J.; Goller, E.; Schweinsberg, F.; Scmidt, V. (1991). Morphological and toxicological findings after intravenous injection of metallic mercury. *Deutsche Medizinische Wochenshrift,* 116(36):1342-1346.

Hartman, N.; Kreek, M.J. (1983). Narcotic poisoning. *Current Therapy,* 896-898.

Haskell, L.P.; Glicklich, D.; Senitzer, D. (1988). HLA associations in heroin-associated nephropathy. *American Journal of Kidney Diseases,* 12(1):45-50.

Hill, M.D.; Cooper, P.W.; Perry, J.R. (2000). Chasing the dragon—Neurological toxicity associated with inhalation of heroin vapour: case report. *CMAJ*, 162(2): 236-238.

Hillstrom, R.P.; Cohn, A.M.; McCarroll, K.A. (1990). Vocal cord paralysis resulting from neck injections in the intravenous drug use population. *Laryngoscope*, 100:503-506.

Howard, J.D.; Reay, D.T. (1998). Positional asphyxia [letter]. *Annals of Emergency Medicine*, 32(1):116-117.

Hwang, S.W.; Lebow, J.M.; Bierer, M.F.; O'Connell, J.J.; Orav, E.J.; Brennan, T.A. (1998). Risk factors for death in homeless adults in Boston. *Archives of Internal Medicine*, 158:1454-1460.

Inturrisi, C.E.; Max, M.B.; Foley, K.M.; Schultz, M.; Shin, S.U.; Houde, R.W. (1984). The pharmacokinetics of heroin in patients with chronic pain. *New England Journal of Medicine*, 310(19):1213-1217.

Kaplan, J.L.; Marx, J.A.; Calabro, J.J.; Gin-Shaw, S.L.; Spiller, J.D.; Spivey, W.L.; Gaddis, G.M.; Zhao, N.; Harchelroad, F.P. (1999). Double-blind, randomized study of nalmefene and naloxone in emergency department patients with suspected narcotic overdose. *Annals of Emergency Medicine*, 34(1):42-50.

Karch, S.B. (1998). Diphenhydramine toxicity: Comparisons of postmortem findings in diphenhydramine-, cocaine-, and heroin-related deaths. *The American Journal of Forensic Medicine and Pathology*, 19(2):143-147.

Karch, S.B.; Stephens, B.G. (1999). Drug abusers who die during arrest or in custody. *Journal of the Royal Society of Medicine*, 92:110-113.

Karch, S.B.; Stephens, B.G. (2000). Toxicology and pathology of deaths related to methadone: Retrospective review. *Western Journal of Medicine*, 172:11-14.

Karne, S.; D'Ambrosio, C.; Einarsson, O.; O'Connor, P.G. (1999). Hypersensitivity pneumonitis induced by intranasal heroin use. *The American Journal of Medicine*, 107:392-395.

Kenner, C.; D'Apolito, K. (1997). Outcomes for children exposed to drugs in utero. *JOGNN*, 26:595-603.

Klockgether, T.; Weller, M.; Haarmeier, T.; Kaskas, B.; Maier, G.; Dichgans, J. (1997). Gluteal compartment syndrome due to rhabdomyolysis after heroin abuse. *Neurology*, 48:275-276.

Kreek, M.J. (1973a). Medical safety and side effects of methadone in tolerant individuals. *The Journal of the American Medical Association*, 223(6):665-668.

Kreek, M.J. (1973b). Physiological implications of methadone treatment. Appendix D, *Methadone Treatment Manual*, U. S. Department of Justice, USGPO #2700-00227, 85-91.

Kreek, M.J. (1973c). Plasma and urine levels of methadone: Comparison following four medication forms used in chronic maintenance treatment. *New York State Journal of Medicine*, 73(23):2773-2777.

Kreek, M.J. (1987). Multiple drug abuse patterns and medical consequences. In: Meltzer, H.Y. (ed.), *Psychopharmacology: The Third Generation of Progress* (pp. 1597-1604). New York: Raven Press.

Kreek, M.J. (1990a). Immune functions in heroin addicts and former heroin addicts in treatment: Pre- and post-AIDS epidemic. *NIDA Research Monograph,* 96: 192-219.

Kreek, M.J. (1990b). Immunological function in active heroin addicts and methadone-maintained former addicts: Observations and possible mechanisms. *NIDA Research Monograph,* 105:75-80.

Kreek, M.J. (1996). Opiates, opioids, and addiction. *Molecular Psychiatry,* 1:232-254.

Kreek, M.J. (2000). Methadone-related opioid agonist pharmacotherapy for heroin addiction: History, recent molecular and neurochemical research and future in mainstream medicine. *Annals of the New York Academy of Sciences,* 909:186-216.

Kreek, M.J.; Dodes, L.; Kane, S.; Knobler, J.; Martin, R. (1972). Long-term methadone maintenance therapy: Effects on liver function. *Annals of Internal Medicine,* 77(4):598-602.

Kreek, M.J.; Garfield, J.W.; Gutjahr, C.L.; Giusti, L.M. (1976). Rifampin-induced methadone withdrawal. *New England Journal of Medicine,* 294:1104-1106.

Kreek, M.J.; Khuri, E.; Fahey, L.; Miescher, A.; Arns, P.; Spagnoli, D.; Craig, J.; Millman, R.; Harte, E.H. (1986). Long-term followup studies of the medical status of adolescent former heroin addicts in chronic methadone maintenance treatment: Liver disease and immune status. *NIDA Research Monograph,* 67:307-309.

Kreek, M.J.; Khuri, E.; Flomenberg, N.; Albeck, H.; Ochshorn, M. (1990). Immune status of unselected methadone maintained former heroin addicts. *Progress in Clinical and Biological Research,* 328:445-448.

Kreigstein, A.R.; Armitage, B.A.; Millar, W.S.; Shungu, D.C.; Brust, J.C.M.; Goldman, J.E.; Lynch, T. (1998). Toxic heroin-induced spongiform leukoencephalopathy in two American patients [abstract]. *Neurology,* 50:A81-A82.

Kringsholm, B.; Christoffersen, P. (1987). Lung and heart pathology in fatal drug addiction: A consecutive autopsy study. *Forensic Science International,* 34: 39-51.

Kumar, R.; West, D.M.; Jingree, M.; Laurence, A.S. (1999). Unusual consequences of heroin overdose: Rhabdomyolysis, acute renal failure, paraplegia, and hypercalcaemia. *British Journal of Anaesthesia,* 83:496-498.

Lafont, A.; Olive, A.; Gelman, M.; Roca-Burniols, J.; Cots, R.; Carbonell, J. (1994). *Candida albicans* spondylocystitis and vertebral osteomyelitis in patients with intravenous heroin drug addiction: Report of 3 new cases. *Journal of Rheumatology,* 21:953-956.

Lazzarin, A.; Mella, L.; Trombini, M.; Uberti-Foppa, C.; Franzetti, F.; Mazzoni, G.; Galli, M. (1984). Immunological status in heroin addicts: Effects of methadone maintenance treatment. *Drug and Alcohol Dependence,* 13(2):117-123.

Levenson, T.; Greenberger, P.A.; Donoghue, E.R.; Lifschultz, B.D. (1996). Asthma deaths confounded by substance abuse: An assessment of fatal asthma. *Chest,* 110:604-610.

Liang, B.T.; Gross, G.J. (1999). Direct preconditioning of cardiac myocytes via opioid receptors and K_{ATP} channels. *Circulation Research,* 84:1396-1400.

Lossos, I.S.; Yossepowitch, O.; Kandel, L.; Yardeni, D.; Arber, N. (1998). Septic arthritis of the glenohumeral joint. *Medicine,* 77:177-187.

Lynn, K.L.; Pickering, W.; Gardner, J.; Bailey, R.R.; Robson, R.A. (1998). Intravenous drug use and glomerular deposition of lipid-like material. *Nephron,* 80: 274-276.

Mathew, J.; Addai, T.; Anand, A.; Morrobel, A.; Maheshwari, P.; Freels, S. (1995). Clinical features, site of involvement, bacteriologic findings, and outcome of infective endocarditis in intravenous drug users. *Archives of Internal Medicine,* 155:1641-1648.

McCance-Katz, E.F.; Rainey, P.M.; Jatlow, P.; Friedland, G. (1998). Methadone effects on zidovudine disposition (AIDS Clinical Trials Group 262). *Journal of Acquired Immune Deficiency Syndromes and Human Retrovirology,* 18(5):435-443.

Melman, A.; Gingell, J.C. (1999). The epidemiology and pathophysiology of erectile dysfunction. *The Journal of Urology,* 161:5-11.

Mendelson, J.H.; Mello, N.K. (1978). Plasma testosterone levels during chronic heroin use and protracted abstinence: A study of Hong Kong addicts. *NIDA Research Monograph,* (19):142-148.

Miller, A.; Taub, H.; Spinak, A.; Pilipski, M.; Brown, L.K. (1991). Lung function in former intravenous drug abusers: The effect of ubiquitous cigarette smoking. *The American Journal of Medicine,* 90:678-684.

Modahl, L.E.; Young, K.C.; Varney, K.F.; Khayam-Bashi, H.; Murphy, E.L. (1997). Are HTLV-II—Seropositive injection drug users at increased risk of bacterial pneumonia, abscesses, and lymphadenopathy? *Journal of Acquired Immune Deficiency Syndromes and Human Retrovirology,* 16:169-175.

Muga, R.; Roca, J.; Egea, J.M.; Tor, J.; Sirera, G.; Rey-Joly, C.; Munoz, A. (2000). Mortality of HIV-positive and HIV-negative heroin abusers as a function of duration of injecting drug use. *JAIDS Journal of Acquired Immune Deficiency Syndromes,* 23:332-338.

Neugarten, J.; Gallo, G.R.; Buxbaum, J.; Katz, L.A.; Rubenstein, J.; Baldwin, D.S. (1986). Amyloidosis in subcutaneous heroin abusers ("skin poppers' amyloidosis"). *The American Journal of Medicine,* 81:635-640.

Niehaus, L.; Meyer, B.U. (1998). Bilateral borderzone brain infarctions in association with heroin abuse. *Journal of the Neurological Sciences,* 160:180-182.

Novick, D.M.; Farci, P.; Croxson, T.S.; Taylor, M.B.; Schneebaum, C.W.; Lai, M.E.; Bach, N.; Senie, R.T.; Gelb, A.M.; Kreek, M.J. (1988). Hepatitis D virus and human immunodeficiency virus antibodies in parenteral drug abusers who are hepatitis B surface antigen positive. *The Journal of Infectious Diseases,* 158(4):795-803.

Novick, D.M.; Haverkos, H.W.; Teller, D.W. (1997). The medically ill substance abuser. In: Lowinson, J.H.; Ruiz, P; Millman, R.B.; Langrod. J.G. (eds.), *Substance Abuse: A Comprehensive Textbook,* Third Edition (pp. 534-550). Baltimore: Williams and Wilkins.

Novick, D.M.; Khan, I.; Kreek, M.J. (1986). Acquired immunodeficiency syndrome and infection with hepatitis viruses in individuals abusing drugs by injection. *Bulletin on Narcotics,* 38(1/2):15-25.

Novick, D.M.; Kreek, M.J. (1992). Methadone and immune function [letter]. *The American Journal of Medicine,* 92:113-114.

Novick, D.M.; Ochshorn, M.; Ghali, V.; Croxson, T.S.; Mercer, W.D.; Chiorazzi, N.; Kreek, M.J. (1989). Natural killer cell activity and lymphocyte subsets in parenteral heroin abusers and long-term methadone maintenance patients. *The Journal of Pharmacology and Experimental Therapeutics,* 250(2):606-610.

Novick, D.M.; Richman, B.L.; Friedman, J.M.; Friedman, J.E.; Fried, C.; Wilson, J.P.; Townley, A.; Kreek, M.J. (1993). The medical status of methadone maintenance patients in treatment for 11-18 years. *Drug and Alcohol Dependence,* 33:235-245.

O'Donnell, A.E.; Selig, J.; Aravamuthan, M.; Richardson, M.S.A. (1995). Pulmonary complications associated with illicit drug use: An update. *Chest,* 108:460-463.

Otero, A.; Esteban, J.; Martinez, L.; Cejudo, C. (1992). Rhabdomyolysis and acute renal failure as a consequence of heroin inhalation. *Nephron,* 62:245.

Pare, J.P.; Cote, G.; Fraser, R.S. (1989). Long-term follow-up of drug abusers with intravenous talcosis. *American Review of Respiratory Diseases,* 139:233-241.

Peces, R.; Diaz-Corte, C.; Baltar, J.; Seco, M.; Alvarez-Grande, J. (1998). Haemolytic-uraemic syndrome in a heroin addict. *Nephrology Dialysis Transplantation,* 13:3197-3199.

Pena, J.; Aranda, C.; Luque, E.; Vaamonde, R. (1990). Heroin-induced myopathy in rat skeletal muscle. *Acta Neuropathologica,* 80(1):72-76.

Pena, J.; Luque, E.; Aranda, C.; Jimena, I.; Vaamonde, R. (1993). Experimental heroin-induced myopathy: Ultrastructural observations. *Journal of Submicroscopic Cytology and Pathology,* 25(2):279-284.

Perret, G.; Deglon, J.J.; Kreek, M.J.; Ho, A.; LaHarpe, R. (2000). Lethal methadone intoxications in Geneva, Switzerland from 1994-1998. *Addiction,* 95(11):1647-1653.

Perrone, J.; Shaw, L.; De Roos, F. (1999). Laboratory confirmation of scopolamine co-intoxication in patients using tainted heroin. *Clinical Toxicology,* 37(4):491-496.

Piccolo, P.; Borg, L.; Lin, A.; Khuri, E.T.; Wells, A.; Melia, D.; Kreek, M.J. (2000). Prevalence of hepatitis C and HIV-1 in former opioid addicts in methadone maintenance treatment [abstract]. *Problems of Drug Dependence, 2000: Proceedings of the 62nd Annual Scientific Meeting for the College on Problems on Drug Dependence.* National Institute of Drug Abuse Research Monograph Series. Washington, DC: U. S. Government Printing Office.

Pons-Llado, G.; Carreras, F.; Borras, X.; Cadafalch, J.; Fuster, M.; Guardia, J.; Casas, M. (1992). Findings on Doppler echocardiography in asymptomatic intravenous heroin users. *The American Journal of Cardiology,* 69:238-241.

Pope-Harman, A.L.; Davis, W.B.; Allen, E.D.; Christofordis, A.J.; Allen, J.N. (1996). Acute eosinophilic pneumonia: A summary of 15 cases and review of the literature. *Medicine,* 75(6):334-342.

Quigley, E.M.M. (1999). Gastroduodenal motility. *Current Opinion in Gastroenterology,* 15:481-491.

Rabl, W.; Markwalder, C. (1996). Fatal posture- and heroin-related intestinal infarction and leg muscle necrosis after snorting heroin—A case report. *American Journal of Forensic Medicine and Pathology,* 17(2):163-166.

Ramos, A.; Vinhas, J.; Carvalho, M.F. (1994). Mixed cryoglobulinemia in a heroin addict. *American Journal of Kidney Diseases,* 23(5):731-734.

Remskar, M.; Noc, M.; Leskovsek, B.; Horvat, M. (1998). Profound circulatory shock following heroin overdose. *Resuscitation,* 38(1):51-53.

Richards, J.R. (2000). Rhabdomyolysis and drugs of abuse. *The Journal of Emergency Medicine,* 19(1):51-56.

Rizzuto, N.; Morbin, M.; Ferrari, S.; Cavallaro, T.; Sparaco, M.; Boso, G.; Gaetti, L. (1997). Delayed spongiform leukoencephalopathy after heroin abuse. *Acta Neuropathologica,* 94:87-90.

Sanders, M.M.; Marshall, A.P. (1989). Acute and chronic toxic nephropathies. *Annals of Clinical and Laboratory Science,* 19(3):216-220.

Santen, F.J.; Sofsky, J.; Bilic, N.; Lippert, R. (1975). Mechanisms of action of narcotics in the production of menstrual dysfunction in women. *Fertility and Sterility,* 26(6):538-548.

Savige, J.A.; Dowling, J.; Kincaid-Smith, P. (1989). Superimposed glomerular immune complexes in anti-glomerular basement membrane disease. *American Journal of Kidney Diseases,* 14(2):145-153.

Scheidegger, C.; Zimmerli, W. (1989). Infectious complications in drug addicts: Seven-year review of 269 hospitalized narcotics abusers in Switzerland. *Reviews of Infectious Diseases,* 11(3):486-493.

Shapiro, R.L.; Hatheway, C.; Swerdlow, D.L. (1998). Botulism in the United States: A clinical and epidemiological review. *Annals of Internal Medicine,* 129(3):221-228.

Singhal, P.C.; Kapasi, A.A.; Franki, N.; Reddy, K. (2000). Morphine-induced macrophage apoptosis: The role of transforming growth factor-β. *Immunology,* 100:57-62.

Singhal, P.C.; Kapasi, A.A.; Reddy, K.; Franki, N.; Gibbons, N.; Ding, G. (1999). Morphine promotes apoptosis in Jurkat cells. *Journal of Leukocyte Biology,* 66:650-658.

Singhal, P.C.; Pan, C.Q.; Sagar, S.; Gibbons, N.; Valderrama, E. (1995). Morphine enhances deposition of ferritin-antiferritin complexes in the glomerular mesangium. *Nephron,* 70:229-234.

Sjogren, P.; Thunedborg, L.P.; Christrup, L.; Hansen, S.H.; Franks, J. (1998). Is development of hyperalgesia, allodynia, and myoclonus related to morphine metabolism during long-term administration? *Acta Anaesthesiologica Scandinavica,* 42:1070-1075.

Sloan, M.A.; Kittner, S.J.; Feeser, B.R.; Gardner, J.; Epstein, A.; Wozniak, M.A.; Wityk, R.J.; Stern, B.J.; Price, T.R.; Macko, R.F.; et al. (1998). Illicit drug-associated ischemic stroke in the Baltimore-Washington Young Stroke Study. *Neurology,* 50:1688-1693.

Smith, W.R.; Glauser, F.L.; Dearden, D.C.; Wells, I.D.; Novey, H.S.; McRae, D.M.; Reid, J.S.; Newcomb, K.A. (1978). Deposits of immunoglobulin and complement in the pulmonary tissue of patients with "heroin lung." *Chest,* 73(4):471-476.

Spirito, P.; Rapezzi, C.; Bellone, P.; Betocchi, S.; Autore, C.; Conte, M.R.; Bezante, G.P.; Bruzzi, P. (1999). Infective endocarditis in hypertrophic cardiomyopathy: Prevalence, incidence, and indications for antibiotic prophylaxis. *Circulation,* 99:2132-2137.

Sporer, K.A. (1999). Acute heroin overdose. *Annals of Internal Medicine,* 130:584-590.

Sun, K.O.; Chan, Y.W.; Cheung, R.T.F.; So, P.C.; Yu, Y.L.; Li, P.C.K. (1994). Management of tetanus: A review of 18 cases. *Journal of the Royal Society of Medicine,* 87:135-137.

Surks, M.I.; Sievert, R. (1995). Drugs and thyroid function. *The New England Journal of Medicine,* 333(25):1688-1694.

Tagliaro, F.; Capra, F.; Dorizzi, R.; Luisetto, G.; Accordini, A.; Renda, E.; Parolin, A. (1984). High serum calcitonin levels in heroin addicts. *Journal of Endocrinological Investigation,* 7:331-333.

Talan, D.A.; Moran, G.J. (1998). Tetanus among injecting-drug users—California, 1997. *Annals of Emergency Medicine,* 32:385-386.

Thomas, J.A.; Shahid-Salles, K.S.; Donovan, M.P. (1977). Effects of narcotics on the reproductive system. *Advances in Sex Hormone Research,* 3:169-195.

Thomas, P.T.; House, R.V.; Bhargava, H.N. (1995). Direct cellular immunomodulation produced by diacetylmorphine (heroin) or methadone. *General Pharmacology,* 26(1):123-130.

Tong, T.G.; Pond, S.M.; Kreek, M.J.; Jaffery, N.F.; Benowitz, N.L. (1981). Phenytoin-induced methadone withdrawal. *Annals of Internal Medicine,* 94: 349-351.

Tooley, A.; Rostami-Hodjegan, A.; Lennard, M.S.; Tucker, G.T. (1999). Acute inhibition of methadone metabolism by ritonavir: Projection of interindividual variability from in vitro data. *Journal of Clinical Pharmacology,* 48:883P-884P.

Tsao, J.W.; Garlin, A.B.; Marder, S.R.; Haber, R.J. (1999). Mycotic aneurysm presenting as Pancoast's syndrome in an injection drug user. *Annals of Emergency Medicine,* 34(4):546-549.

Utecht, M.J.; Stone, A.F.; McCarron, M.M. (1993). Heroin body packers. *The Journal of Emergency Medicine,* 11:33-40.

Vance, J.C.; Chant, D.C.; Tudehope, D.I.; Gray, P.H.; Hayes, A.J. (1997). Infants born to narcotic dependent mothers: Physical growth patterns in the first 12 months of life. *Journal of Paediatrics and Child Health,* 33:504-508.

Wetli, C.V.; Rao, A.; Rao, V.J. (1997). Fatal heroin body packing. *American Journal of Forensic Medicine and Pathology,* 18(3):312-318.

Yeager, M.P.; Colacchio, T.A.; Yu, C.T.; Hildebrandt, L.; Howell, A.L.; Weiss, J.; Guyre, P.M. (1995). Morphine inhibits spontaneous and cytokine-enhanced natural killer cell cytotoxicity in volunteers. *Anesthesiology,* 83:500-508.

Yuan, C.S.; Foss, J.F.; O'Connor, M.; Osinski, J.; Karrison, T.; Moss, J.; Roizen, M.F. (2000). Methylnaltrexone for reversal of constipation due to chronic methadone use. *JAMA,* 283(3):367-372.

Chapter 8

Medical Consequences of the Use of Cocaine and Other Stimulants

Aaron Schneir
Anthony S. Manoguerra

OVERVIEW

Once thought to be a benign, nonaddicting drug, cocaine now has well-recognized adverse effects. These adverse effects are manifested in nearly all organ systems of the body. It is important to realize that an organ system breakdown in classifying the adverse effects of cocaine is artificial and that multiple organs are often affected by similar mechanisms. In particular, the effects of cocaine on the cardiovascular system help to explain many of the effects on other organs throughout the body. In addition, certain adverse effects may be dependent on the route of administration, or dose of cocaine. The adverse effects of two other stimulant drugs, methamphetamine and phenylpropanolamine, will be summarized at the end of this chapter.

HISTORY

The history of cocaine use has been well described by a number of authors (Karch, 1999; Warner, 1993). Peruvian Indians have a long history of chewing coca leaves to achieve euphoria, combat fatigue, and increase stamina. Sigmund Freud used cocaine and also prescribed it as treatment for alcohol or opiate addiction. At one time, cocaine was a common ingredient in many commercial products, including teas and patent medicines. Although no longer the case, when first introduced, Coca-Cola was formulated using extracts from coca leaves and actually contained a small amount of cocaine. In the late nineteenth century, cocaine use was popular and reports of addiction and adverse effects became known. The Harrison Narcotic Tax Act of 1914 prohibited the importation of cocaine and coca leaves, except for pharmaceutical purposes. This legislation helped curtail much of the burgeoning cocaine use. In 1970, passage of the Controlled Substances Act prohibited the manufacture, distribution, and possession of cocaine, except for limited medical purposes. However, within the past twenty years, the use of cocaine has made a huge resurgence, especially with the advent of crack cocaine. This epidemic has further revealed many adverse effects of cocaine, yet its use remains very popular.

FORMS OF COCAINE

Many review articles describe in depth the various forms and properties of cocaine (Boghdadi and Henning, 1997; Warner, 1993; Cregler and Mark, 1986). Cocaine is an alkaloid extracted from the leaves of the *Erythroxylon coca* plant, grown predominantly in Central and South America. The two different chemical forms in which cocaine is abused are cocaine hydrochloride and cocaine alkaloid. Cocaine hydrochloride is produced by adding hydrochloric acid to cocaine base. The result is a water-soluble salt that is typically insufflated, but may also be administered intravenously. Freebase and crack cocaine are both cocaine alkaloids that are smoked, but are produced by different techniques. Freebase is a colorless, crystalline substance that is made by dissolving cocaine hydrochloride in water, alkalinizing the solution, and then adding ether as a solvent. Cocaine base dissolves in the ether layer and is extracted by evaporating the ether. Many adulterants are removed by this process, but the remaining flammable ether predisposes the user to burns. Crack cocaine is made by a simpler process that allows more adulterants to remain, but does not require the use of ether. Crack is made by dissolving cocaine hydrochloride in water, adding baking soda, and slowly heating it to allow the alkaloidal cocaine to precipitate. The name crack stems from the popping sound that is made when crack is smoked (see Brick and Erickson, 1999, for a review).

All forms of cocaine produce the desired effect of euphoria. However, the onset and duration of effect differs between the different cocaine forms and mode of administration. Both smoking and intravenous use of cocaine produce a rapid euphoria. Cocaine smoke is rapidly absorbed by the pulmonary vasculature, reaching the brain in six to eight seconds and producing a euphoric effect for about twenty minutes. When used intravenously cocaine reaches the brain in about double the time of smoked cocaine. The euphoria achieved with cocaine insufflation takes longer (three to five minutes), but lasts one to two hours. With insufflation, cocaine causes local vasoconstriction of the nasal mucosa which both delays and prolongs its absorption. Coadministration of cocaine with alcohol also prolongs the euphoria since an active metabolite named cocaethylene is produced when they are used together. Although this metabolite does not seem to produce a greater euphoric effect, it does have a long half-life and may result in a more prolonged euphoria (Hart et al., 2000).

Prior to the late 1970s, cocaine hydrochloride was primarily used by nasal insufflation. At that time, intravenous use of cocaine hydrochloride became popular as well as smoking of freebase cocaine. Smoking of cocaine became even more popular with the introduction of crack cocaine in the 1980s.

PHYSIOLOGIC EFFECTS

The mechanism of action of cocaine helps to explain both the desired effects by users and also many of the adverse effects observed with use. The effects of cocaine are mediated through both the central and peripheral nervous system and have been reviewed in depth (Boghdadi and Henning, 1997; Warner, 1993).

Centrally, cocaine blocks the reuptake of the neurotransmitters dopamine and serotonin into presynaptic neurons, which leads to their accumulation in synaptic clefts. Dopamine and serotonin receptors are stimulated and the desired effects of euphoria, enhanced alertness, increased energy, diminished appetite, and increased self-confidence are achieved. By suppressing activity of two specific parts of the brain, the pontine nucleus and locus ceruleus, cocaine also suppresses feelings of fear and panic. When used repetitively, however, dopamine stores become depleted, leading to the compensatory increased production of dopamine receptors. It is believed that the ensuing cocaine craving experienced by the chronic user results from the "starvation" of these receptors for dopamine.

In the peripheral nervous system, cocaine blocks the reuptake of catecholamines, specifically norepinephrine, by sympathetic nerve terminals, leading to accumulation in the synaptic cleft. Norepinephrine acts on both alpha- and beta-adrenergic receptors located on the heart and blood vessels. Stimulation of alpha-adrenergic receptors leads to constriction and in some cases spasm of blood vessels, whereas stimulation of beta-adrenergic receptors on the heart leads to increased heart rate. These effects of norepinephrine on the heart and blood vessels combined with other systemic effects are referred to as the sympathomimetic effect. The term sympathomimetic derives from the "fight or flight" effect of the sympathetic nervous system. The resulting sympathomimetic presentation may include hypertension (elevated blood pressure), tachycardia (elevated heart rate), hyperthermia (elevated temperature), mydriasis (dilated pupils), and diaphoresis (sweating).

The local anesthetic effect of cocaine is also well known. In fact, cocaine was introduced as the first local anesthetic in Vienna, Austria, in 1884. Cocaine competitively inhibits fast sodium channels in neurons that normally allow sodium to enter cells to initiate the propagation of neural impulses. Blockade of these channels prevents nerve impulse formation and explains the anesthetic effect of cocaine. This effect is still used therapeutically with the use of topical cocaine used to provide local anesthesia to mucous membranes and to reduce bleeding through local vasoconstriction. Sodium channels are also located in the cells of the heart and blockage may result in conduction delays and dysrhythmias (abnormal heart rhythms).

ADVERSE EFFECTS OF COCAINE

Cocaine is one of the most frequently abused illicit drugs and the adverse effects of cocaine use have been well summarized (Boghdadi and Henning, 1997; Warner, 1993; Cregler, 1989; Cregler and Mark, 1986). According to the 1997 National Household Survey on Drug Abuse (NHSDA) an estimated 1.5 million Americans were current cocaine users (National Institute on Drug Abuse, 1999). Of patients presenting to the emergency department following cocaine use, cardiopulmonary, neurologic, and psychiatric presentations have been shown to be the most common (Rich and Singer, 1991; Brody et al., 1990). Although the overall morbidity and mortality of patients presenting with cocaine-associated complaints appears to be low (Brody et al., 1990), devastating effects, including death, do occur. Of New York City residents who died between 1990 and 1992 from intentional or unintentional injury, evidence of recent cocaine use was found in one-fourth of cases. Of these deaths, one-third were attributed to cocaine intoxication and two-thirds to traumatic injury (Marzuk et al., 1995). The psychiatric adverse effects of cocaine are likely contributory to trauma-related deaths.

Cardiovascular

The most significant adverse effects from cocaine use involve the cardiovascular system. In addition, many of the adverse effects in other organ systems are mediated through the effects of cocaine on the cardiovascular system. Adverse effects include myocardial infarction, dysrhythmias, cardiomyopathies, aortic dissection, and endocarditis.

Various pathophysiologic mechanisms help explain the adverse effect cocaine has on the heart. Cocaine-induced ischemia of the cardiac muscle results in the myocardial infarctions seen in cocaine users. The production of tachycardia, hypertension, accelerated atherosclerosis of the coronary arteries, and enhanced platelet aggregation (Heesch et al., 2000) from cocaine use, may contribute to ischemia (Pitts et al., 1997). Vasospasm of the coronary arteries likely explains why, in some cases, cocaine associated myocardial infarctions occur in the absence of coronary artery disease (Howard et al., 1985; Zimmerman et al., 1987; Minor et al., 1991). Cocaine-induced myocardial ischemia may precipitate dysrhythmias (Hollander and Hoffman, 1992) and in addition, the sodium-channel-blocking effect of cocaine may also contribute to conduction disturbances and dysrhythmias (Tanen et al., 2000). Myocardial infarctions and dysrhythmias may be one of the major causes of sudden death related to cocaine use. Chronic myocardial ischemia and systemic hypertension from cocaine may also explain the reported cases of cardiomyopathy (Weiner et al., 1986). The acute hypertension seen with cocaine use has also been implicated in the development of aortic dissections (Fisher and Holroyd, 1992; Chang and Rossi, 1995). The higher than expected incidence of endocarditis from intravenous cocaine administration suggests that by an as yet unknown mechanism, cocaine increases the likelihood of this potentially devastating condition (Chambers et al., 1987).

Many of the most serious cardiovascular complications seem to be rare, considering the relatively common use of cocaine. However, these adverse effects occur with use of cocaine, can be life-threatening, and must be taken seriously. For example, the presence of cocaine-associated chest pain in an otherwise healthy young patient should be taken very seriously by the treating physician.

Neurologic

The adverse effects of cocaine on the neurologic system include all forms of stroke, convulsions, headache, and movement disorders. A retrospective study conducted by researchers at San Francisco General Hospital detailed that convulsions and focal neurological symptoms and signs were the two major presenting acute neurological complications of cocaine use (Lowenstein et al., 1987). Many of these complications can be severe and result in long-term morbidity and death.

A particularly devastating neurologic effect of cocaine use is stroke. Cocaine-related strokes have mostly been reported in patients younger than fifty, an age group that otherwise has a very low incidence of strokes. All types of strokes including subarachnoid hemorrhage, intracerebral hemorrhage, and ischemic infarcts have been reported from cocaine use. In addition, all major vascular territories of the brain have been involved and all routes of cocaine administration have been implicated (Rowbotham and

Lowenstein, 1990). Various etiologies have been postulated. The pharmacologic effect of cocaine to acutely increase blood pressure seems especially likely as an etiology resulting in hemorrhage. The rapid increase in blood pressure may rupture both normal and preexisting abnormal cerebrovasculature (Lichtenfeld et al., 1984; Aggarwal et al., 1996; Wojak and Flamm, 1987; Nolte et al., 1996). Vasospasm, platelet aggregation, and vasculitis may also be contributory to both ischemic and hemorrhagic infarctions (Daras, Tuchman, et al., 1994; Fredericks et al., 1991).

Generalized convulsions are another adverse effect associated with cocaine use (Myers and Earnest, 1984). The local anesthetic effect of cocaine seems a likely etiology and unlike many other adverse effects of cocaine, convulsions appear to be dose related (Rowbotham and Lowenstein, 1990).

Various movement disorders have been associated with cocaine use. The association of choreiform movements with crack cocaine use led to the term "crack dancing" (Daras, Koppel, et al., 1994). Cocaine use may worsen preexisting movement disorders (Daniels et al., 1996), increase the risk of acute dystonic reactions in patients taking dopamine-blocking agents, and occasionally induce an acute dystonic reaction without other contributing factors (Catalano et al., 1997; Farrel and Diehl, 1991). The mechanism by which cocaine induces these effects remains unclear but is thought to be related to dopamine dysregulation (Catalano et al., 1997).

Pulmonary

Pulmonary symptoms are a common presenting complaint of cocaine users and a wide variety of adverse pulmonary effects of cocaine use have been reported. In contrast to the adverse effects on many other organs, the route of cocaine administration seems particularly important in producing pulmonary problems. The vast majority of adverse effects reported result from smoking cocaine either as freebase or crack (Perper and Van Thiel, 1992). Adverse effects range from acute respiratory irritation to asthma exacerbation, pulmonary edema, eosinophilic lung disease, granulomatous lung disease, barotrauma, pulmonary hypertension, and possibly a persistent gas-exchange abnormality.

Cough, hemoptysis, and shortness of breath are common acute respiratory symptoms after smoking cocaine. Often these symptoms are not the result of significant pulmonary damage and are likely from the local irritant effect of cocaine (Perper and Van Thiel, 1992). However, this irritant effect of cocaine has also been implicated in causing more serious pathology. Severe asthma exacerbations have been associated with cocaine smoking (Rebhun, 1988; Rome et al., 2000), and some evidence indicates the increasing incidence of death from asthma may, in part, be related to cocaine use (Levenson et al., 1996). The fact that inhaled but not intravenous cocaine administration induces bronchoconstriction supports a local irritant effect (Tashkin et al., 1996). The irritant effect has also been implicated in the hypersensitivity-related eosinophilic lung disorder referred to as "crack lung," which involves diffuse alveolar infiltrates associated with fever and eosinophilia (Forrester et al., 1990; Kissner et al., 1987). The presence of cutting agents in cocaine may also cause irritation to the lungs and result in granulomatous lung disease. Both cellulose and talc granulomas in the lung have resulted from nasal insufflation of cocaine (Cooper et al.,1983; Oubeid et al., 1990).

Pulmonary barotrauma including pneumediastinum (Morris and Schuck, 1985), pneumothorax (Chan et al., 1997; Shesser et al., 1981), and pneumopericardium (Adrouny and Magnusson, 1985), have all been reported in association with cocaine inhalation. Pneumomediastinum has also been reported with cocaine insufflation (Shesser et al., 1981). Prolonged and repeated Valsalva maneuvers performed by individuals attempting to heighten the effect of the drug are thought to induce alveolar rupture. The escaped air then can induce a pneumothorax or move to the mediastinum or, rarely, the pericardium. The fact that similar barotrauma has been reported with the use of other drugs suggests that the etiology is not the result of an intrinsic property of cocaine (Miller et al., 1972).

Much still remains to be learned about the effect of cocaine on the lungs. The etiology of noncardiogenic pulmonary edema seen in association with cocaine use is unknown. The majority of cases have occurred from smoking cocaine (Cucco et al., 1987; Hoffman and Goodman, 1989), but one report exists of fatal pulmonary edema from intravenous administration of "freebase" cocaine (Allred and Ewer, 1981). Cocaine may alter pulmonary diffusion capacity but studies are conflicting (Tashkin et al., 1997; Susskind et al., 1991). Cocaine has also been shown to decrease the effectiveness of alveolar macrophages, but the clinical significance of this has yet to be determined (Baldwin et al., 1997).

Psychiatric

Various psychiatric problems occur with cocaine use. Exactly what effect is observed depends on whether a patient is acutely intoxicated, in a state of withdrawal, or suffering chronic effects from the drug. The exact mechanisms by which cocaine produces such effects are unclear.

Cocaine intoxication may be complicated by poor judgment, delirium, and, in severe cases, psychosis. Psychosis from cocaine use may occur both with acute intoxication with high doses and also more insidiously with chronic use. Psychosis with acute intoxication has been noted to often be associated with violent behavior (Manschreck et al., 1988). Cocaine use in individuals with a predisposition for or preexisting psychiatric illness may certainly make an accurate diagnosis difficult (Mendoza et al., 1992).

Long thought not to occur, a tri-phasic abstinence syndrome observed in outpatients following chronic cocaine abuse has been described. Phase one of the withdrawal involves the "crash" of mood and energy following cocaine binge cessation. It is marked by dysphoria, anxiety, depression, and profound exhaustion, and may last for days. Cocaine craving is also typical. The crash is thought to reflect acute neurotransmitter depletion caused by cocaine. Following the crash, phase two, or cocaine withdrawal ensues. In contrast to the withdrawal associated with many other abused drugs, with cocaine there are no gross physiological alterations. However, significant dysphoria, anhedonia, and amotivation are noted. Memories of cocaine euphoria may prompt the individual to reuse cocaine. Finally, phase three (extinction) occurs, which may last years, in which anhedonia and further craving may prompt reuse (Gawin and Kleber, 1986). It must be noted that additional inpatient studies on cocaine withdrawal did not reveal distinct phases, but a gradually resolving dysphoria. It is currently thought that the characteristics of withdrawal differ from an outpatient to inpatient setting and may rest with the presence or absence of triggering cues which can prompt cravings (Weddington, 1993; Withers et al., 1995).

Genitourinary

Adverse effects of cocaine use on the genitourinary system are significant. Adverse effects include acute renal failure, renal infarction, and progression of chronic renal failure. In addition, various sexual dysfunctions have been described.

Cocaine-induced rhabdomyolysis (muscle breakdown) is well documented and may lead to acute renal failure (Welch et al., 1991; Roth et al., 1988; Herzlich et al., 1988; Merigram and Roberts, 1987). The mechanism by which cocaine induces rhabdomyolysis is unclear and may be multifactorial. Although often associated with convulsions and hyperthermia, rhabdomyolysis associated with cocaine use has been documented without either of these conditions being present (Welch et al., 1991; Roth et al., 1988). A direct toxic effect of cocaine on skeletal muscle, increased muscular activity, and cocaine-induced vasospasm with resultant ischemia have all been suggested mechanisms (Richards, 2000). It is thought that renal damage occurs from the toxic effect of myoglobin on the renal tubules (Richards, 2000). Acute renal failure may also be the result of the severe hypertension precipitated by cocaine use (Thakur et al., 1996). Hypertension from cocaine use may also accelerate the progression of chronic renal failure (Dunea et al., 1995). It is not surprising that reports of renal infarction exist with cocaine use (Wohlman, 1987; Goodman and Rennie, 1995), with the pathophysiology likely similar to that associated with myocardial infarction involving accelerated atherosclerosis, vasospasm, and enhanced platelet aggregation (Nzerue et al., 2000).

At low doses, cocaine can delay ejaculation and orgasm, which combined with its euphoric effects may be used to heighten the sexual experience (Smith et al., 1984). However, chronic cocaine use has been associated with sexual dysfunction. Male users have difficulty maintaining erection and ejaculating (Cregler, 1989). In addition, cocaine use has been associated with priapism (Altman et al., 1999). The mechanisms responsible for sexual dysfunction and priapism remain unclear.

Gastrointestinal

Compared with the effect of cocaine use on other organ systems, there are relatively few reported adverse effects on the gastrointestinal tract (Hoang et al., 1998). However, serious adverse effects of cocaine on the gastrointestinal tract have been observed, and include intestinal ischemia, intestinal infarction, and ulcer perforation. A particular problem with cocaine, related to the gastrointestinal tract, is the ingestion of cocaine in an effort to either hide evidence ("body stuffers") or transport large amounts of it ("body packers") (Hollander and Hoffman, 1998).

The occurrence of intestinal ischemia from cocaine use has been well documented and has occurred from all routes of exposure, including insufflation, intravenous injection, smoking, and ingestion (Herrine et al., 1998; Myers et al., 1996; Hon et al., 1990; Nalbandian et al., 1985). Ischemia in both the large and small intestine has been reported and has progressed to infarction and death in some cases (Hoang et al., 1998). In many of the reported cases, the intestinal vasculature was normal on examination, suggesting vasospasm as the etiology of ischemia and infarction (Herrine et al., 1998; Mustard et al., 1992; Freudenberger et al., 1990). In some cases, however, abnormalities have been documented in the arteries. Damage to small caliber arterioles has been observed, suggesting that the cocaine may have caused endothelial damage (Garfia et al., 1990). Thrombosis in the major mesenteric arteries has also been demonstrated angiographically (Myers et al., 1996). In some cases of gastrointestinal infarction, perforation of the gastrointestinal tract has occurred (Brown et al., 1994). Perforations of gastric and duodenal ulcers are also known to occur in temporal relation to crack use (Sharma et al., 1997; Lee et al., 1990; Feliciano et al., 1999). The mechanism for this remains unknown but may also be related to the vasoconstrictive effect of cocaine on the stomach and duodenum (Sharma et al., 1997; Feliciano et al., 1999).

A particular problem frequently encountered is the individual who has swallowed large amounts of cocaine. This may have been done in an attempt to conceal evidence during imminent arrest, or as a means of concealment for drug smuggling (Caruana et al., 1984). When done for drug smuggling the cocaine is often packaged in balloons or condoms (Suarez et al., 1977). Although many people pass the packets uneventfully, rupture of one or more of the packets has caused convulsions and death (Suarez et al., 1977; Fishbain and Wetli, 1981).

Liver

Liver damage is a relatively uncommon reported adverse effect associated with cocaine use (Mallat and Dhumeaux, 1991). However, liver damage, and in some cases liver failure, have been reported (Perino et al., 1987; Wanless et al., 1990; Silva et al., 1991; Kanel et al., 1990). In addition, the lifestyle of cocaine users and the intravenous route of cocaine administration may predispose users to various viral causes of hepatitis (Van Thiel and Perper, 1992).

The mechanism for cocaine-induced liver damage is probably multifactorial (Mallat and Dhumeaux, 1991) and liver damage often occurs in the setting of cocaine-induced hyperthermia and shock, which are known causes of liver injury (Silva et al., 1991). Furthermore, the metabolism of cocaine may lead to toxic metabolites which may be directly injurious to liver cells. The majority of cocaine is metabolized in the blood by pseudocholinesterase and in the liver by hepatic esterase to nontoxic metabolites. Within the liver, the cytochrome P450 system metabolizes the remaining cocaine (Van Thiel and Perper, 1992) through a minor pathway which produces metabolites such as norcocaine nitroxide, a free radical that may initiate liver damage (Ndikum-Moffor et al., 1998; Kloss et al., 1984).

Pancreas

One study from Brazil associated chronic cocaine smoking with the development of pancreatic adenocarcinoma. Further study is required to confirm this association (Duarte et al., 1999).

Head and Neck, Nose and Throat

Head and neck complications from cocaine use are intimately related to the route of drug administration. Adverse effects include chronic rhinitis, nasal septal perforations, destructive facial processes, sinusitis, dental erosions, and thermal injuries.

Chronic nasal insufflation of cocaine may lead to various local effects to the nares. Rebound hyperemia after drug discontinuation may lead to a condition of chronic rhinitis similar to rhinitis medicamentosa (Schwartz et al., 1989). Nasal septal perforation is a well-known adverse effect of chronic cocaine insufflation that in some cases has progressed to nasal cartilage collapse and saddle-nose deformity (Deutsch and Millard, 1989; Vilensky, 1982). An even more devastating condition is an aggressive destructive facial process that may simulate Wegener's granulomatosis, neoplasms, or chronic infections (Carter and Grossman, 2000; Sittel and Eckel, 1998; Dagget et al., 1990). A similar condition resulted when an individual was assaulted and had crack cocaine forcibly impacted in the nostrils (Tierney and Stadelmann, 1999). Nasal septal perforation and the more devastating conditions associated with chronic nasal insufflation all involve the progressive destruction of tissue. This is likely the result of a combination of chronic cocaine-induced vasoconstriction, irritation, and local trauma from nasal picking. Irritation from adulterants in the insufflated cocaine may also be contributory (Carter and Grossman, 2000; Dagget et al., 1990). Insufflation has also been associated with bacterial sinusitis, including an unusual case in which the causative organism was *Clostridium botulinum* (Kudrow et al., 1988).

Dental erosions have been reported with insufflation and with an abuser who applied cocaine topically (Krutchkoff et al., 1990). Rapid gingival recession has also been reported in an individual who regularly applied cocaine to his gums (Kapila and Kashani, 1997).

Thermal injuries from smoking both freebase and crack have resulted in burns to the upper respiratory tract and esophagus (Meleca et al., 1997). Both the hot cocaine vapors and metal from the pipes used to smoke the cocaine have been implicated. One of the potentially life-threatening thermal injuries described is epiglottitis (Mayo-Smith and Spinale, 1997; Savitt and Colagiovanni, 1991). In one case, passive inhalation of crack smoke in a child was implicated in thermal epiglottitis (Karasch et al., 1990). Hot cocaine vapor has also caused loss of eyelash and eyebrow hair (Tames and Goldenring, 1986).

Ocular

Relatively few adverse effects of cocaine use on the eyes have been reported. The adverse effects include corneal epithelial defects, preseptal cellulitis, optic neuropathy, precipitation of acute angle-closure glaucoma, opsoclonus, and impaired color vision.

Corneal epithelial defects resulting from crack smoking have led to the term "crack eye" (McHenry et al., 1989). Multiple mechanisms postulated include a direct toxic effect of the cocaine alkaloid and a local anesthetic effect that disrupts normal blink mechanisms and causes an exposure keratopathy (Sachs et al., 1993). In some cases, the injuries led to a secondary bacterial infection (Zagelbaum et al., 1991). Another infection, preseptal cellulitis, has been reported in the setting of cocaine-induced bony orbit destruction (Underdahl and Chiou, 1998). The ability of chronic cocaine use to cause an osteolytic sinusitis leading to bilateral optic neuropathy has also been reported (Newman et al., 1988).

Nasal insufflation of cocaine has precipitated narrow angle-closure glaucoma. It is thought that cocaine may reach the eye by retrograde delivery via the nasolacrimal system or by inadvertent rubbing of the eye. The mydriatic (pupil-dilating) effect of cocaine appears to be a precipitating factor (Mitchell and Schwartz, 1996; Hari et al., 1999).

Opsoclonus, an abnormal movement disorder of the eye that involves rapid, irregular, nonrhythmic movements in horizontal and vertical directions, has been reported with cocaine use. The mechanism is unclear (Elkardoudi-Pijnenburg and Van Vliet, 1996). Studies have also shown impaired color vision in patients recovering from cocaine use. It is postulated that cocaine interferes with the retinal dopamine system, which affects retinal neurotransmission (Desai et al., 1997).

Pregnancy

Cocaine use during pregnancy is associated with various adverse effects both to the mother and fetus including an increased incidence of placental abruption, prematurity, intrauterine growth retardation, and microcephaly (small brain size). Various neurologic, cardiac, ophthalmic, and gastrointestinal defects have occurred in children who were exposed in utero to cocaine (Plessinger and Woods, 1998). A detailed review of the effects of cocaine on the fetus appears in Chapter 9.

OTHER STIMULANTS

Methamphetamine

Amphetamine was first synthesized in 1887 and introduced in the 1930s in the form of inhalers for treating rhinitis and asthma. Amphetamines and amphetamine derivatives are still prescribed for the treatment of attention deficit disorder and for the treatment of narcolepsy. Multiple drugs, both legal and illegal, have been synthesized by various modifications to the structure of amphetamine. Therapeutic medications include phenylpropanolamine and ephedrine. Illicit drugs include methamphetamine and the "designer" drug, Ecstasy (3,4-methylenedioxymethamphetamine), also known as MDMA (Derlet and Heischober, 1990).

Both amphetamine and methamphetamine have become common drugs of abuse. Methamphetamine differs from amphetamine by the presence of a methyl group on the amine portion of the molecule, which affords improved central nervous system penetration. Amphetamines are abused by various routes of administration including intravenous, oral, insufflation, and inhalation (Albertson et al., 1999). Amphetamine and methamphetamine exert their clinical effects primarily by releasing the catecholamines dopamine and norepinephrine from presynaptic nerve terminals. The resulting clinical effects are very similar to cocaine with a few notable exceptions. The duration of effect of amphetamines is up to twenty-four hours, which is much longer than cocaine. In addition, amphetamines lack the sodium-channel-blocking effect of cocaine and therefore may be less likely to precipitate cardiac dysrhythmias (Chiang, 1991).

As predicted by the very similar mechanism of action and physiological response with cocaine, many of the reported associated adverse effects with amphetamines are also similar (Albertson et al., 1999). Associated cardiovascular adverse effects include hypertension, tachycardia, myocardial infarction (Bashour, 1994; Packe et al., 1990), cardiomyopathy (Hong et al., 1991), and aortic dissection (Davis and Swalwell, 1994). Central nervous system effects include intracerebral hemorrhages (Imanse and Vanneste, 1990), intracerebral ischemic strokes (Rothrock et al., 1988), seizures, psychosis, and choreoathetoid movements (Lundh and Tunving, 1981). Ischemic colitis (Johnson and Berenson, 1991), rhabdomyolysis (Richards et al., 1999), hepatotoxicity (Jones et al., 1994), and various fetal anomalies (Plessinger, 1998) have also been reported. The medical literature detailing the associated adverse effects of cocaine use is much more extensive than the literature detailing amphetamine use. Only time and, unfortunately, continued abuse of amphetamines, will reveal if this is truly the case.

Phenylpropanolamine

Phenylpropanolamine is a synthetic stimulant that has a very similar structure to amphetamine. Until recently it was present in a multitude of both over-the-counter and prescription-only cold preparations, as well as weight loss formulations (Pentel, 1984). Adverse effects associated with its use, misuse, and intentional overdose have been known for many years, leading many to recommend removing it from the market. In 2000, the FDA began taking steps to remove phenylpropanolamine from all drug products and requested that all drug companies discontinue marketing products containing the drug (FDA Talk Paper, 2000).

The major adverse effects associated with phenylpropanolamine are neurologic, particularly hemorrhagic, strokes that have been lethal (Forman et al., 1989; Lake et al., 1990; Glick et al., 1987). Less commonly reported adverse effects include hypertension (Lake et al., 1988), myocardial infarction (Leo et al., 1996; Oosterbaan and Burns, 2000), dysrhythmias (Conway et al., 1989), ischemic bowel (Johnson et al., 1985), seizures, and psychosis (Marshall and Douglas, 1994). Most of the adverse effects are explained by the pharmacologic action of phenylpropanolamine. Phenylpropanolamine primarily works as a direct alpha-one agonist causing constriction of arterioles. Through this mechanism the commonly desired therapeutic effect of nasal decongestion is achieved. With slightly higher than therapeutic doses, however, the alpha-one agonism can cause potentially severe hypertension which may require treatment and lead to lethal complications such as hemorrhagic stroke (Pentel, 1984).

Summary

Cocaine use is fairly common in the United States and is associated with a variety of serious adverse effects. Many of these effects seem to occur by means of the physiological effects of cocaine on the cardiovascular system. Methamphetamine is becoming a more popular drug of abuse whose mechanism of action and adverse effects are very similar to those of cocaine. Phenylpropanolamine is an amphetamine derivative that until recently was found in numerous over-the-counter and prescription medications. Recent recognition that the drug is associated with severe neurological effects led to recommendations that its use be limited.

REFERENCES

Adrouny, A.; Magnusson, P. (1985). Pneumopericardium from cocaine inhalation (letter). *New England Journal of Medicine* 313:48-49.

Aggarwal, S.K.; Williams, V.; Levine, S.R.; Cassin, B.J.; Garcia, J.H. (1996). Cocaine-associated intracranial hemorrhage: Absence of vasculitis in 14 cases. *Neurology* 46:1741-1743.

Albertson, T.E.; Derlet, R.W.; Van Hoozen, B.E. (1999). Methamphetamine and the expanding complications of amphetamines. *Western Journal of Medicine* 170:214-219.

Allred, R.J.; Ewer, S. (1981). Fatal pulmonary edema following intravenous "free-base" cocaine use. *Annals of Emergency Medicine* 10:441-442.

Altman, A.L.; Seftel, A.D.; Brown, S.L.; Hampel, N. (1999). Cocaine associated priapism. *Journal of Urology* 161:1817-1818.

Baldwin, G.C.; Tashkin, D.P.; Buckley, D.M.; Park, A.N.; Dubinett, S.M.; Roth, M.D. (1997). Marijuana and cocaine impair alveolar macrophage function and cytokine production. *American Journal of Respiratory and Critical Care Medicine* 156:1606-1613.

Bashour, T.T. (1994). Acute myocardial infarction resulting from amphetamine abuse: A spasm-thrombus interplay? *American Heart Journal* 128:1237-1239.

Boghdadi, M.S.; Henning, R.J. (1997). Cocaine: Pathophysiology and clinical toxicology. *Heart and Lung* 26:466-483.

Brick, J.; Erickson, C. (1999). *Drugs, the Brain, and Behavior: The Pharmacology of Abuse and Dependence.* Binghamton, NY: The Haworth Medical Press.

Brody, S.L.; Slovis, C.M.; Wrenn, K.D. (1990). Cocaine-related medical problems: Consecutive series of 233 patients. *American Journal of Medicine* 88:325-331.

Brown, D.N.; Rosenholtz, M.J.; Marshall, J.B. (1994). Ischemic colitis related to cocaine abuse. *The American Journal of Gastroenterology* 89:1558-1560.

Carter, E.L.; Grossman, M.E. (2000). Cocaine-induced centrofacial ulceration. *Cutis* 65:73-76.

Caruana, D.S.; Weinbach, B.; Goerg, D.; Gardner, L.B. (1984). Cocaine-packet ingestion. *Annals of Internal Medicine* 100:73-74.

Catalano, G.; Catalano, M.C.; Rodriguez, R. (1997). Dystonia associated with crack cocaine use. *Southern Medical Journal* 90:1050-1052.

Chambers, H.F.; Morris, D.L.; Tauber, M.G.; Modin, G. (1987). Cocaine use and the risk for endocarditis in intravenous drug users. *Annals of Internal Medicine* 106:833-836.

Chan, L.; Pham, H.; Reece, E.A. (1997). Pneumothorax in pregnancy associated with cocaine use. *American Journal of Perinatology* 14:385-388.

Chang, R.A.; Rossi, N.F. (1995). Intermittent cocaine use associated with recurrent dissection of the thoracic and abdominal aorta. *Chest* 108:1758-1762.

Chiang, W.K. (1991). Amphetamines. In Goldfrank, L.R.; Flomenbaum, N.E.; Lewin, N.A.; Weisman, R.S.; Howland, M.A.; Hoffman, R.S. (eds.), *Goldfrank's Toxicological Emergencies* (pp. 1091-1103). Stamford, CT: Simon and Schuster.

Conway, E.E.; Walsh, C.A.; Palomba, A.L. (1989). Supraventricular tachycardia following the administration of phenylpropanolamine in an infant. *Pediatric Emergency Care* 5:173-174.

Cooper, C.B.; Bai, T.R.; Heyderman, E. (1983). Cellulose granulomas in the lungs of a cocaine sniffer. *British Medical Journal* 286:2021-2022.

Cregler, L.L. (1989). Adverse health consequences of cocaine abuse. *Journal of the National Medical Association* 81:27-38.

Cregler, L.L.; Mark, H. (1986). Medical complications of cocaine abuse. *New England Journal of Medicine* 315:1495-1500.

Cucco, R.A.; Yoo, O.H.; Cregler, L.; Chang, J.C. (1987). Nonfatal pulmonary edema after "freebase" cocaine smoking. *American Review of Respiratory Diseases* 136:179-181.

Dagget, R.B.; Haghighi, P.; Terkeltaub, R.A. (1990). Nasal cocaine abuse causing an aggressive midline intranasal and pharyngeal destructive process mimicking midline reticulosis and limited Wegener's granulomatosis. *Journal of Rheumatology* 17:838-840.

Daniels, J.; Baker, D.G.; Norman, A.B. (1996). Cocaine-induced tics in untreated Tourette's syndrome (letter). *American Journal of Psychiatry* 153:965.

Daras, M.; Koppel, B.S.; Atos-Radzion, E. (1994). Cocaine-induced choreoathetoid movements ("crack dancing"). *Neurology* 44:751-752.

Daras, M.; Tuchman, A.J.; Koppel, B.S.; Samkoff, L.M.; Weitzner, I.; Marc, J. (1994). Neurovascular complications of cocaine. *Acta Neurologica Scandinavica* 90:124-129.

Davis, G.G.; Swalwell, C.I. (1994). Acute aortic dissections and ruptured berry aneurysms associated with methamphetamine abuse. *Journal of Forensic Sciences* 39:1481-1485.

Derlet, R.W.; Heischober, B. (1990). Methamphetamine: Stimulant of the 1990s? *Western Journal of Medicine* 153:625-628.

Desai, P.; Roy, M.; Roy, A.; Brown, S.; Smelson, D. (1997). Impaired color vision in cocaine-withdrawn patients. *Archives of General Psychiatry* 54:696-699.

Deutsch, H.L.; Millard, R. (1989). A new cocaine abuse complex. *Archives of Otolaryngology Head and Neck Surgery* 115:235-237.

Duarte, J.G.C.; Pantoja, A.F.; Pantoja, J.G.; Chaves, C.P. (1999). Chronic inhaled cocaine abuse may predispose to the development of pancreatic adenocarcinoma. *American Journal of Surgery* 178:426-427.

Dunea, G.; Arruda, J.; Bakir, A.A.; Share, D.S.; Smith, E.C. (1995). Role of cocaine in end-stage renal disease in some hypertensive African Americans. *American Journal of Nephrology* 15:5-9.

Elkardoudi-Pijnenburg, Y.; Van Vliet, A. (1996). Opsoclonus: A rare complication of cocaine misuse (letter). *Journal of Neurology, Neurosurgery, and Psychiatry* 60:592.

Farrel, P.E.; Diehl, A.K. (1991). Acute dystonic reaction to crack cocaine. *Annals of Emergency Medicine* 20:322.

FDA Talk Paper (2000). FDA issues public health warning on phenylpropanolamine. November 6.

Feliciano, D.V.; Ojukwu, J.C.; Rozycki, G.S.; Ballard, R.B.; Ingram, W.L.; Salomone, J.; Narnias, N.; Newman, P.G. (1999). The epidemic of cocaine-related juxtapyloric perforations. *Annals of Surgery* 229:801-806.

Fishbain, D.A.; Wetli, C.V. (1981). Cocaine intoxication, delirium, and death in a body packer. *Annals of Emergency Medicine* 10:531-532.

Fisher, A.; Holroyd, B.R. (1992). Cocaine-associated dissection of the thoracic aorta. *Journal of Emergency Medicine* 10:723-727.

Forman, H.P.; Levin, S.; Stewart, B.; Patel, M.; Feinstein, S. (1989). Cerebral vasculitis and hemorrhage in an adolescent taking diet pills containing phenylpropanolamine: Case report and review of literature. *Pediatrics* 83:737-741.

Forrester, J.M.; Steele, A.W.; Waldron, J.A.; Parsons, P.E. (1990). Crack lung: An acute pulmonary syndrome with a spectrum of clinical and histopathologic findings. *American Review of Respiratory Diseases* 142:462-467.

Fredericks, R.K.; Lefkowitz, D.S.; Challa, V.R.; Troost, T. (1991). Cerebral vasculitis associated with cocaine abuse. *Stroke* 22:1437-1439.

Freudenberger, R.S.; Cappell, M.S.; Hutt, D.A. (1990). Intestinal infarction after intravenous cocaine administration. *Annals of Internal Medicine* 113:715-716.

Garfia, A.; Valverde, J.L.; Borondo, J.C.; Candenas, I.; Lucena, J. (1990). Vascular lesions in intestinal ischemia induced by cocaine-alcohol abuse: Report of a fatal case due to overdose. *Journal of Forensic Sciences* 35:740-745.

Gawin, F.H.; Kleber, H.D. (1986). Abstinence symptomatology and psychiatric diagnosis in cocaine abusers. *Archives of General Psychiatry* 43:107-113.

Glick, R.; Hoying, J.; Cerullo, L.; Perlman, S. (1987). Phenylpropanolamine: An over-the-counter drug causing central nervous system vasculitis and intracerebral hemorrhage. Case report and review. *Neurosurgery* 20:969-974.

Goodman, P.E.; Rennie, P.M. (1995). Renal infarction secondary to nasal insufflation of cocaine. *American Journal of Emergency Medicine* 13:421-423.

Hari, C.K.; Roblin, D.G.; Clayton, M.I.; Nair, R.G. (1999). Acute angle closure glaucoma precipitated by intranasal application of cocaine. *Journal of Laryngology and Otology* 113:250-251.

Hart, C.L.; Jatlow, P.; Sevarino, K.A.; McCance-Katz, E.F. (2000). Comparison of intravenous cocaethylene and cocaine in humans. *Psychopharmacology* 149: 153-162.

Heesch, C.M.; Wilhelm, C.R.; Ristich, J.; Bontempo, F.A.; Wagner, W.R. (2000). Cocaine activates platelets and increases the formation of circulating platelet containing microaggregates in humans. *Heart* 83:688-695.

Herrine, S.K.; Park, P.K.; Wechsler, R.J. (1998). Acute mesenteric ishchemia following intranasal cocaine use. *Digestive Diseases and Sciences* 43:586-589.

Herzlich, B.C.; Arsura, E.L.; Pagala, M.; Grob, D. (1988). Rhabdomyolysis related to cocaine abuse. *Annals of Internal Medicine* 109:335-336.

Hoang, M.P.; Lee, E.L.; Anand, A. (1998). Histologic spectrum of arterial and arteriolar lesions in acute and chronic cocaine-induced mesenteric ischemia. *The American Journal of Surgical Pathology* 22:1404-1410.

Hoffman, C.K.; Goodman, P.C. (1989). Pulmonary edema in cocaine smokers. *Radiology* 172:463-465.

Hollander, J.E.; Hoffman, R.S. (1992). Cocaine-induced myocardial infarction: An analysis and review of the literature. *Journal of Emergency Medicine* 10:169-177.

Hollander, J.E.; Hoffman, R.S. (1998). Cocaine. In Goldfrank, L.R.; Flomenbaum, N.E.; Lewin, N.A.; Weisman, R.S.; Howland, M.A.; Hoffman, R.S. (eds.), *Goldfrank's Toxicologic Emergencies* (pp. 1072-1089). Stamford, CT: Simon and Schuster.

Hon, D.C.; Salloum, L.J.; Hardy, H.W.; Barone, J.E. (1990). Crack-induced enteric ischemia. *New Jersey Medicine* 87:1001-1002.

Hong, R.; Matsuyama, E.; Nur, K. (1991). Cardiomyopathy associated with the smoking of crystal methamphetamine. *Journal of the American Medical Association* 265:1152-1154.

Howard, R.E.; Heuter, D.C.; Davis, G.J. (1985). Acute myocardial infarction following cocaine abuse in a young woman with normal coronary arteries. *Journal of the American Medical Association* 254:95-96.

Imanse, J.; Vanneste, J. (1990). Intraventricular hemorrhage following amphetamine abuse. *Neurology* 40:1318-1319.

Johnson, D.A.; Stafford, P.W.; Volpe, R.J. (1985). Ischemic bowel infarction and phenylpropanolamine use. *Western Journal of Medicine* 142:399-400.

Johnson, T.D.; Berenson, M.M. (1991). Methamphetamine-induced ischemic colitis. *Journal of Clinical Gastroenterology* 13:687-689.

Jones, A.L.; Jarvie, D.R.; McDermid, G.; Proudfoot, A.T. (1994). Hepatocellular damage following amphetamine intoxication. *Clinical Toxicology* 32:435-444.

Kanel, G.C.; Cassidy, W.; Shuster, L.; Reynolds, T.B. (1990). Cocaine-induced liver cell injury: Comparison of morphological features in man and in experimental models. *Hepatology* 11:646-651.

Kapila, Y.L.; Kashani, H. (1997). Cocaine-associated rapid gingival recession and dental erosion. A case report. *Journal of Periodontology* 68:485-488.

Karasch, S.; Vinci, R.; Reece, R. (1990). Esophagitis, epiglottitis, and cocaine alkaloid ("crack"): "Accidental" poisoning or child abuse? *Pediatrics* 86:117-119.

Karch, S.B. (1999). Cocaine: History, use, abuse. *Journal of the Royal Society of Medicine* 92:393-397.

Kissner, D.G.; Lawrence, W.D.; Selis, J.E.; Flint, A. (1987). Crack lung: Pulmonary disease caused by cocaine abuse. *American Review of Respiratory Diseases* 136:1250-1252.

Kloss, M.W.; Rosen, G.M.; Rauckman, E.J. (1984). Cocaine-mediated hepatotoxicity: A critical review. *Biochemical Pharmacology* 33:169-173.

Krutchkoff, D.J.; Eisenberg, E.; O'Brien, J.E.; Ponzillo, J.J. (1990). Cocaine-induced dental erosions (letter). *New England Journal of Medicine* 320:408.

Kudrow, D.B.; Henry, D.A.; Haake, D.A.; Marshall, G.; Mathisen, G. (1988). Botulism associated with *Clostridium botulinum* sinusitis after intranasal cocaine abuse. *Annals of Internal Medicine* 109:984-985.

Lake, C.R.; Gallant, S.; Masson, E.; Miller, P. (1990). Adverse drug effects attributed to phenylpropanolamine: A review of 142 case reports. *American Journal of Medicine* 89:195-208.

Lake, C.R.; Zaloga, G.; Clymer, R.; Quirk, R.; Chernow, B. (1988). A double dose of phenylpropanolamine causes transient hypertension. *American Journal of Medicine* 85:339-343.

Lee, H.S.; LaMaute, H.R.; Pizzi, W.F.; Picard, D.L.; Luks, F.I. (1990). Acute gastroduodenal perforations associated with use of crack. *Annals of Surgery* 211:15-17.

Leo, P.J.; Hollander, J.E.; Shih, R.D.; Marcus, S.M. (1996). Phenylpropanolamine and associated myocardial injury. *Annals of Emergency Medicine* 28:359-362.

Levenson, T.; Greenberger, P.A.; Donoghue, E.R.; Lifschultz, B.D. (1996). Asthma deaths confounded by substance abuse. *Chest* 110:604-610.

Lichtenfeld, P.J.; Rubin, D.B.; Feldman, R.S. (1984). Subarachnoid hemorrhage precipitated by cocaine snorting. *Archives of Neurology* 41:223-224.

Lowenstein, D.H.; Massa, S.M.; Rowbotham, M.C.; Collins, S.D.; McKinney, H.E.; Simon, R.P. (1987). Acute neurologic and psychiatric complications associated with cocaine abuse. *American Journal of Medicine* 83:841-846.

Lundh, H.; Tunving, K. (1981). An extrapyramidal choreiform syndrome caused by amphetamine addiction. *Journal of Neurology, Neurosurgery, and Psychiatry* 44:728-730.

Mallat, A.; Dhumeaux, D. (1991). Cocaine and the liver. *Journal of Hepatology* 12: 275-278.

Manschreck, T.C.; Laughery, J.A.; Weisstein, C.C.; Allen, D.; Humblestone, B.; Neville, M.; Podlewski, H.; Mitra, N. (1988). Characteristics of freebase cocaine psychosis. *Yale Journal of Biology and Medicine* 61:115-122.

Marshall, R.D.; Douglas, C.J. (1994). Phenylpropanolamine-induced psychosis: Potential predisposing factors. *General Hospital Psychiatry* 16:358-360.

Marzuk, P.M.; Tardiff, K.; Leon, A.C.; Hirsch, C.S.; Stajic, M.; Portera, L.; Hartwell, N.; Iqbal, I. (1995). Fatal injuries after cocaine use as a leading cause of death among young adults in New York City. *New England Journal of Medicine* 332:1753-1757.

Mayo-Smith, M.F.; Spinale, J. (1997). Thermal epiglottitis in adults: A new complication of illicit drug abuse. *Journal of Emergency Medicine* 15:483-485.

McHenry, J.G.; Zeiter, J.H.; Mandion, M.P.; Cowden, J.W. (1989). Corneal epithelial defects after smoking crack cocaine. *American Journal of Ophthalmology* 108:732.

Meleca, R.J.; Burgio, D.L.; Carr, R.M.; Lolachi, C.M. (1997). Mucosal injuries of the upper aerodigestive tract after smoking crack or freebase cocaine. *Laryngoscope* 107:620-625.

Mendoza, R.; Miller, B.L.; Mena, I. (1992). Emergency room evaluation of cocaine-associated neuropsychiatric disorders. *Recent Developments in Alcoholism* 10:73-87.

Merigram, K.S.; Roberts, J.R. (1987). Cocaine intoxication: Hyperpyrexia, rhabdomyolysis and acute renal failure. *Clinical Toxicology* 25:135-148.

Miller, W.E.; Spiekerman, R.E.; Hepper, N.G. (1972). Pneumomediastinum resulting from performing Valsalva maneuvers during marijuana smoking. *Chest* 62: 233-234.

Minor, R.L.; Scott, B.D.; Brown, D.D.; Winniford, M.D. (1991). Cocaine-induced myocardial infarction in patients with normal coronary arteries. *Annals of Internal Medicine* 115:797-806.

Mitchell, J.D.; Schwartz, A.L. (1996). Acute angle-closure glaucoma associated with intranasal cocaine abuse. *American Journal of Ophthalmology* 122:425-426.

Morris, J.B.; Shuck, J.M. (1985). Pneumomediastinum in a young male cocaine user (letter). *Annals of Emergency Medicine* 14:164-166.

Mustard, R.; Gray, R.; Maziak, D.; Deck, J. (1992). Visceral infarction caused by cocaine abuse: A case report. *Surgery* 112:951-955.

Myers, J.A.; Earnest, M.P. (1984). Generalized seizures and cocaine abuse. *Neurology* 34:675-676.

Myers, S.I.; Clagett, P.; Valentine, J.; Hansen, M.; Anand, A.; Chervu, A. (1996). Chronic intestinal ischemia caused by intravenous cocaine use: Report of two cases and review of the literature. *Journal of Vascular Surgery* 23:724-729.

Nalbandian, H.; Sheth, N.; Dietrich, R.; Georgiou, J. (1985). Intestinal ischemia caused by cocaine ingestion: Report of two cases. *Surgery* 97:374-376.

National Institute on Drug Abuse (1999). Research Report Series: Cocaine abuse and addiction. NIH Publication Number 99-4342.

Ndikum-Moffor, F.M.; Schoeb, T.R.; Roberts, S.M. (1998). Liver toxicity from norcocaine nitroxide: An n-oxidative metabolite of cocaine. *The Journal of Pharmacology and Experimental Therapeutics* 284:413-419.

Newman, N.M.; DiLoreto, D.A.; Ho, J.T.; Klein, J.C.; Birnbaum, N.S. (1998). Bilateral optic neuropathy and osteolytic sinusitis complications of cocaine abuse. *Journal of the American Medical Association* 259:72-74.

Nolte, K.B.; Brass, L.M.; Fletterick, C.F. (1996). Intracranial hemorrhage associated with cocaine abuse: A prospective autopsy study. *Neurology* 46:1291-1296.

Nzerue, C.M.; Hewan-Lowe, K.; Riley, L.J. (2000). Cocaine and the kidney: A synthesis of pathophysiologic and clinical perspectives. *American Journal of Kidney Diseases* 35:783-795.

Oosterbaan, R.; Burns, M.J. (2000). Myocardial infarction associated with phenylpropanolamine. *Journal of Emergency Medicine* 18:55-59.

Oubeid, M.; Bickel, J.T.; Ingram, E.A.; Scott, G.C. (1990). Pulmonary talc granulomatosis in a cocaine sniffer. *Chest* 98:237-239.

Packe, G.E.; Garton, M.J.; Jennings, K. (1990). Acute myocardial infarction caused by intravenous amphetamine abuse. *British Heart Journal* 64:23-24.

Pentel, P. (1984). Toxicity of over-the-counter stimulants. *Journal of the American Medical Association* 252:1898-1903.

Perino, L.E.; Warren, G.H.; Levine, J.S. (1987). Cocaine-induced hepatotoxicity in humans. *Gastroenterology* 93:176-180.

Perper, J.A.; Van Thiel, D.H. (1992). Respiratory complications of cocaine abuse. *Recent Developments in Alcoholism* 10:363-377.

Pitts, W.R.; Lange, R.A.; Cigarroa, J.E.; Hillis, L.D. (1997). Cocaine-induced myocardial ischemia and infarction: Pathophysiology, recognition, and management. *Progress in Cardiovascular Diseases* 40:65-76.

Plessinger, M.A. (1998). Prenatal exposure to amphetamines: Risks and adverse outcomes in pregnancy. *Obstetrics and Gynecological Clinics of North America* 25: 119-138.

Plessinger, M.A.; Woods, J.R. (1998). Cocaine in pregnancy: Recent data on maternal and fetal risks. *Obstetrics and Gynecology Clinics of North America* 25:99-118.

Rebhun, J. (1988). Association of asthma and freebase smoking. *Annals of Allergy* 60:339-342.

Rich, J.A.; Singer, D.E. (1991). Cocaine-related symptoms in patients presenting to an urban emergency department. *Annals of Emergency Medicine* 20:616-621.

Richards, J.R. (2000). Rhabdomyolysis and drugs of abuse. *Journal of Emergency Medicine* 19:51-56.

Richards, J.R.; Johnson, E.B.; Stark, R.W.; Derlet, R.W. (1999). Methamphetamine abuse and rhabdomyolysis in the ED: A 5-year study. *American Journal of Emergency Medicine* 17:681-685.

Rome, L.A.; Lippmann, M.L.; Dalsey, W.C.; Taggart, P.; Pomerantz, S. (2000). Prevalence of cocaine use and its impact on asthma exacerbation in an urban population. *Chest* 117:1324-1329.

Roth, D.; Alarcon, F.J.; Fernandez, J.A.; Preston, R.A.; Bourgoignie, J.J. (1988). Acute rhabdomyolysis associated with cocaine intoxication. *New England Journal of Medicine* 319:673-677.

Rothrock, J.F.; Rubenstein, R.; Lyden, P.D. (1988). Ischemic stroke associated with methamphetamine inhalation. *Neurology* 38:589-592.

Rowbotham, M.C.; Lowenstein, D.H. (1990). Neurologic consequences of cocaine use. *Annual Review of Medicine* 41:417-422.

Sachs, R.; Zagelbaum, B.M.; Hersh, P.S. (1993). Corneal complications associated with the use of crack cocaine. *Opthalmology* 100:187-191.

Savitt, D.L.; Colagiovanni, S. (1991). Crack cocaine-related epiglottitis (letter). *Annals of Emergency Medicine* 20:322-323.

Schwartz, R.H.; Estroff, T.; Fairbanks, D.; Hoffmann, N.G. (1989). Nasal symptoms associated with cocaine abuse during adolescence. *Archives of Otolaryngology Head and Neck Surgery* 115:63-64.

Sharma, R.; Organ, C.H.; Hirvela, E.R.; Henderson, V.J. (1997). Clinical observation of the temporal association between crack cocaine and duodenal ulcer perforation. *American Journal of Surgery* 174:629-633.

Shesser, R.; Davis, C.; Edelstein, S. (1981). Pneumomediastinum and pneumothorax after inhaling alkaloidal cocaine. *Annals of Emergency Medicine* 10:213-215.

Silva, M.O.; Roth, D.; Reddy, K.R.; Fernandez, J.A.; Albores-Saavedra, J.; Schiff, E.R. (1991). Hepatic dysfunction accompanying acute cocaine intoxication. *Journal of Hepatology* 12:312-315.

Sittel, C.; Eckel, H.E. (1998). Nasal cocaine abuse presenting as a central facial destructive granuloma. *European Archives of Otorhinolaryngology* 255:446-447.

Smith, D.E.; Wesson, D.R.; Apter-Marsh, M. (1984). Cocaine- and alcohol-induced sexual dysfunction in patients with addictive diseases. *Journal of Psychoactive Drugs* 16:359-361.

Suarez, C.A.; Arango, A.; Lester, L. (1977). Cocaine-condom ingestion. *Journal of the American Medical Association* 238:1391-1392.

Susskind, H.; Weber, D.A.; Volkow, N.D.; Hitzemann, R. (1991). Increased lung permeability following long-term use of free-base cocaine (crack). *Chest* 100: 903-909.

Tames, S.M.; Goldenring, J.M. (1986). Madarosis from cocaine use (letter). *New England Journal of Medicine* 314:1324.

Tanen, D.A.; Graeme, K.A.; Curry, S.C. (2000). Crack cocaine ingestion with prolonged toxicity requiring electrical pacing. *Clinical Toxicology* 38:653-657.

Tashkin, D.P.; Kleerup, E.C.; Hoh, C.K.; Kim, K.J.; Webber, M.M.; Gil, E. (1997). Effects of "crack" cocaine on pulmonary alveolar permeability. *Chest* 112:327-335.

Tashkin, D.P.; Kleerup, E.C.; Koyal, S.N.; Marques, J.A.; Goldman, M.D. (1996). Acute effects of inhaled and IV cocaine on airway dynamics. *Chest* 110:904-910.

Thakur, V.K.; Godley, C.; Weed, S.; Cook, M.E.; Hoffman, E. (1996). Cocaine-associated accelerated hypertension and renal failure. *American Journal of Medical Science* 312:295-298.

Tierney, B.P.; Stadelmann, W.K. (1999). Necrotizing infection of the face secondary to intranasal impaction of "crack" cocaine. *Annals of Plastic Surgery* 43: 640-643.

Underdahl, J.P.; Chiou, A. (1998). Preseptal cellulites and orbital wall destruction secondary to nasal cocaine abuse. *American Journal of Ophthalmology* 125: 266-267.

Van Thiel, D.H.; Perper, J.A. (1992). Hepatotoxicity associated with cocaine abuse. *Recent Developments in Alcoholism* 10:335-341.

Vilensky, W. (1982). Illicit and licit drugs causing perforation of the nasal septum. *Journal of Forensic Sciences* 27:958-962.

Wanless, I.R.; Dore, S.; Gopinath, N.; Tan, J.; Cameron, R.; Heathcote, E.J.; Blendis, L.M.; Levy, G. (1990). Histopathology of cocaine hepatotoxicity report of four patients. *Gastroenterology* 98:497-501.

Warner, E.A. (1993). Cocaine abuse. *Annals of Internal Medicine* 119:226-235.

Weddington, W.W. (1993). Cocaine diagnosis and treatment. *Psychiatric Clinics of North America* 16:87-95.

Weiner, R.S.; Lockhart, J.T.; Schwartz, R.G. (1986). Dilated cardiomyopathy and cocaine abuse. *American Journal of Medicine* 81:699-701.

Welch, R.D.; Todd, K.; Krause, G.S. (1991). Incidence of cocaine-associated rhabdomyolysis. *Annals of Emergency Medicine* 20:154-157.

Withers, N.W.; Pulvirenti, L.; Koob, G.F.; Gillin, J.C. (1995). Cocaine abuse and dependence. *Journal of Clinical Psychopharmacology* 15:63-78.

Wohlman, R.A. (1987). Renal artery thrombosis and embolization associated with intravenous cocaine injection. *Southern Medical Journal* 80:928-930.

Wojak, J.C.; Flamm, E.S. (1987). Intracranial hemorrhage and cocaine use. *Stroke* 18:712-715.

Zagelbaum, B.M.; Tannenbaum, M.H.; Hersh, P.S. (1991). *Candida albicans* corneal ulcer associated with crack cocaine. *American Journal of Ophthalmology* 111:248-249.

Zimmerman, F.H.; Gustafson, G.M.; Kemp, H.G. Jr. (1987). Recurrent myocardial infarction associated with cocaine abuse in a young man with normal coronary arteries: Evidence for coronary artery spasm culminating in thrombosis. *Journal of the American College of Cardiology* 9:964-968.

Chapter 9

The Medical and Developmental Consequences of Prenatal Drug Exposure

Karen K. Howell
Claire D. Coles
Julie Kable

OVERVIEW

This chapter addresses the medical and developmental consequences of prenatal exposure to commonly used drugs during pregnancy, such as nicotine, cocaine, and marijuana. The impact of opiate use during pregnancy is also discussed. Both the direct impact of the teratogenic agent as well as social and environmental factors which influence the expression of these agents are presented. When available, the effects of these substances on the growth, cognition, behavior, and social-emotional development of the prenatally exposed child are addressed.

PRINCIPLES OF TERATOLOGY AND BEHAVIORAL TERATOLOGY

The concepts of teratogen exposure and the factors that influence the expression of the teratogen on offspring are important variables in any discussion of the medical and developmental consequences of prenatal drug exposure. A *teratogen* is defined as a substance that causes fetal malformations. The *teratogenic theory* on the effects of prenatal exposure to drugs explains negative consequences of prenatal exposure in terms of direct damage to the fetus caused by exposure during gestation (Coles, 1995). The general principles and mechanisms of teratogenic response were outlined by Wilson (1977), who described six generalizations. These generalizations or principles outline important concepts regarding prenatal exposure to potential teratogens, such as the interaction between the genotype of the fetus and environmental factors; the issue of critical periods for exposure and its expression; the specificity of teratogenic agents; the final manifestations of teratogenic response; the access and nature of the teratogenic agent; and the dose-response relationship of teratogenic agents (Wilson, 1977). More recently, a parallel set of generalizations has been posited for *behavioral teratogenic responses,* or the postnatal effects on behavior of prenatal exposure to teratogenic agents such as drugs (Vorhees, 1986).

MATERNAL SUBSTANCE USE
AND DEVELOPMENTAL IMPACT: TOBACCO

Epidemiology of Tobacco Use in Pregnancy

According to the latest estimates, approximately 27 to 33 percent of women of childbearing age are smokers (Cnattingus, 1989; Ebrahim et al., 2000; Fingerhut et al., 1990; Williamson et al., 1989). Although increasing pressure is being placed on those who smoke to cease during pregnancy, the majority of expecting mothers fail to do so. The Centers for Disease Control (CDC) reports that 20 to 25 percent of expectant mothers continue their tobacco use during gestation (Ebrahim et al., 2000). In the National Health Interview Survey, only 27 percent of women were able to immediately quit use when told that they were pregnant and an additional 12 percent were able to quit by the third trimester of pregnancy (Fingerhut et al., 1990).

Growth Effects

Tobacco use by pregnant women raises concerns about potential teratogenic effects. Nicotine and its by-product, cotinine, are found in fetal serum and amniotic fluid at 15 percent higher concentrations than in maternal blood and last for 15 to 20 hours (Slotkin, 1998). Large amounts of nicotine and cotinine can be ingested by nursing infants of women who smoke (Polifka, 1998). It has been well documented for many years that tobacco exposure affects fetal growth even after controlling for pertinent demographic and confounding variables (Abel, 1984; Werler et al., 1985). The earliest reported study on human infants who were prenatally exposed to tobacco smoke was done by Simpson (1957). She found that the incidence of low birth weight (<2,599 grams) among infants whose mothers smoked was twice as high as the incidence rate among mothers who did not smoke. The incidence of low birth weight in this study was dose related to the quantity of cigarettes smoked per day. Numerous studies have subsequently investigated the relationship between cigarette smoking and birth weight. In reviews of the effects of maternal smoking during pregnancy, the authors agree that there is overwhelming evidence to support the original finding that low birth weight is associated with maternal cigarette smoking (Abel, 1984; Landesman-Dwyer and Emanuel, 1979; Werler et al., 1985; Witter and King, 1980). In addition, this dose-response relationship is found when controlling for such factors as age, parity, maternal weight gain, pre-pregnancy weight/height ratio, gestational age, socioeconomic status, and race (Abel, 1984; Werler et al., 1985). The risk of having a small-for-gesta-tional-age (SGA) infant is two to four times higher for smokers, with smok-ers' neonates weighing an average of 200 grams to 300 grams less than non-smokers' infants (Kearney, 1999). This effect was not found, however, among smokers who quit during their pregnancy. Hebel et al. (1988) re-ported no effect on birth weight among women who quit before week 30 of gestation. Rantakallio (1978) also reported no differences in birth weight between infants whose mothers quit smoking by the third trimester and in-fants whose mothers did not smoke during pregnancy.

Additional physiological variables that have been linked to tobacco smoke exposure after controlling for pertinent demographic and confound-ing variables include decreased gestational length (Landesman-Dwyer and Emanuel, 1979), increased risk of spontaneous abortion (Himmelberger et al., 1978; Kline et al., 1983), and sudden infant death syndrome (Haglund and Cnattingus, 1990). Among the long-term physiological effects of ma-ternal smoking, increased incidence rates of bronchitis and pneumonia have been found (Colley et al., 1974; Harlap and Davies, 1974). Increased inci-dences of asthma (Kershaw, 1987) and increased severity of asthmatic symptoms (Evans et al., 1987) have also been associated with maternal smoking.

Cognitive Effects

Evidence for a general cognitive deficit during infancy and early child-hood in children borne by mothers who smoked during pregnancy is mixed. General cognitive deficits have been found in some studies (e.g., Fried and Watkinson, 1990; Sexton et al., 1990) but not in others (e.g., Makin et al., 1991; Streissguth et al., 1989). Deficits in learning and achievement have also been posited as being associated with maternal smoking. Data from the National Collaborative Perinatal Project (NCPP) have shown that children of smokers have deficiencies in achievement, particularly in the areas of reading and spelling (Hardy and Mellits, 1972; Naeye and Peters, 1984). No difference in achievement has been found in other studies comparing chil-dren of smokers and nonsmokers (Fergusson and Lloyd, 1991; Makin et al., 1991).

Language Effects

Investigations into verbal ability among children of smokers have yielded mixed results as well. Fried and Watkinson (1990) found a difference between the receptive verbal abilities of children of smokers and nonsmokers, although not the expressive abilities of these two groups. This finding was later replicated, with a significant difference between the receptive language skills of children who were prenatally exposed to nicotine and children who were not (Makin et al., 1991). Although deficits in verbal processing have been found, these skills are known to be highly correlated with general cognitive ability. As such, it is difficult to determine the relative contribution of a general cognitive deficit from a specific deficit in verbal processing.

Auditory Processing Effects

Although there are few studies in this area, the evidence for a negative impact on the early auditory development of the children of women who smoked during pregnancy has been more consistent than that for most other outcomes (Fried, 1998). Poorer auditory habituation on standardized infant assessments has been found repeatedly (Fried and Makin, 1987; Jacobson et al., 1985; Picone et al., 1982; Saxton, 1978). In polygraphic studies of sleep, Franco and colleagues (1999) reported that infants of smokers, both newborns and 12-week-olds, showed decreased arousal to auditory stimuli compared to infants of nonsmokers. The evidence in older infants and children is more limited but consistent (e.g., Fried and Watkinson, 1988; Kristjansson et al., 1989). These findings suggest that an underlying auditory processing deficit is associated with prenatal exposure to tobacco smoke that manifests in delays in early language development and later reading and academic skills.

Attention and/or Activity Level Effects

The role which early tobacco exposure plays in producing attentional deficiencies has been explored by a number of researchers. Results of these studies suggest that children who were exposed to tobacco during early development may have subtle deficits in their ability to control and regulate their behavior to meet environmental demands. Naeye and Peters (1984) examined behavioral ratings of children whose mothers smoked during pregnancy and found that these children were rated as having lower attention spans and greater motor activity. Streissguth et al. (1984) found that maternal cigarette use was significantly related to poorer attention and orientation to a vigilance task in children. Kristjansson et al. (1989) also found deficits in auditory and visual vigilance and greater levels of motor activity among children of smokers.

More recently, a growing number of studies have reported associations between maternal smoking during pregnancy and externalizing behavioral problems during childhood and adolescence (Fergusson et al., 1993; Fergusson et al., 1998; Wakschlag et al., 1997; Weitzman et al., 1992). It remains to be seen whether this possible causal relationship may be the result of uncontrolled confounding variables.

Social and Environmental Considerations

Some evidence suggests that the relationship between early tobacco smoke exposure and behavioral outcomes may be the consequence of a different psychosocial environment created by a parent who chooses to smoke. Differences have been found in the manner in which parents who smoke relate to their children when compared to parents who do not smoke. Fried and Watkinson (1988) found that nicotine use was negatively related to maternal involvement with the child, opportunities for variety in daily routines, emotional/verbal responsivity to the mother, avoidance of restriction and punishment, organization of the physical and temporal environment, and provision of appropriate play materials. Furthermore, researchers have hypothesized that important personality characteristics, behaviors, and lifestyle variables differentiate smokers and nonsmokers. Smokers differ from nonsmokers on measures of anxiety, extroversion, nurturance, and deference. They report more symptoms of psychopathology, have more hospitalizations, lower status occupations, and more job changes than nonsmokers (Eysenck, 1980, 1991; Krogh, 1991; McManus and Weeks, 1982; Schneider and Houston, 1970; Matarazzo and Saslow, 1960; Eysenck et al., 1960; Lilienfeld, 1959). It remains to be seen whether any of these characteristics that exist between smokers and nonsmokers may be capable of mediating the relationship found between tobacco smoke exposure and teratogenic outcome variables.

Summary

No consistent evidence among available studies indicates that smoking during pregnancy is associated with major structural anomalies. Clear associations exist between prenatal cigarette smoking and low birth weight, perinatal death, alterations in fetal cardiorespiratory status, problems with long-term growth, and sudden infant death syndrome (Behnke and Eyler, 1993).

ILLICIT DRUG USE: COCAINE

Epidemiology of Cocaine Use in Pregnancy

Although the epidemic of cocaine and crack use that began in the 1980s has waned, the problem of prenatal exposure to cocaine persists. According to the National Institute on Drug Abuse (NIDA, 1996), approximately 2.3 percent of women of childbearing age have used cocaine in the past year and many of these women continue to use when pregnant. This figure may be higher in certain population subgroups and lower in others. In 1994, using blood drawn from a cohort of neonates, about 0.1 percent of all births were reported to have been exposed to cocaine (Brantley et al., 1996), with a higher incidence among older women, those delivering without prenatal care, and inner-city populations. Most women reporting cocaine use also used tobacco, alcohol, and cocaine, and some combined the use of cocaine or crack with heroin (Day et al., 1993).

Because of concerns raised during the "crack baby" period (Coles, 1993), extensive examination occurred of the teratogenic potential of this drug in both animal models and clinical studies. Although in 1993 one could conclude that inadequate data existed to support conclusions about the effects of this drug (e.g., Coles and Platzman, 1993), during the latter half of the 1990s many studies were published that provide considerable understanding of this area, at least during infancy and the preschool period (see Eyler and Behnke, 1999; Tronick and Beeghly, 1999, for reviews).

Growth Effects

Cocaine exposure has been associated with lower gestational age and reduced growth parameters at birth in a number of studies (Chouteau et al., 1988; Kliegman et al., 1994). Because cocaine users have many other characteristics that may be associated with such outcomes, interpretation of these effects can be difficult (Holtzman and Paneth, 1994). However, Kliegman and colleagues (1994) found that cocaine exposure was associated with preterm birth as well as lower birth weight even when associated factors were controlled for statistically. Richardson et al. (1999) controlled for the effects of prenatal care by comparing the effects of cocaine use for both those who had prenatal care and those who did not. They found that cocaine had a significant impact on both gestational age and birth weight in each group even when the effects of alcohol, marijuana, and tobacco were controlled. Even when growth effects are observed, interpreting the relationship may not be straightforward. While examining the relationship between gestational age and cocaine exposure in neonates, Brown and colleagues (1998) found that lower birth weight was characteristic only of full-term cocaine-exposed infants, suggesting that such effects occurred in the third trimester. In contrast, Richardson and colleagues (1999) found that growth effects in their sample were attributable to exposure during the first and second trimesters. Finally, even when statistically significant effects are found during the neonatal period, cocaine-exposed children do not have "clinically significant" growth failure and often appear to have a postnatal "catch-up" in growth. For instance, while comparing preterm and full-term cocaine-exposed infants to socioeconomic status (SES)-matched contrast groups, Coles and colleagues (2000) found that growth differences could no longer be observed by eight weeks of age and there were no differences in growth rate over 24 months for weight, length, or ponderal index.

Motor Development

Early studies of cocaine effects identified reflexive behavior and motor development as areas of concern. Schneider and Chasnoff (1992) compared 30 full-term four-month-old infants exposed to cocaine (and other drugs) to 50 unexposed infants using the Movement Assessment of Infants (MAI). Exposed infants were found to have higher risk scores on motor tone, primitive reflexes, and volitional movements. Swanson and colleagues (1999) found poorer mean scores on the volitional movements subscale of the MAI as well as the total risk score among four-month-old exposed infants compared to controls. Fetters and Tronick (1996) followed 28 cocaine-exposed and 22 control infants to 15 months and found a negative drug effect on motor performance at this age. The authors note, however, that both cocaine-exposed and contrast groups of children performed more poorly than would be expected from the age norms.

Arendt and his colleagues (1999) used the Psychomotor Index of the Bayley Scales of Infant Development (BSID) (Bayley, 1993) and the MAI as well as other measures of sensorimotor development in a sample of inner-city children exposed to cocaine. They found small but significant effects of cocaine and other drug exposure on a variety of motor indicators both early in infancy and at 12 months. At 24 months, children from this sample were reassessed using the Peabody Developmental Motor Scales with the cocaine-exposed group performing significantly lower on both fine and gross motor development indices. The effects appeared to be more significant in the fine motor rather than the gross motor area.

Later in infancy (e.g., Chasnoff et al., 1992; Jacobson et al., 1996) motor differences are not described by most investigators. This discrepancy may be the result of differences in the measurement tools used. Those studies reporting effects often used the MAI, while those that did not used the BSID. As more longitudinal data is published, it will be possible to evaluate the implications of observed differences in motor function for later development.

Behavioral Effects

Initially, severe consequences were anticipated in this area of development (Coles, 1993), although the evidence to support such effects was not strong. Studies of newborns provided conflicting information about the immediate impact of maternal cocaine use during gestation. In a meta-analysis, Held and colleagues (1999) critically reviewed Brazelton Neurobehavioral Assessment Scale (BNBAS) studies of infants (Brazelton, 1984). It was concluded that while effects could be found reliably on motor performance, abnormal reflexes, orientation, and autonomic regulation, the effect size was small and tended to diminish over the first month of life. As well-controlled studies of later development are reported, evidence of direct teratogenic effects on cognition have been limited (Hurt et al., 1997; Tronick and Beeghly, 1999), although children born to drug-using mothers in low SES populations continue to be at risk for nonoptimal development in many domains. For instance, in a follow-up study that examined outcomes at four to six years, Chasnoff and colleagues (1998) reported that differences in developmental functioning in their clinical samples can be accounted for by environmental factors, principally, caregiver behavior. Singer et al. (1997) reported that prenatal cocaine and alcohol exposure as well as maternal postpartum psychological distress directly impacted the BSID Mental Development Index (MDI) while Psychomotor Index (PI) scores were affected only by cocaine. Kilbride and colleagues (2000) reported that at 36 months no effects on cognition, psychomotor skills, or language were observed in exposed children who had received case management services, compared to those who did not receive services and a nonexposed contrast group. Kilbride et al. also found that those exposed children who remained with their mothers and did not receive services had lower verbal scores on intelligence tests and measures of language development. In contrast, Richardson (1998) found that in three-year-olds, cocaine exposure was associated with lower scores on some of the subtests of the Stanford-Binet (fourth edition), including composite IQ scores and short-term memory scores, although all children scored within the typical range of development. A previous study of a different cohort of children by the same author (Richardson et al., 1996) did not show effects on cognition, demonstrating the extent to which these outcomes are dependent on sampling and other methodological considerations.

Language Development

A number of studies have identified deficiencies in the early language development of children born to cocaine-using women. Bland-Stewart et al. (1998) compared semantic content category in a small sample of low-SES infants exposed to cocaine with a contrast group matched for social class and ethnicity and found some restriction in the development of semantic representations (meaning) in the children of cocaine users. No effect was observed in the structural features of language, that is, mean length of utterance (MLU) and utterance type, or for general language and cognitive functioning. In contrast, Hurt and colleagues (1997) found no differences in language functioning at two-and-a-half years when cocaine-exposed and contrast children from the same SES group were compared using the Preschool Language Scale (PLS), a standardized measure of early language development. In reviewing the literature in this area, Mentis (1998) suggested that there is not yet sufficient evidence for definitive statements about the language development of this group of children. While language development may be disrupted, the factors affecting such development are numerous and their interaction is complex. She also suggested that deficits may be specific to certain areas of language function and are only evident under stressful conditions.

Play Behavior

Play behavior is often assessed as an indicator of children's functional status that does not require standardized testing. Play behavior has been examined in a number of studies of cocaine- and polydrug-exposed children that followed an initial study by Rodning et al. (1989) that reported alterations in the usual play patterns. Subsequent studies have been inconsistent in reported outcomes. Metosky and Vondra (1995) reported differences in play analogous to Rodning and colleagues (1989), while several other investigators have not found evidence of differences in the play of toddlers that can be attributed to the direct effects of cocaine (e.g., Beeghley et al., 1995; Hagen and Myers, 1997; Hurt et al., 1992) when associated factors are controlled. These outcomes suggest that such behavioral observations may be accounted for by environmental factors or group differences.

Arousal Regulation and Attention

The most persuasive evidence for a behavioral effect of cocaine concerns the impact on physiological arousal (e.g., heart rate, respiration) in early infancy and, by extension, on temperament and social/emotional development. Mayes (1999) provides an animal model of this phenomenon that suggests that dopamine regulation has been impacted. Several investigators have identified increased irritability in young infants and alterations in psychophysiology, including heart rate and respiration (Brown et al., 1998; DiPietro et al., 1994). These effects appear to persist beyond the neonatal period. At eight weeks, Bard and colleagues (2000) identified cocaine-related alterations in baseline heart rate and respiration as well as differences in response to moderate stress that appeared to be drug-related. Karmel, Gardner, and their colleagues (Karmel and Gardner, 1996; Karmel et al., 1996) identified cocaine-related differences in attention and arousal modulation in newborns that persisted through four months of age. At four months, Bendersky and Lewis (1998) found that exposed infants were less able to modulate arousal. Other systems, such as sleep (Coles et al., 2000), appear to be impacted during the toddler period. That cognition may also be affected in some manner is suggested by reported effects on early attention. Mayes et al. (1995) reported that cocaine exposure affected three-month-old children's ability to complete a procedure measuring attention. Coles and colleagues (1999) found differences in attentional response associated with prenatal cocaine, but not other drug exposure at eight weeks. However, as these authors note, the caregiving instability associated with maternal drug use independently accounted for more variance in attentional response than did the direct effect of cocaine. These findings raise concerns about the vulnerability of exposed children. In addition to physiological dysregulation associated with prenatal exposure to cocaine and other drugs, exposed children are clearly also at environmental risk to an increased incidence of developmental psychopathology.

Summary

Prenatal cocaine exposure is a marker for a number of risk factors that appear to have negative consequences for the infant and developing child. No specific "cocaine syndrome" has yet emerged and many of the problems previously anticipated have not manifested. However, the weight of the evidence suggests that cocaine exposure may produce an increased vulnerability to certain environmental stressors. The interactions of these factors may have long-term negative consequences for children.

MARIJUANA

Epidemiology of Marijuana Use in Pregnancy

In a recent NIDA survey (1996) of the prevalence and patterns of substance use among pregnant women, 2.8 percent reported marijuana use during their first trimester of pregnancy. This indicates that marijuana is the most commonly used illicit drug and, after alcohol and tobacco, the most commonly used drug during pregnancy (Goldschmidt et al., 2000). As Fried observed (1996), this makes the paucity of objective information on the relationship between marijuana use during pregnancy and the impact of such use upon the outcome of the child all the more striking.

Growth Effects

Of the longitudinal studies of marijuana use during pregnancy, most find few significant effects on growth parameters. Day and colleagues (1991) obtained neonatal outcome data on more than 500 infants born prenatally exposed to varying amounts of marijuana in utero. There were few significant effects of marijuana use during pregnancy on birth weight, head or chest circumference, gestational age, or growth retardation. There was a small but significant negative effect of marijuana use during the first two months of pregnancy on birth length and a positive effect of marijuana use during the third trimester on birth weight. In a more recent study of growth from birth to early adolescence in offspring prenatally exposed to marijuana, this exposure was not significantly related to any growth measure (Fried et al., 1999).

Behavioral Effects

Much of the existing information concerning the behavioral effects of prenatal exposure to marijuana comes from reports of the Ottawa Prenatal Prospective Study (OPPS) (Fried, 1996) and the work of Nancy Day and her colleagues (1991). The first report from the Ottawa study examined four-day-old infants born to regular marijuana users and found that prenatal exposure to marijuana was associated with decreased rates of visual habituation and increased tremors. Similar observations were also noted at nine and 30 days of age (Fried and Makin, 1987). When these same children were examined at one year of age, no adverse effects of prenatal marijuana exposure were noted (Fried and Watkinson, 1988). Fried et al. (1992) noted the difficulty in unraveling the long-term consequences of in utero marijuana exposure. Although some observations of a neurobehavioral effect on verbal ability and memory of four-year-old subjects was noted, this relationship did not persist at ages two, three, five, or six years after statistically adjusting for other important variables such as ratings of the home environment.

Arousal Regulation and Attention

A few research findings indicate that prenatal marijuana exposure has an effect on child behavior problems at preschool and school age. In a prospective study of the effects of prenatal marijuana exposure on child behavior problems at age ten, prenatal marijuana exposure in the first and third trimesters predicted significantly increased hyperactivity, inattention, and impulsivity symptoms (Goldschmidt et al., 2000). These results are consistent with the work of O'Connell and Fried (1991) who found a significant tendency for mothers who used marijuana heavily during pregnancy to rate their children as being more impulsive or hyperactive. The authors note, however, that it remains to be seen whether these results indicate a true behavioral difference in the attention-related domain or a lowered parental tolerance.

Social and Environmental Considerations

According to Goldschmidt et al. (2000), it is difficult to isolate the effects of marijuana exposure from its correlates and from environmental risk factors. Variables such as socioeconomic status, access to medical and social services, and the presence or absence of a male figure in the household have a significant influence on child development. Maternal mental health, social support networks, stressful life events such as exposure to violence or domestic abuse are also important variables that impact long-term developmental outcomes. Many of these environmental risk factors are directly associated with maternal marijuana use, making it difficult to identify the impact of prenatal exposure in isolation.

Summary

After statistically controlling for maternal personality and home environment conditions, many of the neurobehavioral consequences of prenatal exposure to marijuana do not remain significant. According to Fried (1996), the only definitive statement regarding prenatal exposure to marijuana would be that, if there are long-term consequences of prenatal exposure to marijuana, such effects are very subtle. At this point there are few human studies on the effects of marijuana use during pregnancy and no precise mechanism of action has been substantiated (Behnke and Eyler, 1993).

OPIATES

Epidemiology of Opiate Use in Pregnancy

The literature regarding developmental outcomes for infants prenatally exposed to opiates is relatively sparse and was primarily generated in the 1970s and early 1980s. The literature is also made more problematic by the issue of polysubstance abuse, as research investigating prenatal opiate exposure includes exposure to heroin, methadone, or both, and may also include exposure to amphetamines, barbiturates, benzodiazepines, cocaine, alcohol, and nicotine (Kaltenbach, 1996). Recent studies report prevalence for opiate use during pregnancy to range from less than 1 to 2 percent to as high as 21 percent (Chasnoff et al., 1990; McCalla et al., 1991; Ostrea et al., 1992).

Growth/Physiological Effects

The most consistently reported effect of prenatal opiate exposure is associated with fetal growth retardation and neonatal abstinence syndrome (Behnke and Eyler, 1993). Neonatal abstinence is described by Kaltenbach and Finnegan (1986) as a generalized disorder characterized by signs and symptoms of central nervous system hyperirritability, gastrointestinal dysfunction, respiratory distress, and vague autonomic symptoms that include yawning, sneezing, mottling, and fever. These early neurobehavioral outcomes do not persist, however (Finnegan, 1979; Householder et al., 1982).

Within the past decade, methadone maintenance has become accepted as the standard of care for opiate addiction during pregnancy (Kandall et al., 1999). Methadone treatment stabilizes maternal drug levels and reduces the amount of polydrug use and associated complications (Kearney, 1997). According to Kandall and colleagues (1999), no study has yet reported either a higher rate of malformations compared with control populations or an increase in any specific dysmorphic syndrome which could be related to maternal methadone use during pregnancy. Methadone treatment during pregnancy is associated with increased fetal growth and higher birth weights in offspring compared with heroin-exposed infants in earlier studies (Connaughton et al., 1975; Zelson, 1973), although these findings have not been supported by more recent studies (Householder et al., 1982; Zuckerman and Bresnahan, 1991).

Cognitive Effects

Studies on the early development of methadone-exposed offspring indicate relatively normal development, at least during infancy (de Cubas and Field, 1993). In studies by Hans and her colleagues, no differences in mental development were found at four months, 12 months, and 24 months of age when comparing opiate-exposed and nonexposed children (Hans, 1989; Hans and Marcus, 1983). Kaltenbach and Finnegan (1986) found no differences in mental development scores at six months, 12 months, and 24 months when the two groups were compared. Between three and six years of age, heroin-exposed children performed more poorly than their peers on a cognitive index in one study, but the same on behavior and skills in another study (Kearney, 1999). Kaltenbach (1996) concludes her review of the effects of prenatal opiate exposure by stating that opiate-exposed infants through two years of age function well within the normal range of development and that children between two and five years of age do not differ in cognitive function from other high-risk populations.

Social and Environmental Considerations

Illicit drug use is associated with late and inadequate prenatal care, poverty, poor nutrition, domestic and stranger violence, and other severe threats to maternal and infant health (Frohna et al., 1999). It is especially difficult to identify the impact of a specific illicit substance such as heroin due to the issue of polysubstance abuse. As with cocaine exposure, outcomes of heroin and methadone exposure are more strongly related to home and parenting environment variables than to direct drug effects (Hans, 1996; Kaltenbach, 1996).

SUMMARY: IMPACT OF MATERNAL SUBSTANCE USE

Children of mothers who abuse drugs during pregnancy are affected by a range of biological and environmental factors. At the present time, it is clear that there are negative effects of substance abuse on fetal development and family function and that these consequences must be addressed. The physical and behavioral problems seen in children with prenatal exposure to drugs are the result of many related factors such as poverty, exposure to violence, and lack of access to medical and social services. These factors likely interact with the initial prenatal drug exposure to negatively impact long-term developmental outcomes for the child.

REFERENCES

Abel, E.L. (1984). Smoking and pregnancy. *Journal of Psychoactive Drugs, 16,* 327-338.

Arendt, R.; Angelopoulos, J.; Salvator, A.; Singer, L. (1999). Motor development of cocaine-exposed children at age two years. *Pediatrics, 103,* 86-92.

Bard, K.A.; Coles, C.D.; Platzman, K.A.; Lynch, M.A. (2000). The effects of prenatal drug exposure, term status, and caregiving on arousal and arousal modulation in 8-week-old infants. *Developmental Psychobiology, 36,* 194-212.

Bayley, N. (1993). *Bayley Scales of Infant Development.* San Antonio, TX: Psychological Corporation.

Beeghly, M.; Tronick, E.; Brilliant, G.; High, A.; Flaherty, C.; Cabral, H.; Frank, D. (1995). *Object play and affect of in-utero cocaine exposed and nonexposed infants at 1 year: Characteristics and context effects* (abstract). Presented at the biennial meeting of the Society for Research on Child Development. Providence, RI, April.

Behnke, M.; Eyler, F.D. (1993). The consequences of prenatal substance use for the developing fetus, newborn, and young child. *The International Journal of the Addictions, 28*(13), 1341-1391.

Bendersky, M.; Lewis, M. (1998). Arousal modulation in cocaine-exposed infants. *Developmental Psychology, 34,* 555-564.

Bland-Stewart, L.M.; Seymour, H.N.; Beeghly, M.; Frank, D.A. (1998). Semantic development of African-American children prenatally exposed to cocaine. *Seminars in Speech and Language, 19,* 167-187.

Brantley, M.; Rochat, R.; Floyd, V.; Norris, D.; Franko, E.; Blake, P.; Toomey, K.; Mayer, L.; Ziegler, B.; Fernhoff, P.M. (1996). Population-based prevalence of perinatal exposure to cocaine—Georgia, 1994. *Morbidity and Mortality Weekly Report, 41,* 887-891.

Brazelton, T.B. (1984). *Neonatal Behavioral Scales.* Vol. 88 of *Clinics in Developmental Medicine.*

Brazelton, T.B.; Nugent, J.K. (1995). *Neonatal assessment* (Third edition). Clinics in Developmental Medicine, Cambridge: McKeith Press.

Brown, J.V.; Bakeman, R.; Coles, C.D.; Sexson, W.R.; Demi, A. (1998). Maternal drug use, fetal growth, and newborn behavior: Are preterms and fullterms affected differently? *Developmental Psychology, 34*(3), 540-554.

Chasnoff, I.J.; Anson, A.; Hatcher, R.; Stenson, H.; Iaukea, K.; Randolph, L.A. (1998). Prenatal exposure to cocaine and other drugs: Outcome at four to six years. *Annals of the New York Academy of Sciences, 846,* 314-328.

Chasnoff, I.J.; Griffith, D.R.; Freier, C.; Murray, J. (1992). Cocaine/polydrug use in pregnancy: Two year follow-up. *Pediatrics, 89*(2), 284-289.

Chasnoff, I.J.; Landress, H.J.; Barrett, M.E. (1990). The prevalence of illicit-drug or alcohol use during pregnancy and discrepancies in mandatory reporting in Pinellas County, Florida. *New England Journal of Medicine, 322,* 1202-1206.

Chouteau, M.; Namerow, P.B.; Leppert, P. (1988). The effect of cocaine abuse on birth weight and gestational age. *Obstetrics and Gynecology, 72,* 351-354.

Cnattingus, S. (1989). Smoking habits in early pregnancy. *Addictive Behaviors, 14,* 453-457.

Coles, C.D. (1993). Saying "goodbye" to the "crack baby." *Neurotoxicology and Teratology, 5,* 290-292.

Coles, C.D. (1995). Children of parents who abuse drugs and alcohol. In Smith, G.H.; Coles, C.D.; Poulsen, M.K.; Cole, C.K. (eds.), *Children, Families, and Substance Abuse: Challenges for Changing Educational and Social Outcomes* (pp. 3-23). Baltimore: Paul H. Brookes.

Coles, C.D.; Bard, K.A.; Bakeman, R.; Platzman, K.A.; Lynch, M.E.; Moretto, S. (2000). *Neurodevelopment and growth in drug-exposed and preterm infants.* Poster presented at the International Conference on Infancy Studies. Brighton, UK, July.

Coles, C.D.; Bard, K.A.; Platzman, K.A.; Lynch, M.E. (1999). Attentional response at 8 weeks in prenatally drug-exposed and preterm infants. *Neurotoxicology and Teratology, 21*(5), 527-537.

Coles, C.D.; Platzman, K.A. (1993). Behavioral development in children prenatally exposed to drugs and alcohol. *The International Journal of the Addictions, 28,* 1393-1433.

Colley, J.R.; Holland, W.W.; Corkhill, R.T. (1974). Influence of passive smoking and parental phlegm on pneumonia and bronchitis in early childhood. *Lancet, 2,* 1031-1034.

Connaughton, J.F.; Finnegan, L.P.; Schut, J.; Emich, J.P. (1975). Current concepts in the management of the pregnant opiate addict. *Addictive Diseases, 2,* 21-35.

Day, N.L.; Cottreau, C.M.; Richardson, G.A. (1993). The epidemiology of alcohol, marijuana, and cocaine use among women of child-bearing age and pregnant women. *Clinical Obstetrics and Gynecology, 36,* 232-245.

Day, N.; Sambamoorthi, U.; Taylor, P.; Richardson, G.; Robles, N.; Jhon, Y.; Scher, M.; Stoffer, D.; Cornelius, M.; Jasperse, D. (1991). Prenatal marijuana use and neonatal outcome. *Neurotoxicology and Teratology, 13,* 329-334.

de Cubas, M.M.; Field, T. (1993). Children of methadone-dependent women: Developmental outcomes. *American Journal of Orthopsychiatry, 63*(2), 266-276.

DiPietro, J.A.; Caughy, M.O.; Cusson, R.; Fox, N.A. (1994). Cardiorespiratory functioning of preterm infants: Stability and risk associations for measures of heart rate variability and oxygen saturation. *Developmental Psychobiology, 27,* 137-152.

Ebrahim, S.H.; Floyd, R.L.; Merritt, R.K.; Decoufle, P.; Holtzman, D. (2000). Trends in pregnancy-related smoking rates in the United States, 1987-1996. *Journal of the American Medical Association, 283*(3), 361-366.

Evans, D.; Levison, M.J.; Feldman, C.H.; Clark, N.M.; Wasilewski, Y.; Levin, B.; Mellins, R.B. (1987). The impact of passive smoking on emergency room visits of urban children with asthma. *American Journal of Respiratory Disease, 135,* 567-572.

Eyler, F.D.; Behnke, M. (1999). Early development of infants exposed to drugs prenatally. *Clinics in Perinatology, 26*(1), 107-150.

Eysenck, H.J. (1980). *The causes and effects of smoking.* London: Maurice Temple Smith.

Eysenck, H.J. (1991). *Smoking, personality, and stress: Psychosocial factors in the prevention of cancer and coronary heart disease.* New York: Springer-Verlag.

Eysenck, H.J.; Tarrant, M.; Woolf, M.; England, L. (1960). Smoking and personality. *British Medical Journal, 1,* 1456-1460.

Fergusson, D.M.; Horwood, L.J.; Lynskey, M.T. (1993). Maternal smoking before and after pregnancy: Effects on behavioral outcomes in middle childhood. *Pediatrics, 92,* 815-822.

Fergusson, D.M.; Lloyd, M. (1991). Smoking during pregnancy and its effects on child cognitive ability from the ages of 8 to 12 years. *Pediatric and Perinatal Epidemiology, 5,* 189-200.

Fergusson, D.M.; Woodward, L.J.; Horwood, L.J. (1998). Maternal smoking during pregnancy and psychiatric adjustment in late adolescence. *Archives of General Psychiatry, 55*(8), 721-727.

Fetters, L.; Tronick, E.Z. (1996). Neuromotor development of cocaine-exposed and control infants from birth through 15 months: Poor and poorer performance. *Pediatrics, 98,* 938-943.

Fingerhut, L.A.; Kleinman, J.C.; Kendrick, J.S. (1990). Smoking before, during, and after pregnancy. *American Journal of Pharmacy, 80,* 541-544.

Finnegan, L.P. (1979). Pathophysiological and behavioral effects of the transplacental transfer of narcotic drugs to the fetuses and neonates of narcotic-dependent mothers. *Bulletin of Narcotics, 31*(3), 1-58.

Franco, P.; Groswasser, J.; Hassid, S.; Lanquart, J.P.; Scaillet, S.; Kahn, A. (1999). Prenatal exposure to cigarette smoking is associated with a decrease in arousal in infants. *Journal of Pediatrics, 135,* 34-38.

Fried, P. A. (1996). Behavioral outcomes in preschool and school-age children exposed prenatally to marijuana: A review and speculative interpretation. In Wetherington, C.L.; Smeriglio, V.L.; and Finnegan, L.P. (eds.), *Behavioral Studies of Drug-Exposed Offspring: Methodological Issues in Human and Animal Research* (pp. 242-260). Rockville, MD: NIDA.

Fried, P.A. (1998). Cigarette smoke exposure and hearing loss. *Journal of the American Medical Association, 280,* 963.

Fried, P.A.; Makin, J.E. (1987). Neonatal behavioral correlates of prenatal exposure to marijuana, cigarettes, and alcohol in a low risk population. *Neurotoxicology and Teratology, 9,* 1-7.

Fried, P.A.; Watkinson, B. (1988). Twelve- and twenty-four-month neurobehavioral follow-up of children prenatally exposed to marijuana, cigarettes, and alcohol. *Neurotoxicology and Teratology, 10,* 305-313.

Fried, P.A.; Watkinson, B. (1990). Thirty-six- and forty-eight-month neurobehavioral follow-up of children prenatally exposed to marijuana, cigarettes, and alcohol. *Developmental and Behavioral Pediatrics, 11,* 49-58.

Fried, P.A.; Watkinson, B.; Gray, R. (1992). A follow-up study of attentional behavior in 6-year-old children exposed prenatally to marijuana, cigarettes, and alcohol. *Neurotoxicology and Teratology, 14,* 299-311.

Fried, P.A.; Watkinson, B.; Gray, R. (1999). Growth from birth to early adolescence in offspring prenatally exposed to cigarettes and marijuana. *Neurotoxicology and Teratology, 21*(5), 513-525.

Frohna, J.G.; Lantz, P.M.; Pollack, H. (1999). Maternal substance abuse and infant health: Policy options across the life course. *The Milbank Quarterly, 77*(4), 531-570.

Goldschmidt, L.; Day, N.L.; Richardson, G.A. (2000). Effects of prenatal marijuana exposure on child behavior problems at age 10. *Neurotoxicology and Teratology, 22*, 325-336.

Hagan, R.; Myers, B.J. (1997). Mother-toddler play interaction: A contrast of substance exposed and nonexposed children. *Infant Mental Health Journal, 18*(1), 40-57.

Haglund, B.; Cnattingus, S. (1990). Cigarette smoking as a risk factor for sudden infancy death syndrome: A population-based study. *American Journal of Health, 80*, 29-32.

Hans, S.L. (1989). Developmental consequences of prenatal exposure to methadone. *Annals of the New York Academy of Science, 562*, 195-207.

Hans, S.L. (1996). Prenatal drug exposure: Behavioral functioning in late childhood and adolescence. In Wetherington, C.L.; Smeriglio, V.L.; and Finnegan, L.P. (eds.), *Behavioral Studies of Drug-Exposed Offspring: Methodological Issues in Human and Animal Research* (pp. 261-276). Rockville, MD: NIDA.

Hans, S.L.; Marcus, J. (1983). Motor and attentional behavior in infants of methadone maintained women. In Harris, L. (ed.), *Problems of Drug Dependence*. Rockville, MD: NIDA.

Hardy, J.B.; Mellits, E.D. (1972). Does maternal smoking during pregnancy have a long-term effect on the child? *Lancet, 1*, 1332-1336.

Harlap, S.; Davies, A.M. (1974). Infant admissions to hospital and maternal smoking. *Lancet, 2*, 529-532.

Hebel, J.R.; Fox, N.L.; Sexton, M. (1988). Dose-response of birth weight to various measures of maternal smoking during pregnancy. *Journal of Clinical Epidemiology, 41*, 483-489.

Held, J.R.; Riggs, M.L.; Dorman, C. (1999). The effect of prenatal cocaine exposure on neonatal outcome. *Neurotoxicology and Teratology, 21*, 619-625.

Himmelberger, D.U.; Brown, B.W.; Cohen, E.N. (1978). Cigarette smoking during pregnancy and the occurrence of spontaneous abortion and congenital abnormality. *American Journal of Epidemiology, 108*, 470-479.

Holtzman, C.; Paneth, N. (1994). Maternal cocaine use during pregnancy and perinatal outcomes. *Epidemiological Review, 16*, 315-320.

Householder, J.; Hatcher, R.; Burns, W.; Chasnoff, I. (1982). Infants born to narcotic-addicted mothers. *Psychological Bulletin, 92*, 453-468.

Hurt, H.; Brodsky, N.L.; Giannetta, J. (1992). Comparison of play behaviors in cocaine exposed and control toddlers: A prospective study. *Pediatric Research, 11A*, 31.

Hurt, H.; Malmud, E.; Betancourt, L.; Braitman, L.E.; Brodsky, N.L.; Giannetta, J. (1997). Children with in utero cocaine exposure do not differ from control subjects on intelligence testing. *Archives of Pediatric and Adolescent Medicine, 151,* 1237-1241.

Jacobson, J.L.; Jacobson, S.W.; Sokol, R.J.; Martier, S.S.; Chiodo, L.M. (1996). New evidence for neurobehavioral effects of in utero cocaine exposure. *Journal of Pediatrics, 129*(4), 581-590.

Jacobson, S.W.; Fein, G.G.; Jacobson, J.L.; Schwartz, P.M.; Dowler, J.K. (1985). The effect of PCB exposure on visual recognition memory. *Child Development, 56,* 853-860.

Kaltenbach, K.A. (1996). Exposure to opiates: Behavioral outcomes in preschool and school-age children. In Wetherington, C.L.; Smeriglio, V.L.; and Finnegan, L.P. (eds.), *Behavioral Studies of Drug-Exposed Offspring: Methodological Issues in Human and Animal Research* (pp. 230-241). Rockville, MD: NIDA.

Kaltenbach, K.A.; Finnegan, L.P. (1986). Neonatal abstinence syndrome: Pharmacotherapy and developmental outcome. *Neurobehavioral Toxicology and Teratology, 8,* 353-355.

Kandall, S.R.; Doberczak, T.M.; Jantunen, M.; Stein, J. (1999). The methadone-maintained pregnancy. *Clinics in Perinatology, 26*(1), 173-183.

Karmel, B.Z.; Gardner, J.M. (1996). Prenatal cocaine exposure effects on arousal-modulated attention during the neonatal period. *Developmental Psychobiology, 29,* 463-480.

Karmel, B.Z.; Gardner, J.M.; Freedland, R.L. (1996). Arousal-modulated attention at four months as a function of intrauterine cocaine exposure and central nervous system injury. *Journal of Pediatric Psychology, 21,* 821-832.

Kearney, M.H. (1997). Drug treatment for women: Traditional models and new directions. *Journal of Obstetric, Gynecologic, and Neonatal Nursing, 26,* 449-458.

Kearney, M.H. (1999). *Perinatal impact of alcohol, tobacco, and other drugs.* White Plains, NY: March of Dimes Publishing.

Kershaw, C.R. (1987). Passive smoking, potential atopy, and asthma in the first five years. *Journal of the Royal Society of Medicine, 80,* 683-688.

Kilbride, H.; Castor, C.; Hoffman, E.; Fuger, K.L. (2000). Thirty-six-month outcome of prenatal cocaine exposure for term or near-term infants: Impact of early case management. *Developmental and Behavioral Pediatrics, 21,* 19-26.

Kliegman, R.M.; Madura, D.; Kiwi, R.; Eisenberg, I.; Yamashita, T. (1994). Relation of maternal cocaine use to the risks of prematurity and low birth weight. *Journal of Pediatrics, 124,* 751-756.

Kline, J.; Levin, B.; Shrout, P.; Stein, Z.; Susser, M.; Warburton, D. (1983). Maternal smoking and trisomy among spontaneously aborted conceptions. *American Journal of Human Genetics, 35,* 421-431.

Kristjansson, E.A.; Fried, P.A.; Watkinson, B. (1989). Maternal smoking during pregnancy affects children's vigilance performance. *Drug and Alcohol Dependence, 24,* 11-19.

Krogh, D. (1991). *Smoking: The Artificial Passion.* New York: Freeman.

Landesman-Dwyer, S.; Emanuel, I. (1979). Smoking during pregnancy. *Teratology, 19,* 119-126.

Lilienfeld, A.M. (1959). Emotional and other selected characteristics of cigarette smokers and nonsmokers as related to epidemiological studies of lung cancer and other diseases. *Journal of the National Cancer Institute, 22,* 259-282.

Makin, J.; Fried, P.A.; Watkinson, B. (1991). A comparison of active and passive smoking during pregnancy: Long-term effects. *Neurotoxicology and Teratology, 13,* 5-12.

Matarazzo, J.D.; Saslow, G. (1960). Psychological and related characteristics of smokers and nonsmokers. *Psychological Bulletin, 57,* 493-513.

Mayes, L.C. (1999). Developing brain and in utero cocaine exposure: Effects on neural ontogeny. *Development and Psychopathology, 11,* 685-714.

Mayes, L.C.; Bornstein, M.H.; Chawarska, K.; Granger, R.H. (1995). Information processing and developmental assessments in three-month-olds exposed prenatally to cocaine. *Pediatrics, 95,* 539-545.

McCalla, S.; Minkoff, H.L.; Feldman, J.; Delke, I.; Salwin, M.; Valencia, G.; Glass, L. (1991). The biologic and social consequences of perinatal cocaine use in an inner-city population: Results of an anonymous cross-sectional study. *American Journal of Obstetrics and Gynecology, 164,* 625-630.

McManus, I.C.; Weeks, S.J. (1982). Smoking, personality, and reasons for smoking. *Psychological Medicine, 12,* 349-356.

Mentis, M. (1998). In utero cocaine exposure and language development. *Seminars in Speech and Language, 19,* 147-165.

Metosky, P.; Vondra, J. (1995). Prenatal drug exposure and coping in toddlers: A comparison study. *Infant Behavior and Development, 18*(1), 15-25.

Naeye, R.L.; Peters, E.C. (1984). Mental development of children whose mothers smoked during pregnancy. *Obstetrics and Gynecology, 64,* 601-607.

National Institute on Drug Abuse (1996). *National Pregnancy and Health Survey.* Rockville, MD: NIDA.

O'Connell, C.M.; Fried, P.A. (1991). Prenatal exposure to cannabis: A preliminary report of postnatal consequences in school-age children. *Neurotoxicology and Teratology, 13,* 631-639.

Ostrea, E.M.; Brady, M.; Gause, S.; Raymondo, A.L.; Stevens, M. (1992). Drug screening of newborns by meconium analysis: A large-scale, prospective, epidemiologic study. *Pediatrics, 89,* 107-113.

Picone, T.A.; Allen, L.H.; Olsen, P.N.; Ferris, M.E. (1982). Pregnancy outcome in North American women: II. Effects of diet, cigarette smoking, stress, and weight gain on placentas, and on neonatal physical and behavioral characteristics. *The American Journal of Clinical Nutrition, 36,* 1214-1224.

Polifka, J.E. (1998). Drugs and chemicals in breast milk. In Slikker, W.; Chang, L.W. (eds.), *Handbook of developmental neurotoxicology.* San Diego: Academic Press, pp. 383-400.

Rantakallio, P. (1978). Relationship of maternal smoking to morbidity and mortality of the child up to age of five. *Acta Paediatric Scandinavia, 67,* 621-631.

Richardson, G.A. (1998). Prenatal cocaine exposure: A longitudinal study of development. *Annals of the New York Academy of Science, 846,* 144-152.

Richardson, G.A.; Conroy, M.L.; Day, N.L. (1996). Prenatal cocaine exposure: Effects on the development of school-age children. *Neurotoxicology and Teratology, 18,* 627-634.

Richardson, G.A.; Hamel, S.C.; Goldschmidt, L.; Day, N.L. (1999). Growth of infants prenatally exposed to cocaine/crack: Comparison of a prenatal care and a no prenatal care sample. *Pediatrics, 104,* 1-10.

Rodning, C.; Beckwith, L.; Howard, J. (1989). Characteristics of attachment organization and play organization in prenatally drug exposed toddlers. *Development and Psychopathology, 1,* 277-287.

Saxton, D.W. (1978). The behavior of infants whose mothers smoke in pregnancy. *Early Human Development, 2,* 363-369.

Schneider, J.W.; Chasnoff, I.J. (1992). Motor assessment of cocaine/polydrug exposed infants at 4 months. *Neurotoxicology and Teratology, 14,* 91-101.

Schneider, N.G.; Houston, J.P. (1970). Smoking and anxiety. *Psychological Reports, 26,* 941-942.

Sexton, M.; Fox, N.L.; Hebel, J.R. (1990). Prenatal exposure to tobacco: II. Effects on cognitive functioning at age three. *International Journal of Epidemiology, 19,* 72-77.

Simpson, K.J. (1957). A preliminary report of cigarettes and the incidence of prematurity. *American Journal of Obstetric Gynecology, 73,* 808.

Singer, L.; Arendt, R.; Farkas, K.; Minnes, S.; Huang, J.; Yamashita, T. (1997). Relationship of prenatal cocaine exposure and maternal postpartum psychological distress to child developmental outcome. *Development and Psychopathology,* 9(3), 473-489.

Slotkin, T. (1998). Fetal nicotine or cocaine exposure: Which one is worse? *Journal of Pharmacology and Experimental Therapeutics, 285,* 931-945.

Streissguth, A.P.; Barr, H.M.; Sampson, P.D.; Darby, B.L.; Martin, D.C. (1989). IQ at age 4 in relation to maternal alcohol use and smoking during pregnancy. *Developmental Psychology, 25,* 3-11.

Streissguth, A.P.; Martin, D.C.; Barr, H.M.; Sandman, B.M. (1984). Intrauterine alcohol and nicotine exposure: Attention and reaction time in 4-year-old children. *Developmental Psychology, 20,* 533-541.

Swanson, M.W.; Streissguth, A.P.; Sampson, P.D.; Carmichael-Olsen, H. (1999). Prenatal cocaine and neuromotor outcome at four months: Effect of duration of exposure. *Developmental and Behavioral Pediatrics, 20,* 325-334.

Tronick, E.Z.; Beeghly, M. (1999). Prenatal cocaine exposure, child development, and the compromising effects of cumulative risk. *Clinics in Perinatology, 26,* 151-171.

Vorhees, C.V. (1986). Principles of behavioral teratology. In Riley, E.P.; Vorhees, C.V. (eds.), *Handbook of Behavioral Teratology* (pp. 23-48). New York: Plenum Press.

Wakschlag, L.S.; Lahey, B.B.; Loeber, R.; Green, S.M.; Gordon, R.A.; Leventhal, B.L. (1997). Maternal smoking during pregnancy and the risk of conduct disorders in boys. *Archives of General Psychiatry, 54,* 670-676.

Weitzman, M.; Gortmaker, S.; Sobol, A. (1992). Maternal smoking and behavior problems in children. *Pediatrics, 90,* 342-349.

Werler, M.M.; Pober, B.R.; Holmes, L.B. (1985). Smoking and pregnancy. *Teratology, 32,* 473-481.

Williamson, D.F.; Serdula, M.K.; Kendrick, J.S.; Binkin, N.J. (1989). Comparing the prevalence of smoking in pregnant and nonpregnant women, 1985 to 1986. *Journal of the American Medical Association, 261,* 70-74.

Wilson, J.G. (1977). Current status of teratology: General principles and mechanisms derived from animal studies. In Wilson, J.G.; Fraser, F.C. (eds.), *Handbook of Teratology General Principles and Etiology,* Volume 1 (pp. 49-60). New York: Plenum Press.

Witter, F.; King, T.M. (1980). Cigarettes and pregnancy. *Progress in Clinical and Biological Research, 36,* 83-92.

Zelson, C. (1973). Infant of the addicted mother. *New England Journal of Medicine, 288,* 1391-1395.

Zuckerman, B.; Bresnahan, K. (1991). Developmental and behavioral consequences of prenatal drug and alcohol exposure. *Pediatric Clinics of North America, 38,* 1387-1406.

Chapter 10

Inhalant Abuse

Paul Kolecki
Richard Shih

OVERVIEW

The intentional inhalation of fumes derived from solvents (e.g., spray paint, glue, gasoline, nitrous oxide) is extremely common among the youth culture (Spiller and Krenzelok, 1997; Litovitz et al., 2000). Ease of availability, administration, titration, and low cost have all contributed to this widespread and growing epidemic. A recent case series from two poison control centers noted the typical inhalant user to be between the ages of 10 and 24 and typically male. The two most abused inhalants were spray paint and gasoline (Spiller and Krenzelok, 1997). In 1999, the American Association of Poison Control Centers reported more than 20,000 cases of gasoline exposure and numerous other cases of various inhalant exposure (Litovitz et al., 2000). Approximately twenty cases of mortality associated with intentional inhalant abuse were reported (Litovitz et al., 2000). The exact incidence and mortality rate from inhalant abuse, however, is unknown.

Two distinct groups of adolescents who sniff glue have been identified: those who do it for experience and experimentation as part of a peer group, and a smaller group who become dependent, chronic users (Masterton, 1979). Prior physical and/or sexual child abuse is suspected to be one important correlate for extensive involvement of inhalant use (Fendrich et al., 1997). Several studies have reported significant past inhalant abuse among youths in juvenile detention or correctional facilities (Young et al., 1999; McGarvey et al., 1999). A majority of these youths preferred using the inhalants in the presence of friends and abusing inhalants at the home of a friend (McGarvey et al., 1999). Studies also report significant inhalant abuse (e.g., volatile nitrites) among males in their workplace, including homosexual males, Native Americans, and Hispanic youths (Craib et al., 2000; Cohen, 1984).

It is a commonly held belief that most inhalant abusers usually engage in this activity for short periods of time. Some reports, however, cite patients who chronically abuse inhalants, such as prisoners who work with industrial solvents (Lewis et al., 1981; Davies et al., 1985). These workers inhale the fumes of accessible solvents periodically during their daily shifts in an attempt to maintain euphoria throughout the work week (Cohen, 1984). Inhalant abusers have also been reported to proceed to chronic alcohol and illicit drug abuse.

HISTORY

The inhalation of intoxicants is not new. The early Greeks used inhalants to mark the rites of passage of the young. The intentional inhalation of volatile substances (e.g., gasoline) was first observed in the United States before World War II (Morton, 1987; Nicholi, 1983). In the United States, a number of communities in widely separated areas began reporting a relatively high incidence of "glue sniffing" around 1960 (Kupperstein and Susman, 1968). Concern about the abuse of inhalants have since been expressed from many countries around the world (Morton, 1987; Nicholi, 1983).

Inhalation abuse is classically described as "the deliberate inhalation of solvent vapors to induce sensations of euphoria and exhilaration" (Glaser and Massengale, 1962, p. 179). Inhalation is usually continued until the desired sensation is achieved or until all of the toxic fumes have evaporated (Kupperstein and Susman, 1968). "Huffing" and "sniffing" are two of the more common methods of inhaling toxic fumes. Huffing involves nasally inhaling the fumes from a solvent-saturated rag (Barker and Adams, 1963). Sniffing involves the act of directly sniffing the fumes from the container or squeezing the toxic substance onto a rag and nasally sniffing the fumes from the rag. Another method, "bagging," involves the act of transferring the toxic substance into a paper bag, placing the bag over the nose and mouth, and inhaling deeply. Some abusers transfer the toxic substance into a pan or other vessel which is then heated. This results in a more rapid and concentrated vapor (Kupperstein and Susman, 1968). Finally, some toxic substances (e.g., nitrous oxide) are inhaled after being transferred into a balloon. This form of inhalant abuse, called "ballooning," is very common at tailgate parties before and after sporting events and rock concerts.

SUBSTANCES

The inhaled substances of abuse are aromatic and short-chained volatile hydrocarbons that, upon inhalation, have a rapid onset of intoxicating effects (Table 10.1).

The volatilized inhalant used is well absorbed from the lungs and rapidly distributed to the central nervous system. One or two large inhalations of the inebriating substance intoxicates the user very quickly, and the effects can last for hours. Some chronic inhalant abusers maintain a prolonged state of inebriation by periodically inhaling a substance. It is very difficult to clinically differentiate an inhalant-induced inebriation from ethanol-induced inebriation, although toxic inhalation inebriation is usually of shorter duration as compared to alcohol. Two distinguishing signs of inhalant abuse include the smell of solvents on the patient's hands or breath and skin discoloration secondary to paint sniffing (LoVecchio and Gerkin, 1997; Shih, 1998).

TABLE 10.1. Inhalants of Abuse and Their Main Chemical Constituents

Inhalants of abuse	Chemical constituents
Acrylic paint	Toluene
Aerosol propellant	Fluorocarbons
Anesthetics	Chloroform, nitrous oxide
Fire-extinguishing agent	Bromochlorodifluoromethane
Fuel, lighter fluid, torches	Propane, butane
Gasoline	Hydrocarbons, tetraethyl lead
Glues, plastic cement, rubber cement	Benzene, carbon tetrachloride, methylethyl ketone, *n*-hexane, toluene, trichloroethylene, trichloroethane, xylene
Inks	Toluene, xylene
Paint stripper	Methylene chloride
Paints, varnishes, lacquer	Trichloroethylene, toluene
Refrigerants	Fluorocarbons
Shoe polish	Chlorinated hydrocarbons, toluene
Spot remover	Trichloroethane, trichloroethylene, carbon tetrachloride
Typewriter correction fluid (e.g., Wite-Out)	Tetrachloroethylene, trichloroethane, trichloroethylene

Source: Adapted from LoVecchio and Gerkin, 1997.

Toxic Effects by Organ System

Patients who abuse inhalants typically experience the anticipated euphoria and suffer no long-term physiologic consequences. However, the intentional abuse of inhalants is potentially dangerous, as patients can acutely die and/or suffer severe permanent organ damage. The following paragraphs detail both the acute and chronic effects of commonly abused inhalants based on organ system.

Acute Toxic Effects of Inhalant Abuse

Central Nervous System

Patients abuse inhalants for the expected euphoria. This intoxication has been reported as a feeling of lightheadedness, stupor, lethargy, excitation, and occasional hallucinations (e.g., auditory and visual) (Spiller and Krenzelok, 1997). Profound relaxation and deep sleep usually follow this initial euphoric phase (LoVecchio and Gerkin, 1997). Unpleasant symptoms reported after the use of inhalants include agitation, seizures, ataxia, headache, and dizziness (Spiller and Krenzelok, 1997; Shih, 1998).

Pulmonary

Pulmonary effects following inhalant abuse are rare but deadly. High concentrations of an inhalant have resulted in oxygen displacement, hypoxia, asphyxiation, and suffocation (Linden, 1990). Symptoms of hypoxia develop when the inspired oxygen concentration suddenly falls below 17 percent, while loss of consciousness often occurs when inspired oxygen concentrations fall below 10 percent (Linden, 1990). Most victims were found with a paper bag over their head (Press and Done, 1967).

Cardiac

During the 1960s and late 1950s, an epidemic of sudden deaths occurred among teenagers who recently inhaled volatile hydrocarbons. This scenario, termed *sudden sniffing death* (SSD), was initially believed to result from plastic-bag suffocation (Press and Done, 1967). However, a comprehensive review in 1970 questioned this theory (Bass, 1970). In this study, 110 cases of SSD were reviewed. Common scenarios among these patients were the inhalation of a volatile hydrocarbon, then a scream or a vocalized impending sense of doom, followed by the victim running away from the agent of abuse. In many cases, the dead patient was found more than 100 feet from the abused substance or object used to transfer the inhalant (e.g., a paper bag). In this report, fluorocarbon propellants (pressurized aerosol containers) and trichloroethane (spot remover) were the two most common agents associated with SSD (Bass, 1970). Anoxia was thought not to be the cause of death, as many of these patients were well oxygenated after dashing several hundred feet before collapsing. Rather, it was postulated that SSD resulted from the volatile hydrocarbons sensitizing the myocardium to catecholamines, which subsequently produced lethal cardiac arrhythmias (Bass, 1970).

In 1972, a revealing animal study demonstrated that dogs exposed to fluorinated hydrocarbons suffered a chain of arrhythmias (e.g., sinus bradycardia, junctional or ventricular escape, ventricular fibrillation, asystole) and death (Flowers and Horan, 1972). These arrhythmias occurred in the setting of normal oxygenation. In addition, these arrhythmias continued despite halting exposure to the hydrocarbon at the first sign of rhythm change. This data concluded that SSD occurs secondary to cardiac arrhythmias and not anoxia. It has also been suggested that SSD can occur after the inhalant "senses doom" and discontinues the action of abuse (Flowers and Horan, 1972). For example, a typical scenario of SSD postulated by some toxicologists occurs when teenagers are caught abusing inhalants by parents or police. After being caught, a rush of catecholamines occurs in these teenagers as they sense a fear of parental punishment or they run to escape legal complications. It has been suggested that the catecholamine rush then "excessively stimulates" the inhalant-sensitized myocardium, leading to lethal arrhythmias and death in some teenagers.

There are numerous other reports of human SSD associated with the recent abuse of inhalants. Some inhalants reported to cause lethal arrhythmias and SSD include freon, bromochlorodifluoromethane, butane, propane, 1,1,1-trichloroethane, gasoline, and trichloroethylene (Siegel and Wason, 1990; Heath, 1986; King et al., 1985; Smeeton and Clark, 1985; Brady et al., 1994; Morita et al., 1977; Bass, 1978).

Hematologic

Methemoglobinemia and carboxyhemoglobinemia, two abnormal hemoglobin states, are associated with the abuse of certain inhalants. Methemoglobinemia occurs when oxidant stress is placed on the hemoglobin molecule and thus causes the iron moiety of the hemoglobin molecule to exist in the ferric state. When the iron moiety exists in the ferric state, methemoglobinemia occurs and the resulting abnormal hemoglobin molecule known as methemoglobin is unable to bind oxygen. Abuse of alkyl nitrites (amyl, butyl, and isobutyl) have been reported to cause methemoglobinemia and male patients abuse these nitrites mainly for their supposed aphrodisiac properties (Linden, 1990; Cohen, 1979). The aphrodisiac properties reportedly occur because of the vasodilatory effects on the cerebral blood vessels, which subsequently causes an increase in intracranial pressure and a euphoric effect (Haverkos and Dougherty, 1988). In addition, abuse of these alkyl nitrites "slows the sense of time." Abusers inhale these nitrites before sexual climax in an attempt to prolong and enhance the sensation of orgasm (Cohen, 1979). Other reported aphrodisiac properties include penile erection and dilation of the anal sphincter (Forsyth and Moulden, 1991). Amyl nitrite is a yellowish, volatile, flammable liquid with a fruity odor. Amyl nitrite was initially introduced into medical practice as a coronary vasodilator. It is not used for this purpose today, however, and has since been replaced by organic nitrates. Amyl nitrite continues to be marketed as fragile glass pearls covered with a woven absorbent material. These pearls are available in cyanide antidote kits.

When used to treat a cyanide overdose, the pearls are crushed in the hand and the vapors from the liquid are inhaled. Common street names for amyl nitrite pearls are "poppers" and "snappers," derived from the sound made by the pearls when they are broken. Butyl and isobutyl nitrites are volatile hydrocarbons marketed as room odorizers and advertised as aphrodisiacs. They are often sold in "adult bookstores" in bottles containing 10 to 30 ml of liquid. Common names for butyl and isobutyl nitrites are "Bullet," "Rush," and "Satan's Scent" (Linden, 1990).

Carboxyhemoglobinemia occurs when carbon monoxide (CO) binds to hemoglobin and thus impairs further oxygen binding to hemoglobin and oxygen delivery to tissues. Poisoning by CO has frequently been reported after exposure to methylene chloride, a volatile hydrocarbon commonly found in paint strippers. Methylene chloride is metabolized slowly (over a three-to-eight-hour time period) to CO. Methylene chloride poisoning has been frequently reported while the patient was stripping paint in a semienclosed area (Stewart and Hake, 1976; Rioux and Myers, 1989). There are also reports of intentional abuse of methylene chloride products (Sturmann et al., 1985; Horowitz, 1986). Interestingly, methylene chloride exposure has not been associated with lethal arrhythmias in the human or animal literature (LoVecchio and Gerkin, 1997).

Hepatic

Liver injury secondary to hepatocellular necrosis has been reported after exposure to certain chlorinated hydrocarbons, mainly trichloroethylene, carbon tetrachloride, and 1,1,1-trichloroethane. Tricloroethylene (TCE) was originally used as an obstetric general anesthetic but has been banned in the United States because of an association with trigeminal neuropathies (Mitchell and Parsons-Smith, 1969; Cavanagh and Buxton, 1989). TCE is used in typewriter correction fluid, paint remover, spot remover, furniture stripper, and degreasers. Carbon tetrachloride was widely used as a dry-cleaning agent and a constituent of fire extinguishers in the 1930s. Fatalities from thermal decomposition of carbon tetrachloride to phosgene gas led to the banning of its use in fire extinguishers in the 1960s. The FDA banned the use of carbon tetrachloride as a dry-cleaning agent in the 1970s. Presently, carbon tetrachloride is used in the production of solvents, aerosol propellants, and fluorocarbon refrigerants. Although carbon tetrachloride poisoning is commonly associated with chronic abuse, acute poisoning does not frequently occur. 1,1,1-trichloroethane is one of the most commonly abused solvents and presently is used as a metal cleaner, degreaser, aerosol propellant, and pesticide.

Inhalant abusers of these chlorinated hydrocarbons have been labeled as "solvent sniffers." However, reports of hepatic toxicity involve cases not only of inhalational abuse but also from occupational exposure and suicide attempts (Thiele et al., 1982). The histopathologic liver damage associated with certain chlorinated hydrocarbon poisonings is centrolobular hepatic necrosis. This histopathologic pattern is also the pattern seen with severe acetaminophen (Tylenol) and poisonous mushroom *(Amanita phalloides)* toxicity. In all three poisonings (e.g., chlorinated hydrocarbons, acetaminophen, *Amanita phalloides*), the liver damage occurs secondarily to toxic metabolites produced during metabolism of the parent compounds by the cytochrome p450 system. Tetrachloroethylene, the chlorinated hydrocarbon used presently in most dry-cleaning industries, has rarely been reported to cause liver damage (Wax, 1997).

CHRONIC TOXIC EFFECTS OF INHALANT ABUSE

Metabolic/Renal

Metabolic abnormalities have been classically described in patients who abuse toluene. Toluene is a hydrocarbon found in a variety of household products, including adhesives, spray paints, paint thinners, and varnishes.

Chronic toluene abuse may cause metabolic acidosis with and without an anion gap (Taher et al., 1974). The elevated anion gap results from an accumulation of acidic metabolites, mainly hippuric and benzoic acid (Fischman and Oster, 1979). The electrolyte abnormalities include hypokalemia, hypochloremia, and hypophosphatemia. These electrolytes abnormalities occur due to the induction of a distal renal tubular acidosis by toluene (Fischman and Oster, 1979; Kamijo et al., 1998). The hypokalemia may be so great that patients suffer muscle weakness severe enough to cause rhabdomyolysis, paralysis, and respiratory failure (Kao et al., 2000). These metabolic abnormalities typically occur after chronic abuse of toluene. Complete recovery has been reported in patients during periods of avoidance (Taher et al., 1974). Severe hypokalemia and death associated with chronic toluene abuse have been reported (Kirk et al., 1984). Patients suffering the medical consequences of toluene abuse often are found in a severely weakened state with paint still on their face and fingers.

Acute ingestion of toluene has been reported to cause central nervous system depression and diarrhea severe enough to cause a non-anion-gap metabolic acidosis (Caravati and Bjerk, 1997).

Neurologic

Permanent cerebral and cerebellar neurologic disability is a major toxic effect following chronic inhalant abuse (Lazar et al., 1983; Streicher et al., 1981). Long-term abusers or those who have been occupationally exposed have been reported to develop a neurobehavioral syndrome consisting of memory loss, cognitive impairment, sleep disturbance, depression, anxiety, and personality changes (Hormes et al., 1986). In addition, painters chronically exposed to solvents have developed encephalopathy, cerebral atrophy, and abnormal electroenchephalograms (EEGs) (Larsen and Leira, 1988). Permanent cognitive disorders are also well described in patients who chronically sniff gasoline (Poklis and Burkitt, 1977).

Chronic abuse of *n*-hexane and nitrous oxide are well known to cause peripheral neurologic deficits. *n*-hexane is a commonly abused solvent found in glue. Long-term abuse or occupational exposure of *n*-hexane can produce a profound sensorimotor polyneuropathy (Herskowitz et al., 1971; Prockop, 1979). This neuropathy typically begins with sensory involvement in the distal extremities and progresses proximally to the motor system, eventually causing weakness. Many of these effects are reversible over weeks to months with discontinuation of abuse or exposure. Chronic *n*-hexane abuse is also associated with memory loss. Methyl n-butyl ketone, a similar industrial solvent, has also been reported to cause peripheral neuropathy following chronic exposure (Allen et al., 1975).

Nitrous oxide is an anesthetic agent used by medical practitioners, especially dentists, for pain control during procedures. Transient euphoria and CNS depression occur when nitrous oxide is inhaled. Excluding intoxication, the acute side effects are minimal. Chronic inhalation of nitrous oxide can cause significant side effects. With chronic abuse, nitrous oxide can produce a demyelinating polyneuropathy and extremity weakness (Pema et al., 1998; Layzer, 1987). The neurologic sequelae associated with chronic abuse occurs secondary to vitamin B_{12} inactivation (Pema et al., 1998). Nitrous oxide abuse is very common today among younger drug abusers because of its ease of availability. Nitrous oxide abuse is very common at sporting event and rock concert tailgaters parties, where the gas is transferred from large containers into balloons and then inhaled. On a smaller scale, compressed nitrous oxide is present in cartridges for whipped cream dispensers and easily obtained in many supermarkets. Abusers discharge the cartridge into an empty cream dispenser and inhale the nitrous oxide (Lai et al., 1997). The slang term for abuse of nitrous oxide in this fashion is "whippets." Nitrous oxide-induced peripheral neuropathy is reversible following avoidance.

Hematologic

Chronic use and/or abuse of nitrous oxide also can cause hematologic abnormalities, specifically megaloblastic anemia (Lassen et al., 1956; Amess et al., 1978; Amos et al., 1982). This disorder occurs because chronic nitrous oxide abuse inactivates B_{12}, an important vitamin needed in bone marrow for the proper production of red blood cells. This anemia has been reported to reverse with B_{12} replacement therapy and discontinuation of nitrous oxide abuse (Layzer, 1987).

The major organic solvent of paints, paint thinners, and glues used to be benzene. The use of benzene as a solvent has been abandoned because of severe bone-marrow toxicity (e.g., leukemia, aplastic anemia, multiple myeloma) (Vigliani and Saita, 1964; Rinsky et al., 1987; Decouffle et al., 1983). Toluene and *n*-hexane have replaced benzene as a constituent of these compounds (Lazar et al., 1983).

Miscellaneous

Gasoline, a mixture of hydrocarbons with various additives, is frequently inhaled in an attempt to get intoxicated. Patients who chronically abuse leaded gasoline are at risk for the neurologic complications associated with organic lead poisoning. These complications include mental confusion, poor short-term memory, psychosis, and encephalopathy (Law and Nelson, 1968). Elements of inorganic lead poisoning (headache, abdominal pain, hepatic injury, renal damage) have also been reported in patients who chronically inhale gasoline (Robinson, 1978; Hansen and Sharp, 1978).

Treatment

Abuse of inhalants may produce significant morbidity, including respiratory depression and life-threatening arrhythmias. Securing an airway and ensuring adequate ventilation are first priority. The patient also should be placed on a cardiac monitor with the establishment of intravenous access. Gastrointestinal decontamination (gastric lavage and/or activated charcoal) should be considered, if it is suspected that the patient also ingested drugs or toxins. Excluding methylene chloride, patients who are asymptomatic for four to six hours after abusing an inhalant are generally considered safe for medical discharge. Specific management issues of caring for the acute and chronic toxic effects from inhalant abuse, including methylene chloride, are discussed in the following sections.

TREATMENT OF THE ACUTE TOXIC EFFECTS OF INHALANT ABUSE

Central Nervous System and Pulmonary

The main treatment of central nervous system depression is adequate ventilation until the effects of the inhalant terminate. Patients who become aggressive or agitated after abusing an inhalant may need to be physically restrained and pharmacologically sedated. Hypoxic patients need adequate oxygenation and ventilation. If necessary, a definitive airway (e.g., endotracheal or nasotracheal airway) should be established.

Cardiac

SSD (sudden sniffing death) occurs because the inhalants sensitize the myocardium of the patient to catecholamines, which subsequently leads to lethal ventricular arrhythmias and death. In human reports of SSD, standard cardiac pharmacologic treatment and electrotherapy were unsuccessful (King et al., 1985; Smeeton and Clark, 1985). Beta-adrenergic blocking agents have been proposed as a treatment option for life-threatening arrhythmias induced by inhalants (LoVecchio and Gerkin, 1997; Moritz et al., 2000). Should conventional cardiac resuscitation fail in treating inhalant abusers suffering lethal cardiac arrhythmias, the use of beta-adrenergic blocking agents (i.e., esmolol, propanolol) should be considered. Most patients who suffer cardiac consequences of inhalant abuse usually die at the scene or convert back to a normal sinus-cardiac rhythm prior to medical intervention.

Hematologic

Patients who sustain significant methemoglobinemia after alkyl nitrites abuse often suffer from cyanosis. Other signs and symptoms of methemoglobinemia include headache, dyspnea on exertion, tachycardia, tachypnea, confusion, coma, seizures, lethal cardiac arrhythmias, and death. The antidote for methemoglobinemia induced by alkyl nitrite, or by any drug or chemical, is methylene blue.

Methylene chloride, when metabolized, produces carbon monoxide. The production of carbon monoxide occurs over three to eight hours. Signs and symptoms of carbon monoxide poisoning include headache, dizziness, ataxia, seizures, lethal cardiac arrhythmias, coma, and death. A treatment recommended by many physicians for significant carbon monoxide poisoning is hyperbaric oxygen therapy, as there are many reports of successful treatment of methylene chloride-induced carbon monoxide poisoning with hyperbaric oxygen therapy (Rioux and Myers, 1989; Horowitz, 1986; Rudge, 1990). Testing for carbon monoxide poisoning over an eight-hour time is very important in caring for patients exposed to methylene chloride.

Hepatic

Due to the limited number of human cases, there is no standard treatment for chlorinated hydrocarbon-induced hepatotoxicity. *N*-acetylcysteine, an accepted antidote for acetaminophen poisoning, has been recommended as a treatment option for carbon tetrachloride-induced hepatotoxicity (Agency for Toxic Substances and Disease Registry, 1992). Limited data exists showing *N*-acetylcysteine's efficacy in reversing chlorinated hydrocarbon-induced hepatoxicity. Immediate oxygen therapy, including hyperbaric oxygen, has also been recommended for carbon tetrachloride poisoning (Tomaszewski and Thom, 1994; Bernacchi et al., 1984). Again, limited data exists showing oxygen therapy as efficacious in reversing chlorinated hydrocarbon-induced hepatotoxicity.

TREATMENT OF THE CHRONIC TOXIC EFFECTS OF INHALANT ABUSE

Metabolic/Renal

The treatment for chronic toluene-induced electrolyte abnormalities is discontinuation of exposure, airway management if necessary, and fluid and electrolyte replacement. Specific attention to hypokalemia is necessary and significant deficits should be corrected, since metabolic acidosis, rhabdomyolysis, lethal arrhythmias, and death have all been reported secondary to prolonged toluene abuse. Hemodialysis along with aggressive potassium replacement has been reported as a successful treatment option for severe chronic toluene poisoning (Gerkin and LoVecchio, 1998).

Neurologic and Hematologic

The most important treatment option for patients suffering central and peripheral neurologic deficits from chronic inhalant abuse is discontinuation of exposure. Vitamin B_{12} replacement therapy may be helpful for both chronic nitrous oxide-induced peripheral neuropathy and megaloblastic anemia.

Miscellaneous

Standard lead chelation techniques should be considered for chronic gasoline abusers who are suffering signs and symptoms of inorganic lead poisoning.

SUMMARY

Inhalant abuse is a significant problem, especially among the youth population. This form of substance abuse occurs mainly because the common inhalants of abuse are easily attainable, easily administered, and very cheap to buy. Acute abusers of inhalants are at risk for serious pulmonary, cardiac, hematologic, and hepatic toxicity. Chronic abusers of inhalants are potentially at risk of suffering not only severe metabolic abnormalities, but also permanent neurologic and hematologic damage. Knowledge of the pharmacology and toxicology of these inhalants is necessary not only for the successful diagnosis and treatment of poisoned patients, but also for future study of medicinal and addiction therapeutic protocols.

REFERENCES

Agency for Toxic Substances and Disease Registry (1992). Carbon tetrachloride toxicity. *American Family Physician* 46(4):1199-1207.

Allen, N.; Mendell, J.R.; Billmaier, D.J.; Fontaine, R.E.; O'Neill, J. (1975). Toxic polyneuropathy due to methyl n-butyl ketone. *Archives of Neurology* 32:209-218.

Amess, J.A.L.; Burman, J.F.; Rees, G.M.; Nancekievill, D.G.; Mollin, D.L. (1978). Megaloblastic haemopoiesis in patients receiving nitrous oxide. *Lancet* 2(8085): 339-342.

Amos, R.J.; Amess, J.A.L.; Hinds, C.J.; Mollin, D.L. (1982). Incidence and pathogenesis of acute megaloblastic bone-marrow change in patients receiving intensive care. *Lancet* 2(8303):835-838.

Barker, G.H.; Adams, W.T. (1963). Glue sniffers. *Sociology and Social Research* 47(3):45.

Bass, M. (1970). Sudden sniffing death. *JAMA* 212(12):2075-2079.

Bass, M. (1978). Death from sniffing gasoline (Letter). *New England Journal of Medicine* 299:203.

Bernacchi, A.; Myers, R.; Trump, B.F.; Marzella, L. (1984). Protection of hepatocytes with hyperoxia against carbon tetrachloride-induced injury. *Toxicologic Pathology* 12(4):315-323.

Brady, W.J.; Stremski, E.; Eljaiek, L.; Aufderheide, T.P. (1994). Freon inhalational abuse presenting with ventricular fibrillation. *American Journal of Emergency Medicine* 12:533-536.

Caravati, E.M.; Bjerk, P.J. (1997). Acute toluene ingestion toxicity. *Annals of Emergency Medicine* 30(6):838-839.

Cavanagh, B.; Buxton, P.H. (1989). Trichloroethylene cranial neuropathy: Is it really a toxic neuropathy or does it activate latent herpes virus? *Journal of Neurology, Neurosurgery, and Psychiatry* 52:297-303.

Cohen, S. (1979). The volatile nitrite. *JAMA* 241:2077-2078.

Cohen, S. (1984). The hallucinogens and the inhalants. *Psychiatric Clinics of North America* 7(4):681-688.

Craib, K.J.P.; Weber, A.C.; Cornelisse, P.G.A.; Martindale, S.L.; Miller, M.L.; Schechter, M.T.; Strathdee, S.A.; Schilder, A; Hogg, R.S. (2000). Comparison of sexual behaviors, unprotected sex, and substance use between two independent cohorts of gay and bisexual men. *AIDS* 14(3):303-311.

Davies, B.; Thorley, A.; O'Connor, D. (1985). Progression of addiction careers in young adult solvent misusers. *British Medical Journal* 290:109-110.

Decouffle, P.; Blattner, W.A.; Blair, A. (1983). Mortality among chemical workers exposed to benzene and other agents. *Environmental Research* 30:16-25.

Fendrich, M.; Mackesy-Amiti, M.E.; Wislar, J.S.; Goldstein, P.J. (1997). Childhood abuse and the use of inhalants: Differences by degree of use. *American Journal of Public Health* 87(5):765-769.

Fischman, C.M.; Oster, J.R. (1979). Toxic effects of toluene: A new cause of high anion gap metabolic acidosis. *JAMA* 241(16):1713-1715.

Flowers, N.C.; Horan, L.G. (1972). Nonanoxic aerosol arrhythmias. *JAMA* 219(1): 33-37.

Forsyth, R.J.; Moulden, A. (1991). Methaemoglobinaemia after ingestion of amyl nitrite. *Archives of Disease in Childhood* 66:152.

Gerkin, R.D.; LoVecchio, F. (1998). Rapid reversal of life-threatening toluene-induced hypokalemia with hemodialysis. *Journal of Emergency Medicine* 16(4): 723-725.

Glaser, H.H.; Massengale, O.N. (1962). Glue sniffing in children—Deliberate inhalation of vaporized plastic cements. *JAMA* 181:300-303.

Hansen, K.S.; Sharp, F.R. (1978). Gasoline sniffing, lead poisoning, and myoclonus. *JAMA* 240(13):1375-1376.

Haverkos, J.W.; Dougherty, J. (1988). Health hazards of nitrite inhalants. *American Journal of Medicine* 84:479-482.

Heath, M.J. (1986). Solvent abuse using bromochlorodifluoromethane from a fire extinguisher. *Medical Science Law* 26(1):33-34.

Herskowitz, A.; Ishii, N.; Schaumburg, H. (1971). *N*-hexane neuropathy: A syndrome occurring as a result of industrial exposure. *New England Journal of Medicine* 285(2):82-85.

Hormes, J.T.; Filley, C.M.; Rosenberg, N.L. (1986). Neurologic sequelae of chronic solvent abuse. *Neurology* 36:698-702.

Horowitz, B.Z. (1986). Carboxyhemoglobinemia caused by inhalation of methylene chloride. *American Journal of Emergency Medicine* 4(1):48-51.

Kamijo, Y.; Soma, K.; Hasegawa, I.; Ohwada, T. (1998). Fatal bilateral adrenal hemorrhage following acute toluene poisoning: A case report. *Journal of Toxicology—Clinical Toxicology* 36(4):365-368.

Kao, K.-C.; Tsai, Y.-H.; Lin, M.-C.; Huang, C.-C.; Tsao, T.C.-Y.; Chen, Y.-C. (2000). Hypokalemia muscular paralysis causing acute respiratory failure due to rhabdomyolysis with renal tubular acidosis in a chronic glue sniffer. *Journal of Toxicology—Clinical Toxicology* 38(6):679-681.

King, G.S.; Smialek, J.E.; Troutman, W.G. (1985). Sudden death in adolescents resulting from the inhalation of typewriter correction fluid. *JAMA* 253(11):1604-1606.

Kirk, L.M.; Anderson, R.; Martin, K. (1984). Sudden death from toluene abuse. *Annals of Emergency Medicine* 13(1):68-69.

Kupperstein, L.; Susman, R.M. (1968). A bibliography on the inhalation of glue fumes and other toxic vapors—A substance abuse practice among adolescents. *International Journal of the Addictions* 3(1):177-197.

Lai, N.Y.; Silbert, P.L.; Erber, W.N.; Rijks, C.J. (1997). "Nanging": Another cause of nitrous oxide neurotoxicity. *Medical Journal of Australia* 166(3):166.

Larsen, F.; Leira, H.L. (1988). Organic brain syndrome and long-term exposure to toluene: A clinical psychiatric study of vocationally active printing workers. *Journal Occupational Medicine* 30:875-878.

Lassen, H.C.A.; Henriksen, E.; Neukirch, F.; Kristensen, H.S. (1956). Treatment of tetanus. Severe bone-marrow depression after prolonged nitrous-oxide anesthesia. *Lancet* 527-530.

Law, W.R.; Nelson, E.R. (1968). Gasoline-sniffing by an adult. *JAMA* 204(11): 144-146.

Layzer, R.B. (1987). Myeloneuropathy after prolonged exposure to nitrous oxide. *Lancet* 2:1227-1230.

Lazar, R.B.; Ho, S.U.; Melen, O.; Daghestani, A.N. (1983). Multifocal central nervous system damage caused by toluene abuse. *Neurology* 33:1337-1340.

Lewis, J.D.; Moritz, D.; Mellis, L.P. (1981). Long-term toluene abuse. *American Journal of Psychiatry* 138(3):368-370.

Linden, C.H. (1990). Volatile substances of abuse. *Emergency Medicine Clinics of North America* 8(3):559-578.

Litovitz, T.L.; Klein-Schwartz, W.; White, S.; Cobaugh, D.L.; Youniss, J.; Drag, A.; Benson, B.E. (2000). 1999 Annual report of the American Association of Poison Control Centers toxic exposure surveillance system. *American Journal of Emergency Medicine* 8(5):517-566.

LoVecchio, F.; Gerkin, R. (1997). Inhalants of abuse. *Topics in Emergency Medicine* 19(4):44-52.

Masterton, G. (1979). Management of solvent abuse. *Journal of Adolescence* 2: 65-75.

McGarvey, E.L.; Clavet, G.J.; Mason, W. (1999). Adolescent inhalant abuse: Environments of use. *American Journal of Drug and Alcohol Abuse* 25(4):731-741.

Mitchell, A.B.S.; Parsons-Smith, B.G. (1969). Trichloroethylene neuropathy. *British Medical Journal* 1:422-423.

Morita, M.; Miki, A.; Kazama, H.; Sakata, M. (1977). Case report of deaths caused by freon gas. *Forensic Science* 10:253-260.

Moritz, F.; de La Chapelle, A.; Bauer, F.; Leroy, J.-P.; Goullé, J.P.; Bonmarchand, G. (2000). Esmolol in the treatment of severe arrhythmias after acute trichloroethylene poisoning. *Intensive Care Medicine* 26(2):256.

Morton, H.G. (1987). Occurrence and treatment of solvent abuse in children and adolescents. *Pharmacology and Therapeutics* 33:449-469.

Nicholi, A.M. (1983). The inhalants: An overview. *Psychosomatics* 24:914-921.

Pema, P.J.; Horak, H.A.; Wyatt, R.H. (1998). Myelopathy caused by nitrous oxide toxicity. *American Journal of Neuroradiology* 19:894-896.

Poklis, A.; Burkitt, C.D. (1977). Gasoline sniffing: A review. *Clinical Toxicology* 11:35-41.

Press, E.; Done, A.K. (1967). Solvent sniffing: Physiologic effects and community control measure for intoxication from intentional inhalation of organic solvents. *Pediatrics* 39:451-461.

Prockop, L. (1979). Neurotoxic volatile substances. *Neurology* 29:862-865.

Rinsky, R.A.; Smith, A.B.; Hornung, R.; Filloon, T.G.; Young, R.J.; Okun, A.H.; Landrigan, P.J. (1987). Benzene and leukemia: An epidemiologic risk assessment. *New England Journal of Medicine* 316(17):1044-1050.

Rioux, J.P.; Myers, R.A.M. (1989). Hyperbaric oxygen for methylene chloride poisoning: Report on two cases. *Annals of Emergency Medicine* 18:691-695.

Robinson, R.O. (1978). Tetraethyl lead poisoning from gasoline sniffing. *JAMA* 240(13):1373-1374.

Rudge, F.W. (1990). Treatment of methylene chloride induced carbon monoxide poisoning with hyperbaric oxygenation. *Military Medicine* 155:570-572.

Shih, R. (1998). Hydrocarbons. In Goldfrank, L.R.; Flomenbaum, N.E.; Lewin, N.A. (eds.), *Goldfrank's Toxicologic Emergencies,* Sixth Edition. Stamford, CT: Appleton & Lange, pp. 1383-1398.

Siegel, E.; Wason, S. (1990). Sudden death caused by inhalation of butane and propane. *New England Journal of Medicine* 323(23):1638.

Smeeton, W.M.I.; Clark, M.S. (1985). Sudden death resulting from inhalation of fire extinguishers containing bromochlorodifluoromethane. *Medical Science Law* 25(4):258-262.

Spiller, H.A.; Krenzelok, E.P. (1997). Epidemiology of inhalant abuse reported to two regional poison centers. *Journal of Toxicology—Clinical Toxicology* 35(2): 167-173.

Stewart, R.D.; Hake, C.L. (1976). Paint-remover hazard. *JAMA* 235(4):398-401.

Streicher, H.Z.; Gabow, P.A.; Moss, A.H.; Kono, D.; Kaehny, W.D. (1981). Syndromes of toluene sniffing in adults. *Annals of Internal Medicine* 94:758-762.

Sturmann, K.; Mofenson, H.; Caraccio, T. (1985). Methylene chloride inhalation: An unusual form of drug abuse. *Annals of Emergency Medicine* 14:903-905.

Taher, S.M.; Anderson, R.J.; McCartney, R.; Popovtzer, M.M.; Schrier, R.W. (1974). Renal tubular acidosis associated with toluene "sniffing." *New England Journal of Medicine* 290(14):765-768.

Thiele, D.L.; Eigenbrodt, E.H.; Ware, A.J. (1982). Cirrhosis after repeated trichloroethylene and 1,1,1-trichloroethane exposure. *Gastroenterology* 83:925-929.

Tomaszewski, C.A.; Thom, S.R. (1994). Use of hyperbaric oxygen in toxicology. *Emergency Medicine Clinics of North America* 12(2):437-459.

Vigliani, E.C.; Saita, G. (1964). Benzene and leukemia. *New England Journal of Medicine* 217(17):872-876.

Wax, P.M. (1997). Dry cleaners. In Greenberg, M.I.; Hamilton, R.J.; Phillips, S.D.; *Occupational, Industrial, and Environmental Toxicology.* St. Louis, MO: Mosby, 73-82.

Young, S.J.; Longstaffe, S.; Tenebein, M. (1999). Inhalant abuse and the abuse of other drugs. *American Journal of Drug and Alcohol Abuse* 25(2):371-375.

Index

Page numbers followed by the letter "f" indicate figures; those followed by the letter "t" indicate tables.

HANDBOOK OF THE MEDICAL CONSEQUENCES
OF ALCOHOL AND DRUG ABUSE

_____in hardbound at $52.46 (regularly $69.95) (ISBN: 0-7890-1863-2)

_____in softbound at $37.46 (regularly $49.95) (ISBN: 0-7890-1864-0)

Or order online and use special offer code HEC25 in the shopping cart.